T0226846

Surgical Critical Care

Editor

CYNTHIA L. TALLEY

SURGICAL CLINICS
OF NORTH AMERICA

www.surgical.theclinics.com

Consulting Editor
RONALD F. MARTIN

December 2017 • Volume 97 • Number 6

ELSEVIER

1600 John F. Kennedy Boulevard • Suite 1800 • Philadelphia, Pennsylvania, 19103-2899

http://www.surgical.theclinics.com

SURGICAL CLINICS OF NORTH AMERICA Volume 97, Number 6
December 2017 ISSN 0039–6109, ISBN-13: 978-0-323-55300-1

Editor: John Vassallo, j.vassallo@elsevier.com
Developmental Editor: Meredith Madeira

Surgical Clinics of North America (ISSN 0039–6109) is published bimonthly by Elsevier Inc., 360 Park Avenue South, New York, NY 10010-1710. Months of publication are February, April, June, August, October, and December. Business and Editorial Offices: 1600 John F. Kennedy Blvd., Suite 1800, Philadelphia, PA 19103-2899. Periodicals postage paid at New York, NY and additional mailing offices. Subscription prices are $386.00 per year for US individuals, $756.00 per year for US institutions, $100.00 per year for US students and residents, $469.00 per year for Canadian individuals, $958.00 per year for Canadian institutions, $525.00 for international individuals, $958.00 per year for international institutions and $250.00 per year for Canadian and foreign students/residents. To receive student/resident rate, orders must be accompanied by name of affiliated institution, date of term, and the *signature* of program/residency coordinator on institution letterhead. Orders will be billed at individual rate until proof of status is received. Foreign air speed delivery is included in all *Clinics* subscription prices. All prices are subject to change without notice. POSTMASTER: Send address changes to *Surgical Clinics*, Elsevier Health Sciences Division, Subscription Customer Service, 3251 Riverport Lane, Maryland Heights, MO 63043. **Customer Service (orders, claims, online, change of address): Telephone: 1-800-654-2452 (U.S. and Canada); 314-447-8871 (outside U.S. and Canada). Fax: 314-447-8029. E-mail: journalscustomerservice-usa@elsevier.com (for print support); journalsonline support-usa@elsevier.com (for online support).**

Reprints. For copies of 100 or more, of articles in this publication, please contact the Commercial Reprints Department, Elsevier Inc., 360 Park Avenue South, New York, New York 10010-1710. Tel. 212-633-3874, Fax: 212-633-3820, E-mail: reprints@elsevier.com.

The Surgical Clinics of North America is also published in Spanish by McGraw-Hill Interamericana Editores S.A., P.O. Box 5-237 06500 Mexico D.F. Mexico; and in Portuguese by Interlivros Edicoes Ltda., Rua Comandante Coelho 1085, CEP 21250, Rio de Janeiro, Brazil; and in Greek by Paschalidis Medical Publications, Athens Greece.

The Surgical Clinics of North America is covered in *MEDLINE/PubMed (Index Medicus), EMBASE/Excerpta Medica, Current Contents/Clinical Medicine, Current Contents/Life Sciences, Science Citation Index,* and *ISI/BIOMED.*

Contributors

CONSULTING EDITOR

RONALD F. MARTIN, MD, FACS
Colonel (ret.), United States Army Reserve, Department of Surgery, York Hospital, York, Maine, USA

EDITOR

CYNTHIA L. TALLEY, MD, FACS
Program Director, Surgical Critical Care, Section of Trauma and Acute Care Surgery, Associate Professor, Department of Surgery, University of Kentucky HealthCare, Lexington, Kentucky, USA

AUTHORS

BRACKEN A. ARMSTRONG, MD
Clinical Instructors in Surgery, Division of Trauma and Surgical Critical Care, Department of Surgery, Vanderbilt University Medical Center, Nashville, Tennessee, USA

CHRISTOPHER MICHAEL BELL, MD
Surgical Critical Care Fellow, Department of Surgery, The University of Tennessee College of Medicine, Chattanooga, Chattanooga, Tennessee, USA

ANA BERLIN, MD, MPH, FACS
Assistant Professor, Department of Surgery, Rutgers New Jersey Medical School, Newark, New Jersey, USA

ANDREW BERNARD, MD
Professor and Chief, Section on Trauma and Acute Care Surgery, Division of General Surgery, Department of Surgery, University of Kentucky College of Medicine, Lexington, Kentucky, USA

RICHARD D. BETZOLD, MD
Clinical Instructors in Surgery, Division of Trauma and Surgical Critical Care, Department of Surgery, Vanderbilt University Medical Center, Nashville, Tennessee, USA

MARK BLUM, MD
Trauma, Critical Care and Emergency Surgery, Department of Surgery, Virginia Commonwealth University, Richmond, Virginia, USA

BRYAN A. COTTON, MD
Professor, Department of Surgery, The University of Texas, McGovern Medical School at UTHealth, Houston, Texas, USA

JUSTIN R. DAVANZO, MD
Department of Neurosurgery, Milton S. Hershey Medical Center, Penn State College of Medicine, Hershey, Pennsylvania, USA

MACK DRAKE, DO
Clinical Instructor of Surgery, Section on Trauma and Acute Care Surgery, Division of General Surgery, Department of Surgery, University of Kentucky College of Medicine, Lexington, Kentucky, USA

MATTHEW ECKERT, MD, FACS
Madigan Army Medical Center, Tacoma, WA, USA

PAULA FERRADA, MD, FACS
Associate Professor, Trauma, Critical Care and Emergency Surgery, Department of Surgery, Virginia Commonwealth University, Richmond, Virginia, USA

EUGENE HESSEL, MD
Professor, Departments of Anesthesiology and Surgery, University of Kentucky College of Medicine, Lexington, Kentucky, USA

JEREMY L. HOLZMACHER, MD
Center for Trauma and Critical Care, Department of Surgery, The George Washington University, Washington, DC, USA

FAISAL S. JEHAN, MD
Research Fellow, Division of Trauma, Critical Care, Emergency Surgery, and Burns, Department of Surgery, University of Arizona College of Medicine, Tucson, Arizona, USA

BELLAL JOSEPH, MD, FACS
Professor of Surgery, Division of Trauma, Critical Care, Emergency Surgery, and Burns, Department of Surgery, University of Arizona College of Medicine, Tucson, Arizona, USA

KYLE J. KALKWARF, MD
Fellow, Department of Surgery, The University of Texas, McGovern Medical School at UTHealth, Houston, Texas, USA

ANNACHIARA MARRA, MD, PhD(c)
Visiting Research Fellow, Division of Allergy, Pulmonary and Critical Care Medicine, Center for Health Services, Vanderbilt University Medical Center, Nashville, Tennessee, USA; Doctoral Candidate, Department of Neurosciences, Reproductive and Odontostomatological Sciences, University of Naples, Federico II, Naples, Italy

ROBERT A. MAXWELL, MD, FACS
Professor, Department of Surgery, The University of Tennessee College of Medicine, Chattanooga, Chattanooga, Tennessee, USA

ADDISON K. MAY, MD
Ingram Chair in Surgical Sciences and Professor of Surgery and Anesthesiology, Division of Trauma and Surgical Critical Care, Department of Surgery, Vanderbilt University Medical Center, Nashville, Tennessee, USA

ERIN MAYNARD, MD, FACS
Assistant Professor, Department of Surgery, Oregon Health & Science University, Portland, Oregon, USA

NATHAN T. MOWERY, MD
Associate Professor of Surgery, Wake Forest Baptist Medical Center, Winston-Salem, North Carolina, USA

PRATIK P. PANDHARIPANDE, MD, MSCI, FCCM
Professor of Anesthesiology and Surgery, Chief, Division of Anesthesiology Critical Care Medicine, Department of Anesthesiology, Center for Health Services Research, Vanderbilt University Medical Center, Nashville Veterans Affairs Medical Center, Nashville, Tennessee, USA

MAYUR B. PATEL, MD, MPH, FACS
Assistant Professor of Surgery, Neurosurgery, Hearing and Speech Sciences, Division of Trauma, Surgical Critical Care, and Emergency General Surgery, Department of Surgery, Section of Surgical Sciences, Center for Health Services Research, Vanderbilt Brain Institute, Vanderbilt University Medical Center, Nashville Veterans Affairs Medical Center, Nashville, Tennessee, USA

BABAK SARANI, MD, FACS, FCCM
Center for Trauma and Critical Care, Department of Surgery, The George Washington University, Washington, DC, USA

ROWAN SHELDON, MD
Madigan Army Medial Center, Tacoma, WA, USA

EMILY P. SIEG, MD
Department of Neurosurgery, Milton S. Hershey Medical Center, Penn State College of Medicine, Hershey, Pennsylvania, USA

SHELLY D. TIMMONS, MD, PhD, FACS, FAANS
Department of Neurosurgery, Milton S. Hershey Medical Center, Penn State College of Medicine, Hershey, Pennsylvania, USA

Contents

Prevalence of preexisting frailty in patients admitted to the intensive care unit (ICU) is increasing. Critical illness leads to a catabolic state that further diminishes body reserves and contributes to frailty independent of age and prehospital functional status. Because early mobilization of patients in the ICU results in accelerated recovery and improvement in functional status and quality of life, frailty can severely affect the mobility of patients in the ICU ultimately prolonging recovery. Understanding the concept of frailty and the association of frailty and its impact on mobility in the ICU, identifying patients, and timely resource allocation help in optimum care and improve clinical outcomes.

Delirium is one of the most common behavioral manifestations of acute brain dysfunction in the intensive care unit (ICU) and is a strong predictor of worse outcome. Routine monitoring for delirium is recommended for all patients in the ICU using validated tools. In delirious patients, a search for all reversible precipitants is the first line of action and pharmacologic treatment should be considered when all causes have been ruled out, and it is not contraindicated. Long-term morbidity has significant consequences for survivors of critical illness and for their caregivers. Patients in the ICU may develop posttraumatic stress disorder related to their critical illness experience.

Traumatic brain injury remains a serious public health problem, causing death and disability for millions. To maximize outcomes in the face of a complex injury to a complex organ, a variety of advanced neuromonitoring techniques may be used to guide surgical and medical decision making. Because of the heterogeneity of injury types and the plethora of treatment confounders present in this patient population, the scientific study of specific interventions is challenging. This challenge highlights the need for a firm understanding of the anatomy and pathophysiology of brain injuries when making clinical decisions in the intensive care unit.

Death determined by neurologic criteria, commonly referred to as "brain death," occurs when function of the entire brain ceases, including the brain stem. Diagnostic criteria for brain death are explicit, but controversy exists regarding nuances of the evaluation and potential confounders of the examination. Hospitals and ICU teams should carefully consider which clinicians will perform brain death testing and should use standard processes, including checklists to prevent diagnostic errors. Proper diagnosis is essential because misdiagnosis can be catastrophic. Timely, accurate brain death determination and aggressive physiologic support are cornerstones of both good end-of-life care and successful organ donation.

Despite advances in surgical critical care, critical illness remains traumatic and has long-term adverse sequelae. Unrealistic expectations and erroneous assumptions about outcomes acceptable to patients have been identified as drivers of goal-discordant treatment. Goal setting in the ICU begins with compassionately delivered, accurate, and honest prognostic information. Through skilled communication and shared decision making, clinicians forge a mutual understanding of patient values and priorities and the role of therapeutic options in achieving patient goals. Ensuring that treatment is goal-concordant and meets physical, psychosocial, existential, and spiritual needs is crucial for attaining optimal patient and caregiver outcomes, independent of survival.

The use of anticoagulation in the prevention of strokes due to atrial fibrillation or the treatment of venous thromboembolic disease has been on the rise. With the advent and proliferation of direct oral anticoagulation medications, the management of anticoagulation reversal has become increasingly complex, especially when urgent or emergent reversal is required. This article details the commonly used parenteral and oral anticoagulants, the treatment strategies necessary for their reversal, and therapies still in development.

Hemorrhage is the leading cause of preventable deaths in trauma patients. After presenting a brief history of hemorrhagic shock resuscitation, this article discusses damage control resuscitation and its adjuncts. Massively bleeding patients in hypovolemic shock should be treated with damage control resuscitation principles, including limited crystalloid, whole blood, or balance blood component transfusion to permissive hypotension, preventing hypothermia, and stopping bleeding as quickly as possible.

Ultrasound imaging is a user-dependent tool that can help guide therapy. The use of ultrasound to guide central line placement decreases complication rates. Cardiac ultrasound imaging can help with the diagnosis of cases of hypotension. Lung and pleural ultrasound imaging is a useful adjunct for diagnosing causes of desaturation. Abdominal ultrasound imaging can help in rapid visitation of fluid and intraabdominal structures.

Three therapeutic principles most substantially improve organ dysfunction and survival in sepsis: early, appropriate antimicrobial therapy; restoration of adequate cellular perfusion; timely source control. The new definitions of sepsis and septic shock reflect the inadequate sensitivity, specify, and lack of prognostication of systemic inflammatory response syndrome criteria. Sequential (sepsis-related) organ failure assessment more effectively prognosticates in sepsis and critical illness. Inadequate cellular perfusion accelerates injury, and reestablishing perfusion limits injury. Multiple organ systems are affected by sepsis and septic shock, and an evidence-based multipronged approach to systems-based therapy in critical illness results in improve outcomes.

The management of the ventilator in patients with chronic obstructive pulmonary disease (COPD) and acute respiratory distress syndrome (ARDS) has a dramatic effect on the overall outcome. The incidence of COPD is increasing as the US population grows older. The most effective means to deal with pulmonary complications is to avoid them, but both COPD and ARDS have evidence-based interventions that have been shown to improve outcomes. Pulmonary complications affect up to 40% of patients, and their occurrence is associated with an increased duration of hospital stay and an increased mortality.

Acute kidney injury (AKI) occurs frequently in the surgical intensive care unit and results in significant morbidity and mortality. AKI needs to be identified early, and underlying causes need to be treated or eliminated. Sepsis, major surgery such as coronary artery bypass, and hypovolemia are the most common causes, and patients with underlying comorbidities have increased susceptibility. Treatment should begin by ensuring that patients are adequately resuscitated and all contributing causes are replaced or eliminated. After stabilization of hemodynamic status and elimination of contributing causes, treatment becomes largely supportive and may require the use of a renal replacement therapy.

The critically ill patient with decompensated cirrhosis has a unique physiology and alterations in albumin that need to be understood to properly resuscitate them and minimize morbidity and mortality. Little data exist on specific resuscitation of the patient with cirrhosis compared with those patients without liver disease. The effectiveness of albumin administration compared with saline administration in common settings, such as large-volume paracentesis, can be extrapolated to the care of the general surgical patient, but further studies in this area are warranted. This article enhances the understanding of the unique physiology of patients with decompensated cirrhosis to guide their needs in fluid resuscitation in critical illness.

Critical illness and injury affect the gastrointestinal tract almost uniformly. Complications include the sequelae of direct intestinal injury and repair, impaired motility, intraabdominal hypertension, and ulceration, among others. Contemporary clinical practice has incorporated many advances in the prevention and treatment of gastrointestinal complications during critical illness. This article discusses the epidemiology, risk factors, means of diagnosis, treatment, and prevention of some of these compilations.

SURGICAL CLINICS
OF NORTH AMERICA

THE CLINICS ARE AVAILABLE ONLINE!
Access your subscription at:
www.theclinics.com

Foreword

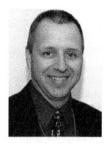

Ronald F. Martin, MD, FACS
Consulting Editor

We are living in turbulent times in the field of medicine. We probably always have been. Still, when scientific turbulence collides with financial turbulence and political turbulence, one is truly in for a wild ride. In very few aspects of medicine are the effects of this uncertainty as keenly felt as they are in the care of the critically ill. As I have stated previously, there are few problems in medicine more streamlined than providing care to the patient who is arresting (we reduce the steps to a laminated card) and few things more complicated than caring for the same patient once the resuscitation has been successful (we fill libraries with books about how to do that). Preventing a patient from arresting is also pretty challenging sometimes—more books. Those who work predominantly in the intensive care units (ICU) live their entire careers on or near this fulcrum, balancing between these worlds of quasi-stability and collapse.

As the role of the acute care hospital changes, we find that forces are trying to drive as much care delivery to the home setting as is possible—and that is probably a very good thing for many reasons. The obvious downstream effect of this is a reduction in the number of people in hospitals who do not require resource-intense care. As the mean acuity of patients in the hospital settings increases, the demand for hospital resources increases, at a time when the desire to provide the funds to hospitals to meet these needs is being challenged daily. As we get better at keeping patients out of the hospitals, the relative and actual cost of taking care of patients in the hospital setting increases, giving at least the appearance, if not the reality, of more expensive care for similar numbers of patients. Under the circumstances, the only way to bend the cost per patient ratio is to increase efficiencies and efficacy.

The ICU environment, while certainly not at risk of being pushed to the home setting at present, does provide the environment where we use the most resources in the most challenging situations. Furthermore, given the nature of the maladies that cause one to be in the ICU, there is a higher likelihood that it may be the last place some will be while they are alive. Even the definition of alive becomes "fluid" in our ICUs. While we have generally accepted medical opinions of what kinds of death there are, society does not always have similar philosophies. On occasion, this focuses the attention of the

Surg Clin N Am 97 (2017) xiii–xiv
https://doi.org/10.1016/j.suc.2017.09.017
0039-6109/17/© 2017 Published by Elsevier Inc.

general population for a period of time with high-profile situations, but resolution and agreement rarely follow.

The fundamental question of how we distinguish what we do for people rather than what we do to people is most evident in the ICU. The ability to set limits and guidelines is always difficult as it frequently requires diametrically opposed plans to shift from the most aggressive treatment we can offer to one with significant limitations or withdrawal of care. Just the emotional energy required on behalf of the families and caregivers alone makes that balancing act challenging.

In the era of value-based medicine, the costs of these extraordinary measures are also under scrutiny; while this scrutiny is necessary and valuable, we don't really have an agreed upon desired end-state shared by all stakeholders, which makes a true value assessment at best compromised and at worst impossible. Patients, families, providers, hospitals, insurers, government, and communities in general all view this value equation through similar but slightly different lenses. Add to that the general disagreement at the federal government level about what system(s) to use in order to finance health care and we get an even less clear set of mutually desirable goals and expectations.

Despite all of the systems and politico-cultural issues surrounding intensive care, there remains a science and art that are deeply embedded in its origins. Those topics are complex by nature and become more complicated as larger fractions of our population suffer from chronic diseases or are treated with medicines that alter their basic physiologic status. Dr Talley and her colleagues have compiled an excellent collection of articles that will help all of us better understand what is becoming not just more possible but also more effective in the understanding and care of critically ill patients. Even if one does not directly care for patients in the ICU, we almost all are involved in some aspect of care of critically ill patients for a portion of our surgical practices. The material contained within the issue will make us better suited to care for our patients as well as be better informed for the discussions within our hospitals and communities in the larger sense. We are all obligated to advocate for our patients at all levels whenever possible. This material should better prepare us to do so. We are deeply indebted to Dr Talley and her colleagues for this excellent material.

Ronald F. Martin, MD, FACS
Colonel (ret.), United States Army Reserve
Department of Surgery
York Hospital
16 Hospital Drive, Suite A
York, ME 03909, USA

E-mail address:
rmartin@yorkhospital.com

Preface

What's New in Surgery Critical Care?

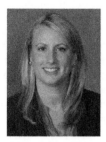

Cynthia L. Talley, MD, FACS
Editor

As a midcareer Associate Professor, I found the articles in this issue to be informative. We as critical care surgeons have committed to life-long learning in order to provide our patients with the very best and up-to-date information. This collection of authors has great experience in their field and embodies the evidence-based medicine philosophy. The authors present a preponderance of data in an ever-changing field of surgical critical care with discussion of landmark research free of opinion and anecdote. The authors are able to organize the evidence clearly and succinctly regarding epidemiology, prevention, diagnosis, and treatment of critical care disease as real take-home points that may guide practice. The articles are presented in part by organ systems as we evaluate our patients in the intensive care unit (ICU).

Drs Joseph and Jehan describe the importance of organizing mobility efforts in the ICU especially for our frail patients. They further describes the pathophysiology of frailty including its impact on patient care, and the importance of organizing mobility efforts in the ICU, especially for our frail patients. Drs Marra, Pandharipande, and Patel present delirium and posttraumatic stress disorder prevention now found to impact ICU patient outcomes significantly. They are able to discern the many evaluation tools for delirium and methods for prevention in order of importance. Drs Davanzo, Sieg, and Timmons introduce traumatic brain injury (TBI) in a sound progression of diagnostic modalities, including clinical and radiologic exams, and the management options, both surgical and medical. Many medical considerations for TBI do not provide a cure but are geared toward mitigating the effects of the primary injury and avoiding secondary injury in order to provide the best chance for neurologic recovery. Drs Drake, Bernard, and Hessel discuss the intricate nuances of brain death determination. The authors steer head-on into the controversies surrounding drug intoxication confounders and the wide variability of practice in US hospitals. Dr Berlin discusses how goal setting in the ICU can be achieved through skilled communication and shared

Surg Clin N Am 97 (2017) xv–xvi
https://doi.org/10.1016/j.suc.2017.09.016
0039-6109/17/© 2017 Published by Elsevier Inc.

surgical.theclinics.com

decision-making to reduce discomfort for both the patient and the caregiver. Drs Holzmacher and Sarani present indications and methods of anticoagulant reversal with a detailed description of traditional and novel anticoagulants and their antidotes. Drs Kalkwarf and Cotton present a history lesson regarding our evolution of hemorrhagic resuscitation and lessons learned. They discuss the best evidence for current treatment strategies, including damage control resuscitation. Drs Blum and Ferrada instruct on the use of ultrasound in the ICU in a stepwise approach with representative images to easily follow along. They also expand on the techniques of the echocardiogram that may be less mainstream in the intensivist's hands. Drs Armstrong, Betzold, and May tackle the complex topic of sepsis, the most expensive and second most common reason for hospitalization. They tease out the vast evidence, including the recent Sepsis-3 guidelines, with new terminology and definitions, the intricate pathophysiology, initial management, and organ system sequelae to create manageable patient care guidelines. Dr Mowery takes chronic obstructive pulmonary disease and acute respiratory distress syndrome, two major pulmonary issues that plague the surgical intensivist, and presents a whole host of ventilator and noninvasive strategies as well as useful adjuncts. Drs Maxwell and Bell describe acute kidney injury in the critically ill regarding its definition, cause, and diagnostics. They also go on to clearly organize the different renal replacement modalities many times deferred to our nephrology colleagues. Dr Maynard addresses the increasing problem of dealing with surgical patients with cirrhosis. How to resuscitate and mitigate against likely mortality is presented in a clear evidence-based path useful to all surgeons in the perioperative period. Drs Sheldon and Eckert discuss the gastrointestinal complications of stress ulceration, enteric fistulae, intestinal ileus, Ogilvie syndrome, and abdominal compartment syndrome, representing some of the more burdensome diseases that surgical intensivists face. I hope you enjoy reading this issue as much as I did.

Cynthia L. Talley, MD, FACS
Section of Trauma and Acute Care Surgery
Department of Surgery
University of Kentucky Healthcare
University of Kentucky
800 Rose Street
UKMC-C224
Lexington, KY 40536-0293, USA

E-mail address:
c.talley@uky.edu

@talleycindy1 (C.L. Talley)

The Mobility and Impact of Frailty in the Intensive Care Unit

Bellal Joseph, MD*, Faisal S. Jehan, MD

KEYWORDS

• Mobility • Frailty • Critically ill patients • ICU

KEY POINTS

- Early mobilization and rehabilitation in ICU patients can reduce the incidence and duration of delirium, shorten ICU and hospital LOS, and lower hospital costs.
- Frailty can significantly compromise and impede the early mobilization of patients in the ICU and thus worsen the ICU course.
- Frailty refers to an increased vulnerability to stressors caused by the lack of physiologic reserves resulting from the age-associated accumulation of deficits in multiple organ systems combined with genetic, environmental, and physical insults.
- Early identification of frail patients and timely resource allocation and interventions to mobilize patient early in their ICU course help improve clinical outcomes and the quality of life.

INTRODUCTION

In the United States, the geriatric population has significantly increased by 21% since 1980.[1] This is because of aging Baby Boomers and increased life expectancy rooted in advances in the standard of living and medical health services. In the United States, those older than the age of 65 now account for 14.5% (46.2 million) of the total population and by 2040, this percentage is expected to increase to approximately 20% (72.1 million).[2] Indeed, geriatric population is the fastest growing subset of the total population. Although the total US population has grown by 39% over the past 30 years, those segments older than 65 and 85 years have grown by almost 89% and 232%, respectively.[3]

Disclosure Statement: The authors have nothing to disclose.
Division of Trauma, Critical Care, Emergency Surgery, and Burns, Department of Surgery, University of Arizona, College of Medicine, 1501 North Campbell Avenue, Room 5334B, PO Box 245063, Tucson, AZ 85724-5063, USA
* Corresponding author.
E-mail address: bjoseph@surgery.arizona.edu

This rapid increase in the elderly population has a significant impact on the US health care system. In 2009 to 2010, for example, persons aged 65 and older made a total of 19.6 million emergency department visits. Their visit rate was 511 per 1000 persons and it increased with age.[4] As a result, older adults will most likely account for an increasing share of hospital and intensive care unit (ICU) use and costs in the coming years.[5] Because increasing age is associated with decreased physiologic reserves and frailty, this will result in admission of more frail patients to the ICU.[6] Premorbid frailty seems to be an independent but potentially modifiable factor associated with less favorable outcomes and greater health services use.[7] Moreover, critical illness leads to a catabolic state that further diminishes body reserves and contributes to frailty independent of age and prehospital functional status. Impairment of mobility is a common manifestation of illness in the frail individual and is therefore a sensitive marker of acute disease. It is one of the major components of frailty and channels the adverse events. Because early mobilization of patients in the ICU results in accelerated recovery and improvement in the functional status and quality of life, frailty can severely affect the mobility and ultimately impede the recovery. It is imperative, therefore, that health care professionals thoroughly understand the particular physiology of this population and the association of frailty and its impact on mobility in the ICU to properly care for them and improve clinical outcomes.

CHALLENGES IN THE CRITICAL CARE OF ELDERLY PATIENTS

For several reasons, the management and care for critically ill elderly patients is far more challenging than their younger counterparts. With advancing age, the response of the body to any stress is diminished and a decline in the functional reserve limits the ability of elderly patients to recover from critical illness. Likewise, increasing age coincides with several comorbidities that can further complicate the primary problem. Furthermore, the immune and inflammatory responses are blunted in the elderly, which results in unreliable signs and symptoms, which can delay the diagnosis and management. Polypharmacy is also commonly encountered in the elderly populations and these drug interactions and masking of symptoms also pose a significant problem.

Similarly, treatment goals for elderly patients may be different than those for younger ones. It is necessary, therefore, for health providers to bear these things in mind throughout the care of such patients. Moreover, elderly patients display great heterogeneity because of each individual's particular physiologic reserve, which is, in turn, determined by several intrinsic host factors (ie, genetics, age, sex, dietary and environmental exposures, long-term patterns of physical activity, hormonal balance, and any pre-existing medical conditions).[8] In short, all of these factors contribute to the frail status of an individual, which increases morbidity and mortality after stressful events.

In the past two decades, as the general paradigm in medicine has shifted to the quality of health care services, it is clear that a better understanding of outcomes in frail and elderly patients admitted to the ICU can advance evidence-based health care and guide patients in making informed decisions about life and death.

AGING AND THE IMPACT OF COMORBIDITES

The process of aging is characterized by the progressive and inevitable loss of function and functional reserve of organ systems and a diminished response of the body in times of physiologic and metabolic stress. This leads to a diminished capability of the body to adapt to changes and vulnerability to several chronic health problems and pathologic processes.[9] With advancing age, the decrease in physiologic reserves, chronic disease, and other health problems collectively complicate the health of an individual and the quality of life. According to the US Census Bureau's American Community Survey, some type of disability (ie, difficulty in hearing, vision, cognition, ambulation, self-care, or independent living) was reported by 36% of people age 65 and older in 2014. Although the gradual decline in function and physiologic reserve somewhat correlates with the increase in age, it also differs from person to person and from one organ-systems to another.[10] Moreover, in geriatric patients, it is challenging to predict who will have an optimal recovery following a stress (surgery or disease) and who will develop a complication that can trigger a cascade of events that may lead to permanent disability or even unexpected death.

INTENSIVE CARE UNIT CARE OF ELDERLY PATIENTS

With the continuous increase in the proportion of the elderly in the general population, the number of elderly patients being admitted to an ICU is also increasing.[11–14] In developed countries, for instance, the proportion of patients older than 80 years has been estimated to be up to 25% of the total ICU admissions.[15–17] This important transformation demands pragmatic decisions regarding appropriate levels of care and the nature of discussions with patients and families about the optimal goals of care. ICU admission can be beneficial to a patient under the following circumstances: the underlying cause of the danger to life is temporary, the patient requires close monitoring, and the patient has the capacity to benefit from an aggressive intervention. However, sometimes it may not be a fruitful decision because it may prolong the dying process, increase the amount of suffering by the patient, and separate the dying patient from his or her family. Risk factors of death in elderly ICU patients include the following:

- Age
- Underlying diagnosis
- Severity of acute illness
- Multiple organ dysfunctions
- Surgical versus nonsurgical diagnosis
- Chronic comorbidities
- Premorbid functional status
- Frail versus nonfrail

MOBILITY IN THE INTENSIVE CARE UNIT

ICU early mobility is a preventive form of physical and cognitive rehabilitation that engages the critically ill patient in activities that assist in the recovery of the cardiopulmonary system, prevent muscle deterioration and joint contractures, and begin the restoration of the patient's autonomy. The term "early" refers to mobilization and rehabilitation that begins immediately after the stabilization of physiologic derangements, often before patients are liberated from mechanical ventilation and low-dose vasopressor infusions. Studies from medical, surgical, and trauma ICUs have reported that almost half of critically ill patients are not able to return to their preillness level of functioning or work. Any critical illness is a complex pathologic state of catabolism and depletion of the body's reserves, often characterized by rapidly developing weakness and fatigue that can last for several years. A prolonged ICU stay and the effects of multiple sedatives can also cause delirium and cognitive changes for most patients. When combined with minimal or no sedation from the start of an ICU stay, mobility is protective and preventative, an essential part of reducing pain, agitation, delirium, and weakness in ICU patients.

Early and progressive mobility and initiation of rehabilitation is safe for ICU patients. It can reduce the incidence and duration of delirium, shorten ICU and hospital length of stay (LOS), and lower hospital costs. Still, developing an ICU system and culture to achieve these benefits is challenging.

Barriers to Early Mobility in the Intensive Care Unit

Several potential barriers can impede implementation of an early mobilization and rehabilitation program in the ICU. A multidisciplinary change in ICU culture to support early mobility and rehabilitation, accompanied by the appropriate required resources, is an essential step to overcome these barriers.[18,19]

- Safety issues
- Frailty status of patient
- Lack of leadership
- Lack of staffing and equipment
- Lack of knowledge and training
- Oversedation
- Delirium
- Fractures or other disabilities
- Patient hemodynamic tolerance and activity
- Patient's attachment to intravenous lines and monitors

Benefits of Early Mobility in the Intensive Care Unit

Mobilizing patients in the ICU can be a cumbersome and labor-intensive process, but the early initiation of daily activities, preferably at the beginning of a patient's ICU stay, can lead to physical independence for patients after discharge.[12,20–22] Some of the benefits of early mobility in the ICU are briefly discussed next.

- Functional mobility and muscle strength: Up to 25% to 50% of ICU patients can develop neuromuscular weakness in the ICU, which can last for years after hospital discharge. Early mobilization therapy is the evidence-based intervention recommended to prevent or ameliorate ICU-acquired weakness. Early mobility and rehabilitation in the ICU improves muscle strength and functional mobility.[21–24] A randomized trial that compared the early institution of physical and occupational therapies with the usual care found that patients who underwent early physical therapies had a higher likelihood of achieving independent functional status, less ICU-acquired weakness, and a greater unassisted walking distance at hospital discharge.[21] Another clinical trial that studied 90 critically ill patients randomized to early bed-cycle ergometer or no intervention found that early exercise in ICU patients enhanced recovery of the functional exercise capacity, self-perceived functional status, and muscle force at hospital discharge.[22] Correspondingly, a quality improvement prospective study at the medical ICU at the Johns Hopkins Hospital showed that early physical therapy, along with reducing heavy sedation, led to marked improvement in physical rehabilitation and functional mobility.[25]
- Quality of life: Early initiation of physical therapy and exercise in the ICU results in improved muscle strength and functional mobility, which leads to physical independence and improved quality of life.[26]

- ICU and hospital LOS and ventilator days: Early initiation of rehabilitation and mobilization in the ICU leads to a faster recovery and early discharge to the floor, which results in a decrease in ventilator days and ICU and hospital LOS.[21,23,27]
- ICU complications: Mobilization early on during the ICU stay also decreases complications, including atelectasis, aspiration and pneumonia, and joint contractures and muscle wasting. Additionally, it decreases the incidence and duration of delirium in the ICU.[28]
- Discharge: Patients who undergo mobilization and rehabilitation early on in the ICU achieve functional mobility and adequate muscle strength. They also have a greater chance to be discharged to home rather than to a skilled nursing facility.
- Readmissions: Early mobilization in the ICU also leads to improved long-term outcomes and decreases the readmission rate. A study that followed patients with acute respiratory failure admitted to the ICU for 1 year found that patients who lacked early ICU mobility had a higher 1-year readmission rate.[29]

Selection of Patient

- Safety: Does the patient have any exclusion criteria?
  - Patient requires significant doses of vasopressors for hemodynamic stability (maintain mean arterial pressure >60 mm Hg)
  - Mechanically ventilated patient who requires fraction of inspired oxygen greater than 0.8 and/or positive end-expiratory pressure greater than 12 mm Hg, or who has acutely worsening respiratory failure
  - Patient maintained on neuromuscular blocking agents
  - Patient in an acute neurologic event (cerebrovascular accident, subarachnoid hemorrhage, intracranial hemorrhage) with reassessment for mobility every 24 hours
  - Patient needs transfer to another hospital
  - Patient unresponsive to verbal stimuli
  - Patient with unstable spine or extremity fractures
  - Patient with a grave prognosis, transferring to comfort care
  - Patient with an open abdomen (risk for dehiscence)

If one of the previously listed factors is present, evaluation of the patient by the physician is required to determine if participation in physical activity is safe before initiation.

- Assessment of the patient's prior activity level
  - Determine the patient's level of activity in the past 2 hours and before the admission
- Assessment of the patient's strength
  - Grossly determine if the patient can lift his or her legs off the bed or bear weight on his or her legs
- Assessment of ability to engage the patient
  - Determine how well the patient can follow commands and if he or she can be engaged in activity

Mobilizing the Patient in the Intensive Care Unit

- Follow a stepwise increase if the patient can tolerate the following:
  - Untangle and secure the lines; connect the portable monitor, if possible
  - Initiate bed exercise; keep monitoring patient, monitor and watch the lines
  - Sit patient on the edge of the bed, if possible; assess for pain and orthostatic blood pressure

- ○ Assist seated patient in standing
- ○ Initiate walking; keep a chair close to the patient; use aides, volunteers, and students to push chair and intravenous poles
- ○ Seat and rest the patient as needed
- Stop and rest the patient if the following occur:
  - ○ Unresponsive
  - ○ Fatigued or becoming pale
  - ○ Respiratory rate consistently greater than 10 beats/min greater than baseline
  - ○ Muscle recruitment decreased
  - ○ Losing balance
  - ○ Weight-bearing ability decreased
  - ○ Diaphoresis present
  - ○ Chest pain
  - ○ Dizzy

FRAILTY

There is no consensus on a single precise and complete definition of frailty.[30] Numerous authors and investigators offer multiple definitions based on their understanding and interpretation of the concept. From a clinical perspective, frailty is defined as a syndrome of decreased physiologic reserve (physical and cognitive) and a decline in the resistance to stressors, which ultimately result in increased vulnerability to poor health outcomes, worsening mobility and disability, hospitalization, and death.[31-33] Alternatively, it is defined as a geriatric syndrome of increased vulnerability to environmental stressors with underlying inherent pathophysiologic mechanisms related to hormonal changes and sarcopenia and nutritional deficiencies.[34] Multiple attempts have also been made to identify the different components and criteria for the diagnosis of frailty. Fried and colleagues[35] defined frailty as the presence of three or more of the following: unintentional weight loss (10 lb in the past year), self-reported exhaustion, weakness (assessed by grip strength), slow walking speed, and low physical activity. Somewhat differently, the Rockwood frailty index uses weight loss, exhaustion or a low level of physical activity, weakness, a low energy and endurance level, and slowness to calculate frailty.[36,37] In addition to physical function, some authors also advocate for including several different other characteristics and domains in the definition of frailty, such as nutrition, psychological characteristics, and psychosocial factors. Although the exact and precise definition and components of frailty are yet to be agreed on by all, there is no doubt that the presence of frailty correlates with poor outcomes. Equally important, it is an indispensable tool for hospital resource allocation and clinical decision-making and family discussions about the goals of care and discharge disposition.

Superiority of Frailty as Compared with Age

Aging and frailty are not synonymous, but frailty becomes increasingly common with advancing age. Although some literature shows that age is an important predictor of worse outcomes, the effect of advanced age on outcomes independent of all the other measured and unmeasured factors (eg, the presence of comorbidities and baseline poor organ function) is not yet well characterized. Indeed, the risk factors for poor outcomes in the elderly are the same as those for younger patients, including comorbidities and prior baseline functional status.[38] Although these factors are more prevalent in the elderly population, they are not uniformly distributed across this population. Consequently, this varied distribution has led to the conception of "heterogeneity of aging," which means that organ function and a decrease in physiologic reserve vary greatly between individuals, and that the age at which these changes begin and the rate of decline also varies. Each organ system experiences a decrease in physiologic reserve at a different rate. Thus, each patient should be approached on a case-by-case basis. Because of these differences, chronologic age cannot accurately predict physiologic reserves. In addition, the commonly used tools to predict complications fail to take into account the physiologic reserves of elderly patients because they are mostly subjective.[39]

In contrast, the "frailty syndrome" refers to an increased vulnerability to stressors caused by the lack of physiologic reserves resulting from the age-associated accumulation of deficits in multiple organ systems combined with genetic, environmental, and physical insults. The advantage of this metric is that it takes into account each patient's physiologic, cognitive, social, and psychological deficits, ultimately leading to more patient-centered decisions resulting in improved outcomes and quality of life. An emerging body of literature suggests the superiority of frailty measurements over chronologic age alone in predicting outcomes.[40–43] Even individual mortality risk, which can be seen as the ultimate outcome of age and frailty,[44] is better predicted by frailty than by chronologic age.[45] Nonetheless, a chronologic age-based criterion is often used to select the geriatric population to determine the risks of any intervention or to predict the hospital course, complications, or mortality. Clearly, however, age alone may not be the best selection criterion because it is not the best predictor of poor outcomes of interventions and treatments.[46–49] Using the concept of decreased physiologic reserve measured by frailty as the criterion to select older persons at risk for interventions may, therefore, be a better tool than selecting geriatric patients based on their chronologic age alone.

Frailty in Intensive Care Unit Patients

The prevalence of frailty in the older population may be as high as 43%.[50,51] Because there is a trend of increased use of ICU resources by older people, the prevalence of pre-existing frailty in patients admitted to the ICU is also increasing.[14] The relevance of frailty in ICU patients, however, is not limited to the admission demographics (age). The development of critical illness may also lead to frailty in vulnerable or prefrail patients. It may also be an important factor impeding recovery and functional independence and autonomy in those already considered frail.[52] Whether it is the premorbid decreased physiologic reserves or the accelerated depletion of reserves as a result of an acute illness, the critically ill patient is vulnerable to adverse clinical outcomes, which may require an increase in the degree of life support, without which such a patient would not survive. In addition, deficits associated with frailty, which typically take years to accumulate in the outpatient geriatric population, rapidly develop in a large proportion of critically ill patients independent of age and illness severity. This may include sarcopenia and clinically significant weakness and poor functional status following discharge from the ICU.[53,54] A study that looked at the functional status immediately after discharge from an ICU showed that reduced grip strength and diminished mobility were correlated with poor functional status shortly after discharge from the ICU.[54] Because critically ill patients share many of the clinical features and characteristics of old, frail patients, the role of frailty has substantial clinical, psychosocial, and economic implications regarding the management of critically ill patients admitted to the ICU. Evaluation of frailty in critically ill patients admitted to the ICU provides information about the prognosis and outcomes. Tailored targeted intervention in these areas may help to improve outcomes and the quality of life.

Impact of Frailty on Mobility

Mobility is one of the major components of many frailty definitions.[36,55] Changes in different health states, such as transitions between different states of mobility, disability, and function, are of great clinical and public health interest. There is a growing consensus that markers of frailty include age-associated declines in lean body mass, muscle mass (sarcopenia), strength, endurance, balance, walking performance, and low activity.[56–59] Multiple of these components must be present clinically to constitute frailty. Frailty may be a precedent stage to disability. A study of 5317 patients aged 65 or more showed that 72% of frail patients reported difficulty in mobility, whereas 60% had difficulty in instrumental activities of daily living.[35] In addition, there was a step-wise increase in disability with increasing frailty status. Similarly, the results of the famous French three-city study showed that frail patients had 2.68 times higher odds of having mobility limitations as compared with the non-frail patients.[60] A novel wearable technology for assessing frailty showed that it can reliably predict and calculate frailty using 20-second trial of elbow flexion, within which patients repetitively flex and extend their dominant elbow to full flexion and extension as quickly as possible.[61] The measurement of frailty using the speed (slowness), power (weakness), and speed reduction (exhaustion) from this wearable technology provides evidence for the strong correlation between frailty and mobility.

Early and progressive mobility in the ICU improve outcomes and quality of life. Critical illness by itself is debilitating and leads to restricted mobility, low energy, and early fatigue. In addition, if the patient is frail or prefail to begin with, the burden of acute illness can significantly compromise the early ICU mobility of patients and thus further worsen the ICU course.

Measurement of Frailty

At least 25 different scales are available to measure frailty. However, there is no consensus on a single scale and the burden of data collection versus reliability/validity of each scale continues to be a consistent problem. The most comprehensive of these measurement tools is the Rockwood frailty model, which uses a judgment-based seven-point Clinical Frailty Scale to measure frailty based on 70 variables that assess the cognitive, physiologic, physical, and social well-being of the individual (**Table 1**).[50] More recently, a modified 50-variable Rockwood frailty index has been shown to reliably predict morbidity in patients undergoing emergency general surgery.[62] A 15-variable Trauma-Specific Frailty Index has also been validated by Joseph and colleagues[63] in geriatric trauma patients (**Table 2**). Another widely used tool is the operational definition described by Fried and colleagues,[35] presented in **Box 1**. All these scores reliably calculate frailty and identify elderly patients at risk of outcomes; however, none of these tests have been used on other subsets of the population to date.[64,65]

Prognostic Implications of Frailty

The modern health care system is evolving and there is a change of focus from health outcomes alone to the quality of health care delivered. In keeping with this aim, frailty is a valuable metric and a major determinant for predicting mortality, hospitalization, discharge disposition, and the quality of life in geriatric patients and is by far superior to the chronologic age alone.[42,45,66] Because frailty deals with physiologic reserves and the ability of the body to respond to stressful conditions, it may also serve as a surrogate for many of the otherwise unmeasurable aspects of a patient's health before the illness. Evidence suggests that physiologic reserve, along with the preillness baseline functional status and the presence of pre-existing comorbidities, may be an important determinant of outcomes and have prognostic value in critically ill patients.[67–70]

Table 1 Clinical Frailty Score		
Score	Status	Description
1	Very fit	People who are robust, active, energetic, and motivated. These people commonly exercise regularly. They are among the fittest for their age.
2	Well	People who have no active disease symptoms but are less fit than those of category 1. Often, they exercise or are active occasionally (that is, seasonally).
3	Managing well	People whose medical problems are well controlled, but are not regularly active beyond routinely walking.
4	Vulnerable	Although not dependent on others for daily help, symptoms often limit activities. A common complaint is being slowed up, and/or being tired during the day.
5	Mildly frail	These people often have more evident slowing, and need help in high-order independent activities of daily living (finances, transportation, heavy housework, medications). Typically, mild frailty progressively impairs shopping and walking outside alone, meal preparation, and housework.
6	Moderately frail	People need help with all outside activities and with keeping house. Inside, they often have problems with stairs and need help with bathing and might need minimal assistance (cuing, standby) with dressing.
7	Severely frail	Completely dependent for personal care, from whatever cause (physical or cognitive). Even so, they seem stable and not at high risk of dying (within ~6 mo)
8	Very severely frail	Completely dependent, approaching the end of life. Typically, they could not recover even from a minor illness.
9	Terminally ill	Approaching the end of life. This category applies to people with a life expectancy <6 mo, who are not otherwise evidently frail.

There are several available scoring systems (based on the acute derangement of hemostasis and vital parameters at admission) to guide decision making, management, and prognostication concerning ICU patients. They include the Acute Physiology and Chronic Health Evaluation II score,[67] the Sequential Organ Failure Assessment score,[71] and the Simplified Acute Physiology Score II. These scoring systems evaluate the severity of the illness to estimate the probability of adverse outcomes and survival[12,72,73]; however, they mostly fail to incorporate the sociodemographic characteristics, prehospital function status, and the presence and severity of other comorbidities and the disability. These limitations are even more relevant when considering quality of life and long-term outcomes following discharge from the ICU. Increasing availability of data on poor, intermediate, and long-term outcomes after critical illness (which comprises not only mortality, but also functional status, disposition to a facility center, and quality of life), coupled with the huge financial cost of critical care therapy, demands the development of better tools to predict those patients who will benefit most from critical care treatment.[74] Currently, however, there is no tool to measure the healing capacity of a patient or to determine his or her physiologic reserves directly; therefore, frailty serves as an invaluable surrogate for these factors in critically ill patients.

A prospective multicenter study in four ICUs showed that frailty was independently associated with increased ICU and 6-month mortalities.[75] It also showed that the

Table 2
Trauma-Specific Frailty Index

Fifteen-variable Trauma-Specific Frailty Index			
Comorbidities			
Cancer history	Yes (1)	No (0)	PCI (0.5)
Coronary heart disease	MI (1) Medication (0.25)	CABG (0.75) None (0)	
Dementia	Severe (1) No (0)	Moderate (0.5)	Mild (0.25)
Daily activities			
Help with grooming	Yes (1)	No (0)	
Help managing money	Yes (1)	No (0)	
Help doing housework	Yes (1)	No (0)	
Help toileting	Yes (1)	No (0)	
Help walking	Wheelchair (1) No (0)	Walker (0.75)	Cane (0.5)
Health attitude			
Feel less useful	Most time (1)	Sometimes (0.5)	Never (0)
Feel sad	Most time (1)	Sometimes (0.5)	Never (0)
Feel effort to do everything	Most time (1)	Sometimes (0.5)	Never (0)
Falls	Within last month (1)	Present not in last month (0.5)	None (0)
Feel lonely	Most time (1)	Sometimes (0.5)	Never (0)
Function			
Sexual active	Yes (0)	No (1)	
Nutrition			
Albumin	<3 (1)	>3 (0)	

Abbreviations: CABG, coronary artery bypass graft; MI, myocardial infarction; PCI, percutaneous coronary intervention.

Clinical Frailty Score predicts outcomes more effectively than the commonly used ICU illness scores. Another study of 421 critically ill adult patients from six hospitals demonstrated that frail patients had an increased risk of an adverse event, mortality, and hospital LOS, and were less likely to be discharged home.[6] Similarly, the

Box 1
Phenotypes of frailty

Criteria:
1. Decreased grip strength
2. Self-reported exhaustion
3. Unintentional weight loss of more than 4.5 kg over the past year
4. Slow walking speed
5. Low physical activity

Definition:
  Positive for frail phenotype: ≥3 criteria present
  Intermediate/prefrail: one or two criteria present
  Nonfrail: no criteria present

readmission rate was also higher in frail patients. Correspondingly, Heyland and colleagues[76] showed that a low frailty index correlated with improved physical recovery and a return to baseline levels of physical function at 1 year in patients aged 80 years or older.

CLINICAL APPLICATIONS OF THIS KNOWLEDGE

Routine assessment of baseline physical function and frailty status could aid in prognostication and informed decision-making for all the critically ill patients, especially the elderly. The measurement and diagnosis of frailty could translate into better-informed decision-making for patients, their families, and clinicians concerning issues related to the provision of advanced life support and designation of the goals of care.

- Informed triage decisions: Knowledge about the frailty status and vulnerability of patients helps to identify patients who are at risk of adverse complications and who would benefit from ICU admission.
- Informed ICU decision-making: It also helps to set realistic goals of care and enhance the discussion with the patient and his or her family about survival, morbidity, disability, being able to be transferred to home versus a skilled nursing facility, the possibility of readmission, and the subsequent quality of life.
- Interventions: The ability to recognize a frail and vulnerable patient on admission augments resource allocation and fosters a focus on maximizing physical recovery, thus limiting the disability. Additionally, an overall effort should also be made to improve the patient's cognitive, psychosocial, and emotional recovery.
- Transition of care: Currently, there is a large body of evidence that demonstrates the existence of serious quality problems for patients undergoing transitions across sites of care. The frailty status of a patient may help in the coordination and continuity of health care during a transfer from one health care setting to another (or to home) and between health care practitioners and settings as the patient's condition and care needs change during the course of acute illness.
- Hospital resources: Frailty is also an important and reliable metric in predicating costs. Increased hospital and ICU LOS among frail patients, for instance, correspond to higher hospital costs.
- Failure to rescue: Failure to rescue (FTR) is defined as death after a major complication. It is an important benchmark of patient safety and health care quality. As a common index of the quality of health care delivery, it shows how well hospitals perform after a patient develops a complication. Several prior studies have found that the in-hospital mortality rate is significantly affected with variation in the management of complications.[41,77] Frailty may also be a valuable patient-level factor that contributes to FTR after a complication. Therefore, the early identification of patients experiencing physical decline and subsequent, appropriate interventions may decrease FTR. Although, there is a paucity of data on the usefulness of frailty in predicting FTR, there is a growing consensus in geriatrics regarding the correlation between the two. There is a solid justification for assessing the impact of frailty on FTR.[78,79]
- End-of-life decision: In patients with a preillness diminished physiologic reserve, the burden of acute illness further dampens the ability to have a meaningful recovery. Therefore, patient preference, the possibility of prolonged measures of life support and extensive rehabilitation, loss of independence, and the quality of life should be discussed with the patient and his or her family to help them make an informed decision and meaningfully participate in the setting up of short- and long-term goals.

SUMMARY

Frailty is a multisystem syndrome reflecting a poor physiologic and functional reserve that also predicts several adverse outcomes. This is especially relevant because the number of frail individuals using ICU resources is increasing with the large, aging Baby Boomer population. Furthermore, a poor frailty syndrome is further exacerbated by the effects of critical illness, which may also be a key factor impeding recovery and functional autonomy in those already considered to be frail. Generally, early and progressive mobility in the ICU assists in the recovery of the patient, prevents muscle deterioration, and improves the quality of life. Frailty can, however, significantly compromise the early ICU mobility of patients and thus further worsen the ICU course. Clearly, therefore, early identification of frail patients and timely resource allocation and interventions help improve clinical outcomes and the quality of life in ICU patients.

REFERENCES

1. Joseph B, Hassan A. Geriatric trauma patients: what is the difference? Curr Surg Rep 2016;4(1):1.
2. Vincent GK, Velkoff VA. The next four decades: the older population in the United States: 2010 to 2050. Washington, DC: US Department of Commerce, Economics and Statistics Administration, US Census Bureau; 2010.
3. Hobbs F, Damon BL. Sixty-five plus in the United States. Washington, DC: US Department of Commerce, Bureau of the Census; 1996.
4. Albert M, McCaig LF, Ashman JJ. Emergency department visits by persons aged 65 and over: United States, 2009–2010. NCHS Data Brief 2013;(130):1–8.
5. Levant S, Chari K, DeFrances CJ. Hospitalizations for patients aged 85 and over in the United States, 2000-2010. NCHS Data Brief 2015;182:1–8.
6. Bagshaw SM, Thomas Stelfox H, McDermid RC, et al. Association between frailty and short-and long-term outcomes among critically ill patients: a multicentre prospective cohort study. Can Med Assoc J 2014;186(2):E95–102.
7. Hope AA, Gong MN, Guerra C, et al. Frailty before critical illness and mortality for elderly Medicare beneficiaries. J Am Geriatr Soc 2015;63(6):1121–8.
8. Degutis LC, Baker C. Trauma in the elderly: a statewide perspective. Conn Med 1987;51(3):161.
9. Beck JC. Geriatrics review syllabus: a core curriculum in geriatric medicine, vol. 3. New York, NY: John Wiley & Sons; 2002.
10. Vijg J, Wei JY. Understanding the biology of aging: the key to prevention and therapy. J Am Geriatr Soc 1995;43(4):426–34.
11. Oeppen J, Vaupel JW. Broken limits to life expectancy. Science 2002;296(5570): 1029–31.
12. Needham DM. Mobilizing patients in the intensive care unit: improving neuromuscular weakness and physical function. Jama 2008;300(14):1685–90.
13. Nguyen Y-L, Angus DC, Boumendil A, et al. The challenge of admitting the very elderly to intensive care. Ann Intensive Care 2011;1(1):29.
14. Bagshaw SM, Webb SA, Delaney A, et al. Very old patients admitted to intensive care in Australia and New Zealand: a multi-centre cohort analysis. Crit Care 2009; 13(2):R45.
15. De Rooij S, Govers A, Korevaar JC, et al. Short-term and long-term mortality in very elderly patients admitted to an intensive care unit. Intensive Care Med 2006;32(7):1039–44.
16. Hamel MB, Davis RB, Teno JM, et al. Older age, aggressiveness of care, and survival for seriously ill, hospitalized adults. Ann Intern Med 1999;131(10):721–8.

17. Somme D, Maillet JM, Gisselbrecht M, et al. Critically ill old and the oldest-old patients in intensive care: short-and long-term outcomes. Intensive Care Med 2003; 29(12):2137–43.
18. Needham DM, Feldman DR, Kho ME. The functional costs of ICU survivorship: collaborating to improve post-ICU disability. Am Thorac Soc 2011;183(8):962–4.
19. Hopkins RO, Spuhler VJ, Thomsen GE. Transforming ICU culture to facilitate early mobility. Crit Care Clin 2007;23(1):81–96.
20. Morris PE, Goad A, Thompson C, et al. Early intensive care unit mobility therapy in the treatment of acute respiratory failure. Crit Care Med 2008;36(8):2238–43.
21. Schweickert WD, Pohlman MC, Pohlman AS, et al. Early physical and occupational therapy in mechanically ventilated, critically ill patients: a randomised controlled trial. Lancet 2009;373(9678):1874–82.
22. Burtin C, Clerckx B, Robbeets C, et al. Early exercise in critically ill patients enhances short-term functional recovery. Crit Care Med 2009;37(9):2499–505.
23. Li Z, Peng X, Zhu B, et al. Active mobilization for mechanically ventilated patients: a systematic review. Arch Phys Med Rehabil 2013;94(3):551–61.
24. Parker A, Needham D. The importance of early rehabilitation and mobility in the ICU. Los Angeles (CA); 2015.
25. Needham DM, Korupolu R, Zanni JM, et al. Early physical medicine and rehabilitation for patients with acute respiratory failure: a quality improvement project. Arch Phys Med Rehabil 2010;91(4):536–42.
26. Kayambu G, Boots R, Paratz J. Physical therapy for the critically ill in the ICU: a systematic review and meta-analysis. Crit Care Med 2013;41(6):1543–54.
27. Malkoc M, Karadibak D, Yldrm Y. The effect of physiotherapy on ventilatory dependency and the length of stay in an intensive care unit. Int J Rehabil Res 2009;32(1):85–8.
28. Brahmbhatt N, Murugan R, Milbrandt EB. Early mobilization improves functional outcomes in critically ill patients. Crit Care 2010;14(5):321.
29. Morris PE, Griffin L, Berry M, et al. Receiving early mobility during an intensive care unit admission is a predictor of improved outcomes in acute respiratory failure. Am J Med Sci 2011;341(5):373–7.
30. Champion HR, Copes WS, Buyer D, et al. Major trauma in geriatric patients. Am J Public Health 1989;79(9):1278–82.
31. Hsia RY, Wang E, Saynina O, et al. Factors associated with trauma center use for elderly patients with trauma: a statewide analysis, 1999-2008. Arch Surg 2011; 146(5):585–92.
32. Fried LP, Kronmal RA, Newman AB, et al. Risk factors for 5-year mortality in older adults: the Cardiovascular Health Study. JAMA 1998;279(8):585–92.
33. Searle SD, Mitnitski A, Gahbauer EA, et al. A standard procedure for creating a frailty index. BMC Geriatr 2008;8(1):24.
34. Ruiz M, Cefalu C, Reske T. Frailty syndrome in geriatric medicine. Am J Med Sci 2012;344(5):395–8.
35. Fried LP, Tangen CM, Walston J, et al. Frailty in older adults evidence for a phenotype. J Gerontol A Biol Sci Med Sci 2001;56(3):M146–57.
36. Rockwood K, Mitnitski A. Frailty in relation to the accumulation of deficits. J Gerontol A Biol Sci Med Sci 2007;62(7):722–7.
37. Mitnitski A, Song X, Rockwood K. Assessing biological aging: the origin of deficit accumulation. Biogerontology 2013;14(6):709–17.
38. Hamel MB, Henderson WG, Khuri SF, et al. Surgical outcomes for patients aged 80 and older: morbidity and mortality from major noncardiac surgery. J Am Geriatr Soc 2005;53(3):424–9.

39. Caterino JM, Valasek T, Werman HA. Identification of an age cutoff for increased mortality in patients with elderly trauma. Am J Emerg Med 2010;28(2):151–8.

40. Joseph B, Pandit V, Zangbar B, et al. Superiority of frailty over age in predicting outcomes among geriatric trauma patients: a prospective analysis. JAMA Surg 2014;149(8):766–72.

41. Jokar TO, Orouji Jokar T, Hassan A, et al. Redefining the association between old age and poor outcomes after trauma: the impact of the frailty syndrome. J Am Coll Surg 2015;221(4):S83–4.

42. Schuurmans H, Steverink N, Lindenberg S, et al. Old or frail: what tells us more? J Gerontol A Biol Sci Med Sci 2004;59(9):M962–5.

43. Makary MA, Segev DL, Pronovost PJ, et al. Frailty as a predictor of surgical outcomes in older patients. J Am Coll Surg 2010;210(6):901–8.

44. Morley J, Perry H, Miller DK. Something about frailty [Editorial]. J Gerontol A Biol Sci Med Sci 2002;57:M698–704.

45. Mitnitski AB, Mogilner AJ, MacKnight C, et al. The mortality rate as a function of accumulated deficits in a frailty index. Mech Ageing Dev 2002;123(11):1457–60.

46. Witz M, Witz S, Shnaker A, et al. Carotid surgery in the octogenarians. Should patients' age be a consideration in carotid artery endarterectomy? Age and ageing 2003;32(4):462–3.

47. Yancik R, Wesley MN, Ries LA, et al. Effect of age and comorbidity in postmenopausal breast cancer patients aged 55 years and older. JAMA 2001;285(7):885–92.

48. Lapierre S, Bouffard L, Dubé M, et al. Aspirations and well-being in old age. 2011.

49. Lamberg L. Illness, not age itself, most often the trigger of sleep problems in older adults. JAMA 2003;290(3):319–23.

50. Rockwood K, Song X, MacKnight C, et al. A global clinical measure of fitness and frailty in elderly people. Can Med Assoc J 2005;173(5):489–95.

51. McDermid RC, Bagshaw SM. Prolonging life and delaying death: the role of physicians in the context of limited intensive care resources. Philos Ethics Humanit Med 2009;4(1):3.

52. McDermid RC, Stelfox HT, Bagshaw SM. Frailty in the critically ill: a novel concept. Crit Care 2011;15(1):301.

53. De Jonghe B, Sharshar T, Lefaucheur JP, et al. Paresis acquired in the intensive care unit: a prospective multicenter study. JAMA 2002;288(22):2859–67.

54. Van der Schaaf M, Dettling DS, Beelen A, et al. Poor functional status immediately after discharge from an intensive care unit. Disabil Rehabil 2008;30(23):1812–8.

55. Mitnitski AB, Mogilner AJ, Rockwood K. Accumulation of deficits as a proxy measure of aging. Scientific World J 2001;1:323–36.

56. Campbell AJ, Buchner DM. Unstable disability and the fluctuations of frailty. Age Ageing 1997;26(4):315–8.

57. Buchner DM, Wagner EH. Preventing frail health. Clin Geriatr Med 1992;8(1):1–17.

58. Fried L, Walston J. Frailty and failure to thrive. In: Hazzard WR, Blass JP, Ettinger WH Jr, et al, editors. Principles of geriatric medicine and gerontology. 4th edition. New York: McGraw Hill; 1998. p. 1387–402.

59. Chandler JM, Hadley EC. Exercise to improve physiologic and functional performance in old age. Clin Geriatr Med 1996;12(4):761–84.

60. Ávila-Funes JA, Helmer C, Amieva H, et al. Frailty among community-dwelling elderly people in France: the three-city study. J Gerontol A Biol Sci Med Sci 2008;63(10):1089–96.

61. Toosizadeh N, Cristine B, Christian B, et al. Assessing upper-extremity motion: an innovative, objective method to identify frailty in older bed-bound trauma patients. J Am Coll Surg 2016;223(2):240–8.
62. Joseph B, Zangbar B, Pandit V, et al. Emergency general surgery in the elderly: too old or too frail? J Am Coll Surg 2016;222(5):805–13.
63. Joseph B, Pandit V, Zangbar B, et al. Validating trauma-specific frailty index for geriatric trauma patients: a prospective analysis. J Am Coll Surg 2014;219(1):10–7.e1.
64. Rockwood K, Mitnitski AB, MacKnight C. Some mathematical models of frailty and their clinical implications. Rev Clin Gerontol 2002;12(02):109–17.
65. Fried LP, Ferrucci L, Darer J, et al. Untangling the concepts of disability, frailty, and comorbidity: implications for improved targeting and care. J Gerontol A Biol Sci Med Sci 2004;59(3):M255–63.
66. Mitnitski AB, Graham JE, Mogilner AJ, et al. Frailty, fitness and late-life mortality in relation to chronological and biological age. BMC Geriatr 2002;2(1):1.
67. Ho K, Finn J, Knuiman M, et al. Combining multiple comorbidities with Acute Physiology Score to predict hospital mortality of critically ill patients: a linked data cohort study. Anaesthesia 2007;62(11):1095–100.
68. Dowdy DW, Eid MP, Sedrakyan A, et al. Quality of life in adult survivors of critical illness: a systematic review of the literature. Intensive Care Med 2005;31(5):611–20.
69. Poses RM, McClish DK, Smith WR, et al. Prediction of survival of critically ill patients by admission comorbidity. J Clin Epidemiol 1996;49(7):743–7.
70. Mata GV, Rivera Fernandez R, Gonzalez Carmona A, et al. Factors related to quality of life 12 months after discharge from an intensive care unit. Crit Care Med 1992;20(9):1257–62.
71. Ferreira FL, Bota DP, Bross A, et al. Serial evaluation of the SOFA score to predict outcome in critically ill patients. JAMA 2001;286(14):1754–8.
72. Knaus WA, Draper EA, Wagner DP, et al. APACHE II: a severity of disease classification system. Crit Care Med 1985;13(10):818–29.
73. Vincent J-L, Moreno R, Takala J, et al. The SOFA (Sepsis-related Organ Failure Assessment) score to describe organ dysfunction/failure. Intensive Care Med 1996;22(7):707–10.
74. Unroe M, Kahn JM, Carson SS, et al. One-year trajectories of care and resource utilization for recipients of prolonged mechanical ventilation cohort study. Ann Intern Med 2010;153(3):167–75.
75. Le Maguet P, Roquilly A, Lasocki S, et al. Prevalence and impact of frailty on mortality in elderly ICU patients: a prospective, multicenter, observational study. Intensive Care Med 2014;40(5):674–82.
76. Heyland DK, Garland A, Bagshaw SM, et al. Recovery after critical illness in patients aged 80 years or older: a multi-center prospective observational cohort study. Intensive Care Med 2015;41(11):1911–20.
77. Green P, Woglom AE, Genereux P, et al. The impact of frailty status on survival after transcatheter aortic valve replacement in older adults with severe aortic stenosis: a single-center experience. JACC Cardiovasc Interv 2012;5(9):974–81.
78. Arya S, Kim SI, Duwayri Y, et al. Frailty increases the risk of 30-day mortality, morbidity, and failure to rescue after elective abdominal aortic aneurysm repair independent of age and comorbidities. J Vasc Surg 2015;61(2):324–31.
79. Bell TM, Zarzaur BL. Insurance status is a predictor of failure to rescue in trauma patients at both safety net and non–safety net hospitals. J Trauma Acute Care Surg 2013;75(4):728–33.

Intensive Care Unit Delirium and Intensive Care Unit–Related Posttraumatic Stress Disorder

CrossMark

Annachiara Marra, MD, PhD(c)[a], Pratik P. Pandharipande, MD, MSCI[b], Mayur B. Patel, MD, MPH[c],*

KEYWORDS

- Intensive care unit • Delirium • Posttraumatic stress disorder • ICU-related PTSD
- Long-term cognitive impairment • Brain dysfunction • Critical illness

KEY POINTS

- Delirium is a strong predictor of increased length of mechanical ventilation, longer intensive care unit (ICU) stays, increased cost, long-term cognitive impairment, and mortality.
- Routine monitoring for delirium is recommended for all ICU patients.
- In delirious patients, pharmacologic treatment should be used only after giving adequate attention to correction of modifiable contributing factors. The ABCDEF (attention to analgesia, both awakening and breathing trials, choosing right sedative, delirium monitoring and management, early exercise, and family involvement) bundle is recommended and associated with improved outcomes, including reduction in delirium.

Continued

Disclosures and Funding: P.P. Pandharipande and M.B. Patel are supported by National Institutes of Health HL111111 and GM120484 (Bethesda, MD). P.P. Pandharipande was supported by the VA Clinical Science Research and Development Service (Washington, DC) and the National Institutes of Health AG027472 and AG035117 (Bethesda, MD). M.B. Patel was supported by the Vanderbilt Faculty Research Scholars Program. P.P. Pandharipande has received research grants from Hospira, Inc. The authors have no other disclosures relevant to this article.

[a] Division of Allergy, Pulmonary and Critical Care Medicine, Center for Health Services Research, University of Naples Federico II, Vanderbilt University Medical Center, 1215 21st Avenue South, Medical Center East, Suite 6100, Nashville, TN 37232-8300, USA; [b] Division of Anesthesiology Critical Care Medicine, Department of Anesthesiology, Center for Health Services Research, Vanderbilt University Medical Center, 1211 21st Avenue South, Medical Arts Building, Suite 526, Nashville, TN 37212, USA; [c] Division of Trauma, Surgical Critical Care, and Emergency General Surgery, Department of Surgery, Section of Surgical Sciences, Center for Health Services Research, Vanderbilt Brain Institute, Vanderbilt University Medical Center, 1211 21st Avenue South, Medical Arts Building, Suite 404, Nashville, TN 37212, USA
* Corresponding author.
E-mail address: mayur.b.patel@Vanderbilt.Edu

Surg Clin N Am 97 (2017) 1215–1235
http://dx.doi.org/10.1016/j.suc.2017.07.008
0039-6109/17/Published by Elsevier Inc.

surgical.theclinics.com

Continued

- Posttraumatic stress disorder (PTSD) is one of many important mental health problems after significant critical illness.
- The incidence of ICU-related PTSD is around 10% and using ICU diaries in routine clinical care may alter PTSD outcomes among both patients and families.

DELIRIUM

One of the most common behavioral manifestations of acute brain dysfunction in intensive care units (ICUs) is delirium. According to the fifth edition of the Diagnostic and Statistical Manual of the American Psychiatric Association (DSM-5), delirium is defined as (1) a disturbance of consciousness (ie, reduced clarity of awareness of the environment) with reduced ability to focus, sustain, or shift attention; (2) a change in cognition (eg, memory deficit, disorientation, language disturbance) or development of a perceptual disturbance that is not better accounted for by a preexisting, established, or evolving dementia; (3) developing over a short period of time, hours to days, and fluctuating over time; (4) with evidence from the history, physical examination, or laboratory findings that the disturbance is caused by a direct physiologic consequence of a general medical condition, an intoxicating substance, medication use, or more than 1 cause[1] (**Fig. 1**).

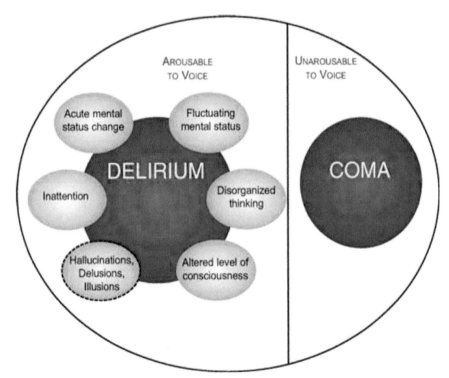

Fig. 1. Cardinal symptoms of delirium. (*From* Morandi A, Pandharipande P, Trabucchi M, et al. Understanding international differences in terminology for delirium and other types of acute brain dysfunction in critically ill patients. Intensive Care Med 2008;34(10):1911; with permission.)

The true prevalence and magnitude of delirium has been poorly documented because a myriad of terms, such as acute confusional state, ICU psychosis, acute brain dysfunction, and encephalopathy, have been used historically to describe this condition.[2] Delirium occurs in up to 60% to 80% of mechanically ventilated medical and surgical ICU patients and 50% to 70% of nonventilated medical ICU patients,[3-7] and should be considered as a significant, serious problem and treated as a possible contributor to mortality risk, increased length of mechanical ventilation, longer ICU stays, increased cost, prolonged neuropsychological dysfunction, and mortality.[8-12]

Numerous risk factors for delirium have been identified, including preexisting cognitive impairment, advanced age, use of psychoactive drugs, mechanical ventilation, untreated pain, heart failure, prolonged immobilization, abnormal blood pressure, anemia, sleep deprivation, and sepsis.[8,13-16] The average medical ICU patient has 11 or more risk factors for developing delirium. These risk factors can be divided into predisposing baseline factors (eg, demographics, comorbidities) and hospital-related factors (eg, acute illness severity, medications, ICU events) (**Table 1**).[17] Delirium prevention in the ICU should focus on reducing the number and duration of potentially modifiable or preventable risk factors. Several mnemonics can aid clinicians in recalling the list of delirium risk factors (**Table 2**).

Many drugs are considered to be risk factors for the development of delirium. Benzodiazepines have shown a strong association with delirium. The class of benzodiazepines does not seem to change the risk profile, with both lorazepam and midazolam being significant risk factors for delirium. The Society of Critical Care Medicine's (SCCM) ICU Pain Agitation Delirium (PAD) guidelines recommend that nonbenzodiazepine sedative options may be preferred to benzodiazepine-based sedative

Table 1
Risk factors for delirium

	Unmodifiable/ Unpreventable Risk Factors	Potentially Modifiable/ Preventable Risk Factors
Baseline Risk Factors	Age and APOE-4 genotype History of hypertension Preexisting cognitive impairment History of alcohol use History of tobacco use History of depression	Sensory deprivation (eg, hearing or vision impairment)
Hospital-related Risk Factors	High severity of illness Respiratory disease Need for mechanical ventilation Number of infusing medications Increased levels of inflammatory biomarkers High LNAA metabolite levels	Anemia Acidosis Hypotension Infection/sepsis Metabolic disturbances Fever Lack of visitors Sedatives/analgesics Immobility Bladder catheters Vascular catheters Gastric tubes Sleep and light deprivation

Abbreviations: APOE-4, apolipoprotien-E4 polymorphism; LNAA, large neutral amino acids.

Adapted from Brummel NE, Girard TD. Preventing delirium in the intensive care unit. Crit Care Clin 2013;29(1):61; with permission.

Table 2
Mnemonics for risk factors for delirium

I Watch Death	Delirium (S)
I: infection: HIV, sepsis, pneumonia	D: drugs
W: withdrawal (alcohol, barbiturate, sedative-hypnotic)	E: eyes, ears, and other sensory deficits
A: acute metabolic (acidosis, alkalosis, electrolyte disturbance, hepatic failure, renal failure)	L: low O_2 states (eg, heart attack, stroke, and pulmonary embolism)
T: trauma (closed head injury, heat stroke, postoperative, severe burns)	I: infection
C: CNS disorder (abscess, hemorrhage, hydrocephalus, subdural hematoma, infection, seizures, stroke, tumors, metastases, vasculitis, encephalitis, meningitis, syphilis)	R: retention (of urine or stool)
H: hypoxia (anemia, carbon monoxide poisoning, hypotension, pulmonary or cardiac failure)	I: ictal state
D: deficiencies (vitamin B_{12}, folate, niacin, thiamine)	U: underhydration/undernutrition
E: endocrinopathies (hyperadrenocorticism/ hypoadrenocorticism, hyperglycemia/ hypoglycemia, myxedema, hyperparathyroidism)	M: metabolic causes (DM, postoperative state, sodium abnormalities)
A: acute vascular (hypertensive encephalopathy, stroke, arrhythmia, shock)	(S): subdural hematoma
T: toxins or drugs (prescription drugs, illicit drugs, pesticides, solvents)	
H: heavy Metals (lead, manganese, mercury)	

Abbreviations: CNS, central nervous system; DM, diabetes mellitus; HIV, human immunodeficiency virus.

Adapted from Saint Louis University Geriatrics Evaluation Mnemonics Screening Tools (SLU GEMS). Developed or compiled by: Faculty from Saint Louis University Geriatrics Division and St. Louis Veterans Affairs GRECC; and http://pda.rnao.ca/content/causes-delirium.

regimens.[18] Pandharipande and colleagues[19] found that every unit dose of lorazepam was associated with a higher risk for daily transition to delirium. Similarly, Seymour and colleagues[20] confirmed that benzodiazepines are an independent risk factor for development of delirium during critical illness even when given more than 8 hours before a delirium assessment. Although targeted pain control has been shown to be associated with improved rates of delirium, Marcantonio and colleagues[21] found that delirium was significantly associated with postoperative exposure to meperidine, although not to other commonly prescribed opiates. Modification of risk factors in the ICU, such as the use of psychoactive drugs, maintenance of sleep/awake cycles, attempts to minimize malnutrition, optimization of the use of restraints, and provision of visual or hearing aids, may decrease the incidence and/or duration of delirium.[22]

The consequences of this brain dysfunction are important. Delirium is a strong predictor of increased length of mechanical ventilation, longer ICU stays, increased cost, long-term cognitive impairment, and mortality.[7,8,22–24] Ely and colleagues[22] showed that more than 80% of mechanically ventilated patients developed delirium during their hospital stays. Most delirium cases occurred initially in the ICU, with an average time of onset between the second and the third day with a mean duration of 3.4 ± 1.9 days. Delirium was the strongest predictor of hospital length of stay, even after adjusting for severity of illness, age, gender, race, and days of psychoactive drug use.

Delirium has been a strong risk factor for mortality.[8,25] Pisani and colleagues[25] pointed out that the number of days of ICU delirium was significantly associated with time to death within 1-year post-ICU admission (hazard ratio, 1.10; 95% confidence interval [CI], 1.02–1.18) and that the cumulative effect of multiple days is multiplicative rather than additive. The relationship between the duration of delirium and mortality was nonlinear, with a greater effect observed earlier in the course of delirium. These data suggest that the harm of delirium may occur early in the period of brain dysfunction for ICU patients.[24] In contrast, Klein Klouwenberg and colleagues[26] speculated that the increased mortality could be mediated through a prolonged ICU length of stay, rather than a direct effect on the daily risk of death, although longer duration of delirium (>2 days) still had some attributable mortality risk. Nonetheless, a meta-analysis of 28 studies with ICU patients consistently showed a higher risk of in-hospital death associated with delirium (risk ratio, 2.19; 95% CI, 1.78–2.70; $P<.001$).[27]

In one of the largest multicenter prospective ICU cohorts to date, a longer duration of ICU delirium was the major independent risk factor for long-term cognitive impairment up to 12 months after surviving a critical illness. This association was independent of severity of illness, sedative or analgesic medication use, age, preexisting cognitive impairment, and comorbid conditions.[28] In this landmark study, the impairment was persistent and no different among medical or surgical ICU populations.[29] This work involved ICU patients without acute structural intracranial injury (eg, no intracranial hemorrhage, no stroke), but they developed long-term cognitive impairment similar to those with Alzheimer disease and moderate traumatic brain injury.[29] Given that delirium is assessable in those with acute structural brain injury (eg, stroke, trauma), further work is being undertaken (ClinicalTrials.gov identifier: https://clinicaltrials.gov/ct2/show/NCT03098459) to understand the interaction between delirium and traumatic brain injury, and their association with long-term cognitive impairment in critically ill trauma survivors.[30–32]

Although the mechanisms by which delirium may predispose patients to long-term cognitive impairment after critical illness have not yet been elucidated, delirium seems associated with inflammation and neuronal apoptosis, which may lead to brain atrophy, particularly in the frontal lobes and hippocampus.[33,34] White-matter disruption has also been associated with cognitive impairment.[35,36] The pathophysiology of delirium is poorly understood, although several different hypotheses exist,[37] involving imbalances in neurotransmitters, neuroinflammation, oxidative stress, neuroendocrine system, diurnal variation, network connectivity, and large amino acids. None of these theories by themselves probably explain the full phenomenon of delirium but possibly 2 or more of these hypotheses, if not all, act together to lead to the biochemical derangement known as delirium.[38]

Delirium assessment is generally considered a 2-step process. The level of arousal to voice is first assessed using a sedation scale, with the particular goal of distinguishing patients who are noncomatose and can then be assessed for delirium (ie, comatose patients are considered unassessable for delirium). The SCCM PAD guidelines recommend the use of the Riker Sedation-Agitation Scale (SAS) or the Richmond Agitation-Sedation Scale (RASS)[18] (**Table 3**). The SAS has 7 individual tiers ranging from 1 (unarousable) to 7 (dangerous agitation),[39] whereas the RASS is a 10-point scale, with 4 levels of escalating agitation (RASS +1 to +4), 1 level denoting a calm and alert state (RASS 0), 3 levels of sedation (RASS −1 to −3), and 2 levels of

Table 3
Richmond Agitation-Sedation Scale and Riker Sedation-Agitation Scale

RASS	SAS
+4: Combative Combative, violent, immediate danger to staff	7: Dangerous agitation Pulling at ETT, trying to remove catheters, climbing over bedrail, striking at staff, trashing side to side
+3: Very agitated Pulls to remove tubes or catheters; aggressive	6: Very agitated Requiring restraint and frequent verbal reminding of limits, biting ETT
+2: Agitated Frequent nonpurposeful movement, fights ventilator	6: Very agitated Requiring restraint and frequent verbal reminding of limits, biting ETT
+1: Restless Anxious, apprehensive, movements not aggressive	5: Agitated Anxious or physically agitated, calms to verbal instructions
0: Alert and calm Spontaneously pays attention to caregiver	4: Calm and cooperative Calm, easily arousable, follows commands
−1: Drowsy Not fully alert, but has sustained awakening to voice; eye opening and contact >10 s	3: Sedated Difficult to arouse but awakens to verbal stimuli or gentle shaking, follows simple commands but drifts off again
−2: Light sedation Briefly awakens to voice; eyes open and contact <10 s	3: Sedated Difficult to arouse but awakens to verbal stimuli or gentle shaking, follows simple commands but drifts off again
−3: Moderate sedation Movement or eye opening to voice; no eye contact	3: Sedated Difficult to arouse but awakens to verbal stimuli or gentle shaking, follows simple commands but drifts off again
−4: Deep sedation No response to voice, but movement or eye opening to physical stimulation	3: Sedated Difficult to arouse but awakens to verbal stimuli or gentle shaking, follows simple commands but drifts off again 2: Very sedated Arouses to physical stimuli but does not communicate or follow commands, may move spontaneously
−5: Unarousable No response to voice or physical stimulation	1: Unarousable Minimal or no response to noxious stimuli, does not communicate or follow commands

Abbreviation: ETT, endotracheal tube.
Data from Khan BA, Guzman O, Campbell NL, et al. Comparison and agreement between the Richmond agitation-sedation scale and the Riker sedation-agitation scale in evaluating patients' eligibility for delirium assessment in the ICU. Chest 2012;142(1):48–54; and http://www.icudelirium.org.

coma (RASS −4 to −5). A unique feature of RASS is that it relies on the duration of eye contact following verbal stimulation. The RASS takes less than 20 seconds to perform, with minimal training, and has been shown high reliability among multiple types of health care providers, with excellent interrater reliability in a broad range of adult medical and surgical ICU patients.[40]

Among noncomatose patients (ie, ≥RASS −3), the next step is to assess for delirium. Several scales have been developed and validated to diagnose delirium in ICU patients[41] (Confusion Assessment Method ICU [CAM-ICU], Delirium Detection Score, Intensive Care Delirium Screening Checklist [ICDSC], Cognitive Test for Delirium, Abbreviated Cognitive Test for Delirium, Neelson and Champagne Confusion Scale [NEECHAM], Nursing Delirium Screening Scale [NuDESC]), but the ICDSC and the CAM-ICU are the tools recommended by the SCCM PAD guidelines for this purpose (Fig. 2, Table 4). The ICDSC checklist is an 8-item screening tool (1 point for each item) that is based on DSM criteria and applied to data that can be collected through medical records or information obtained from the multidisciplinary team.[41] The pooled values for the sensitivity and specificity of the ICDSC are 74% and 81.9%, respectively.[41] The CAM-ICU is composed of 4 features: (1) acute onset of mental status changes or fluctuating course, (2) inattention, (3) disorganized thinking, and (4) altered level of consciousness. If the patient manifests both features 1 and 2, plus either feature 3 or 4, the patient is considered CAM positive, and hence positive for delirium.[42] The overall accuracy of the CAM-ICU is excellent, with pooled values for sensitivity and specificity of 80% and 95.9%, respectively.[41] The CAM-ICU has been modified and validated in pediatric, emergency department, and neurocritical care populations, as well as translated into more than 25 languages.[30–32,43,44]

Delirium can be categorized into subtypes according to psychomotor behavior. Hyperactive delirium is rare in the pure form and is associated with a better overall prognosis and it is characterized by agitation (ie, RASS >0), restlessness, and emotional lability.[45,46] Hypoactive delirium, which is common and often more deleterious for the patient in the long-term, is characterized by decreased responsiveness, sedation (ie, RASS <0), withdrawal, and apathy, and remains unrecognized in 66% to 84% of hospitalized patients.[14,45] Another categorization scheme was proposed by Ouimet and colleagues,[47] who evaluated 600 ICU patients for symptoms of delirium

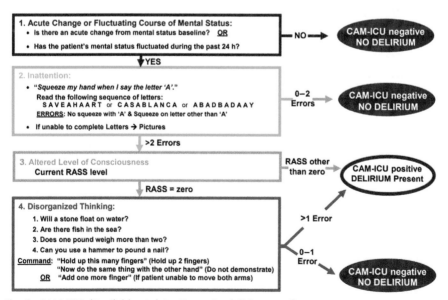

Fig. 2. CAM-ICU. (Available at: http://www.icudelirium.org/.)

	No	Yes
Table 4 **Intensive Care Delirium Screening Checklist**		
ICDSC Worksheet	0	1
1. Altered Level of Consciousness		
Deep sedation/coma over entire shift (SAS = 1, 2; RASS = −4, −5) = not assessable. Agitation (SAS = 5, 6, or 7; RASS = 1–4) at any point = 1 point. Normal wakefulness (SAS = 4; RASS = 0) over the entire shift = 0 points. Light sedation (SAS = 3; RASS = −1, −2, −3) = 1 point (if no recent sedatives) = 0 points (if recent sedatives)		
2. Inattention		
Difficulty following instructions or conversation, patient easily distracted by external stimuli		
Does not reliably squeeze hands to spoken letter A: SAVEA HAART		
3. Disorientation		
In addition to name, place, and date, does the patient recognize ICU caregivers? Does patient know what kind of place the patient is in?		
4. Hallucination, Delusion, or Psychosis		
Ask whether the patient is having hallucinations or delusions (eg, trying to catch an object that is not there). Is the patient afraid of the people or things that are around?		
5. Psychomotor Agitation or Retardation		
Either: (a) hyperactivity requiring the use of sedative drugs or restraints in order to control potentially dangerous behavior (eg, pulling intravenous lines out or hitting staff) or (b) hypoactive or clinically noticeable psychomotor slowing or retardation		
6. Inappropriate Speech or Mood		
Patient displays: inappropriate emotion; disorganized or incoherent speech; sexual or inappropriate interactions; is either apathetic or overly demanding		
7. Sleep-Wake Cycle Disturbance		
Either: frequent awakening or <4 h sleep at night, or sleeping during much of the day		
8. Symptom Fluctuation		
Fluctuation of any of the above symptoms over a 24-h period		
Total shift score (0–8)		

Normal, 0; delirium, 4 to 8; subsyndromal delirium, 1 to 3.

Score the patient over the entire shift. Components do not all need to be present at the same time. Components 1 through 4 cannot be completed when the patient is deeply sedated or comatose (ie, SAS = 1 or 2; RASS = −4 or −5); components 5 through 8 are based on observations throughout the shift. Information from the prior 24 hours should be obtained for components 7 and 8.

Adapted from Bergeron N, Dubois MJ, Dumont M, et al. Intensive care delirium screening checklist: evaluation of a new screening tool. Intens Care Med 2001;27:859–64; and Ouimet S, Riker R, Bergeron N, et al. Subsyndromal delirium in the ICU: evidence for a disease spectrum. Intens Care Med 2007;33:1007–13.

and categorized them according to the number of symptoms present. Patients with no symptoms were considered to have no delirium, those with 4 or more symptoms to have clinical delirium, and those with 1 to 3 symptoms to have subsyndromal delirium.[48] Subsyndromal delirium has also been associated with post-ICU outcomes.[49]

The 2013 PAD guidelines provided an evidence-based road map for clinicians to better manage the intertwined issues of pain, agitation, and delirium in critically ill patients.[18] The treatment of underlying medical conditions and nonpharmacologic issues, like noise, light, sleep, and mobility, are cardinal aspects of delirium management. To improve ICU patient outcomes, including with respect to delirium, an evidence-based organizational approach referred to as the ABCDEF (assess for and manage pain; both spontaneous awakening trials [SATs] and spontaneous breathing trials [SBTs]; choice of appropriate sedation; delirium monitoring, and early mobility and exercise; family engagement) bundle has been proposed.[50]

Assess for and Manage Pain

Pain assessment is the first step in proper pain relief and could be important in patients with delirium. ICUs commonly use patient self-report of pain, like the 1 to 10 numerical rating scale (NRS).[18] If the patient is unable to self-report, observable behavioral and physiologic indicators become important indices for the assessment of pain.[51] The Behavioral Pain Scale (BPS) and the Critical Care Pain Observation Tool (CPOT) are the most valid and reliable behavioral pain scales for ICU patients unable to communicate. According to ICU PAD guidelines, pain medications should be routinely administered in the presence of significant pain (ie, NRS >4, BPS >5, or CPOT >3) and before performing painful invasive procedures.[18]

Both Spontaneous Awakening Trials and Spontaneous Breathing Trials

Protocolized target-based sedation and daily SATs reduce the number of days of mechanical ventilation.[52–54] This strategy also exposes patients to smaller cumulative doses of sedatives. SBTs were shown to be superior to other varied approaches to ventilator weaning.[12] Thus, incorporation of SBTs into practice has reduced the total time of mechanical ventilation. The awakening and breathing controlled trial combined SATs with SBTs, and showed shorter duration of mechanical ventilation, a 4-day reduction in hospital length of stay, a remarkable 15% decrease in 1-year mortality, and no long-term neuropsychological consequences of waking patients during critical illness.[55]

Choice of Appropriate Sedation

The SCCM PAD guidelines emphasize the need for goal-directed delivery of psychoactive medications to avoid oversedation, to promote earlier extubation, and the use of sedation scales (SAS, RASS) to help the medical team agree on a target sedation level for each individual patient.[18] Numerous studies have identified that benzodiazepines are associated with worse clinical outcomes. The Maximizing Efficacy of Targeted Sedation and Reducing Neurological Dysfunction (MENDS) study showed that patients treated with dexmedetomidine had more days alive without delirium or coma (7.0 vs 3.0 days; $P = .01$), with a lower risk for delirium developing on subsequent days.[56] In patients sedated with dexmedetomidine compared with midazolam, the SEDCOM (Safety and Efficacy of Dexmedetomidine Compared with Midazolam) trial showed a reduction in the prevalence of delirium (76.6% vs 54% with risk of difference 22.6%; 95% CI, 14%–33%; $P<.001$), and a reduction in the duration of mechanical ventilation.[57] However, few studies have directly compared dexmedetomidine with propofol. The PRODEX (Propofol versus Dexmedetomidine) study showed no difference in delirium outcomes, although delirium was measured only at a single time point after discontinuation of sedation.[58] In contrast, Djaiani and colleagues[59] recently showed that dexmedetomidine reduced delirium incidence in cardiac surgical patients in the ICU compared with propofol, whereas Su and colleagues[60] showed a reduction in patients treated with dexmedetomidine in non–cardiac surgical patients admitted to the ICU. There is an ongoing trial (MENDS II study) to determine the best sedative medication to reduce delirium and improve survival and long-term brain function in ventilated septic patients (ClinicalTrials.gov identifier: https://clinicaltrials.gov/ct2/show/NCT01739933).

Delirium Management

An important third element in the PAD guidelines is monitoring and management of delirium by using validated tools (CAM-ICU, ICDSC), as described in detail previously.[18] The mnemonic Dr DRE (disease remediation, drug removal, environmental modifications) can aid clinicians in recalling strategies to consider when delirium is present. In delirious patients, a search for all reversible precipitants is the first line of action and pharmacologic treatment should be considered when all other causes are ruled out and it is not contraindicated[22] (**Fig. 3**). The 2013 SCCM PAD guidelines recommend nonpharmacologic approaches to reduce the incidence and duration of ICU delirium, and to improve functional outcomes, such as using early and progressive mobilization; promoting sleep hygiene with control of light, noise, and physical stimuli; and clustering patient care activities.

Antipsychotics, especially haloperidol, are commonly administered for the treatment of delirium in critically ill patients. However, evidence for the safety and efficacy of antipsychotics in this patient population is lacking; hence, the 2013 PAD guidelines did not include specific recommendations for using any particular medication.[18] Because of the lack of evidence about the efficacy of typical versus atypical antipsychotics, Ely and colleagues[61] are conducting the MIND-USA (Modifying the Impact of ICU-induced Neurological Dysfunction–USA) study (ClinicalTrials.gov identifier: https://clinicaltrials.gov/ct2/show/NCT01211522) to define the role of these drugs in the management of delirium and on short-term and long-term clinical outcomes in vulnerable critically ill patients. Delirium prophylaxis with medications is discouraged in the PAD guidelines, but recent small studies on delirium prophylaxis with antipsychotics showed that a low dose of haloperidol may reduce the incidence of delirium in ICU patients.[62,63] By contrast, the HOPE-ICU randomized controlled trial showed no benefit of haloperidol administration for delirium prophylaxis in a mixed population of medical and surgical adult ICU patients.[64]

Exercise and Early Mobility

Early mobility is an integral part of the ABCDEF bundle. During ICU stay, critically ill patients can lose up to 25% of peripheral muscle strength within 4 days when mechanically ventilated and 18% of body weight by the time of discharge, and this process occurs fastest in the first 2 to 3 weeks of immobilization.[65] The consequence of physical dysfunction in critically ill patients can be profound and long-term with significant reduction in functional status being observed even 1 year and 5 years after ICU discharge.[66–68] Morris and colleagues[65] showed that initiating physical therapy early during the patient's ICU stay was associated with decreased length of stay both in the ICU and in the hospital. Schweickert and colleagues[69] showed in mechanically ventilated patients that a daily SAT, plus physical and occupational therapy, resulted in an improved return to independent functional status at hospital discharge, shorter duration of ICU-associated delirium, and more days alive and breathing without assistance. Although all these studies showed the feasibility of physical therapy, it may more effective to start physical therapy early in the ICU course.

A better understanding of the underlying risk factors for disability following critical illness and of the effect that activity, during hospitalization, may have on outcomes

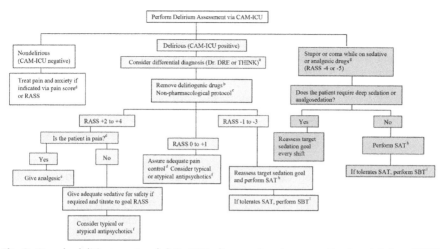

Fig. 3. Sample delirium protocol. [a] Dr DRE: diseases (sepsis, congestive heart failure [CHF], chronic obstructive pulmonary disease); drug removal (SATs and stopping benzodiazepines/narcotics); environment (immobilization, sleep and day/night orientation, hearing aids, eye glasses, noise). THINK: toxic situations (CHF, shock, dehydration, deliriogenic medications [tight titration], new organ failure [eg, liver, kidney]); hypoxemia; infection/sepsis (nosocomial), immobilization; nonpharmacologic interventions[c]; K+ or electrolyte problems. [b] Consider stopping or substituting deliriogenic medications such as benzodiazepines, anticholinergic medications (metoclopramide, H2 blockers, promethazine, diphenhydramine), steroids, and so forth. [c] Nonpharmacologic protocol. Orientation: provide visual and hearing aids, encourage communication and reorient patient repetitively, have familiar objects from patient's home in the room, attempt consistency in nursing staff, family engagement and empowerment. Environment: sleep hygiene (lights off at night, on during day), control excess noise (staff, equipment), earplugs. Early Mobilization and exercise. Music. Saturations greater than 90%. Treat underlying metabolic derangements and infections. ABCDEF bundle. http://www.icudelirium.org/medicalprofessionals.html. [d] If patient is nonverbal assess via CPOT or if patient is verbal assess via visual analog scale. [e] Analgesia: adequate pain control may decrease delirium. Consider opiates, nonsteroidals, acetaminophen, or gabapentin (neuropathic pain). [f] Typical or atypical antipsychotics. There is no evidence that haloperidol decreases the duration of delirium. Atypical antipsychotics may decrease the duration of delirium. Discontinue if high fever, corrected QT prolongation, or drug-induced rigidity. [g] Consider nonbenzodiazepine sedation strategies (propofol or dexmedetomidine). [h] SAT. If meets safety criteria (no active seizures, no alcohol withdrawal, no agitation, no paralytics, no myocardial ischemia, normal intracranial pressure, fraction of inspired oxygen [Fio_2] $\leq$70%). [i] SBT. If meets safety criteria (no agitation, no myocardial ischemia, Fio_2 $\leq$50%, adequate inspiratory efforts, O_2 saturation $\geq$88%, no vasopressor use, positive end-expiratory pressure $\leq$7.5 cm). (*From* http://www.icudelirium.org/.)

is needed. Brummel and colleagues[49] designed the Measuring Outcomes of Activity in Intensive Care (MOSAIC) observational study to evaluate the relationship between activity in the hospital, measured by using a clinical mobility scale and accelerometry, and disability, physical function, and cognitive function in survivors of critical illness 3 and 12 months after ICU discharge (ClinicalTrials.gov identifier: https://clinicaltrials.gov/show/NCT03115840).

Family Engagement

Critical illness usually affects not only individuals but their entire support systems, which may or may not be the nuclear family, or some combination of family and friends or other caregivers who are actively engaged in supportive roles. In light of this, it is crucial not only to recognize the needs of the patient but to identify and address the needs of the patient's family as well. Family members and surrogate decision makers must become active partners in multiprofessional decision making and care.[70]

POSTTRAUMATIC STRESS DISORDER

Posttraumatic stress disorder (PTSD), depression, and anxiety and important mental health problems after critical illness.[71–73] PTSD is a serious psychiatric disorder that can occur in people who have experienced or witnessed a traumatic event (eg, natural disaster, a serious accident, a terrorist act, war/combat, rape or other violent personal assault),[1] like surviving a critical illness. Common screening tools include the PTSD Checklist for DSM-5 (PCL-5), and the Impact of Events Scale (IES), but often require extensive confirmation using diagnostic tools like DSM-5 and Clinician-administered PTSD Scale (CAPS).[74–76] These complexities probably relate to the inconsistent epidemiology of ICU-related PTSD.

The incidence of PTSD, related to the ICU experience and not related to past stressful experiences, has consistently been around 10% in the first year after hospital discharge[73,74,77,78] in the most rigorous studies, despite historically reported higher rates in many other studies.[75,76] It is critically important to recognize that, despite these reports of higher epidemiologic occurrences of PTSD after critical illness,[76] many studies have not distinguished preexisting PTSD from ICU-related PTSD, nor have they used DSM criteria or accounted for the ICU course. Using a multicenter ICU population of US civilians and veterans, the most recent study to clearly identify ICU-related PTSD showed an occurrence of 1 in 10 ICU survivors.[74]

It has been suggested that the quality of cognitive processing at the time of the traumatic event is important in the development of PTSD. Those individuals who report feeling confusion and feeling overwhelmed as they experienced the traumatic situation are more likely to have PTSD.[79] ICU patients may be predisposed to PTSD during the traumatic event, either because of the treatments instituted during the ICU stay or because of the critical illness. Ultimately, their ability to process information is likely to be compromised.[80]

One risk factor for the development of PTSD/PTSD-related symptoms may be early recall of delusional memories. The number of early recall of delusional memories, without any factual memories, has been related to increased risk of developing PTSD and high severity of PTSD-related symptoms.[81,82] Granja and colleagues[80] found that amnesia, for the early period of critical illness, was positively associated with the level of PTSD-related symptoms. However, given that in-ICU amnesia was also associated with longer ICU length of stay, greater illness severity, and greater previous hospital admissions, the investigators suggested that ICU amnesia might be a proxy for trauma severity of disease and that adverse experiences during ICU stay may lead to higher levels of PTSD-related symptoms.[80] Weinert and Sprenkle[83] found that delirious memories were associated with more PTSD-like symptoms, but patients who were the most awake during mechanical ventilation also had the lowest levels of PTSD-like symptoms.

Patients with a history of depression and related disorders may also be at risk of developing PTSD.[74,84] Depression can have emotional, psychological, psychosocial, and physical effects that diminish coping mechanisms. Bienvenu and colleagues[85] and Patel and colleagues[74] both independently found that previous history of depressive illness was a significant predictor of risk for post-ICU PTSD. Similarly, Cuthbertson and colleagues[86] found that treatment-seeking behaviors for psychological distress before ICU admission predicted eventual development of PTSD. However, these studies assessed previous psychiatric history using retrospective accounts, and it could be questioned whether the self-reports of previous mental disorder may have been increased by current psychological distress.[87]

Attention has been focused on the type and duration of ICU sedation, as it relates to risk of post-ICU PTSD, but the data have been conflicting and nonconfirmatory. Particular interest has been placed on the role of benzodiazepines.[19,88] Midazolam,[89] lorazepam,[88] and opiates administered in the ICU have been found to have links to post-ICU PTSD.[85] In contrast, in one of the largest, most comprehensive, and most current ICU-related PTSD studies, no association was found between PTSD and duration of delirium, benzodiazepine dose, or opiate dose.[74] Despite these being modifiable risk factors, especially for ICU providers to consider, the analgosedative classes have no clear relationship with ICU-related PTSD.

The impact of sedation interruption or minimizing sedation on post-ICU PTSD risk remains unclear, but potential benefits of minimizing sedation seem to outweigh the potential harm. Protocol-driven sedation interruptions may reduce PTSD symptoms after ICU care, despite long-standing beliefs to the contrary. The possibility of post-ICU PTSD symptom reduction is promising and provides another reason for physicians to use a goal-directed approach to sedation.[52,55,90]

Exploration of the role of genetics in post-ICU PTSD has provided interesting insights into nonmodifiable factors that potentially influence the occurrence of symptoms among survivors of critical illness. An investigation in cardiac surgery patients requiring ICU care showed increased symptoms of PTSD among individuals homozygous for a single nucleotide polymorphism of the glucocorticoid receptor gene.[91] Another study of mixed ICU patients revealed an association between homozygosity for a single-nucleotide polymorphism of the corticotrophin-releasing hormone binding protein and decreased post-ICU PTSD symptoms.[92] Although genetic polymorphisms are not modifiable, they may offer future targets to assist in identification of patients at higher risk.[93]

Several medications have been studied to potentially prevent PTSD. The protective effects of hydrocortisone[94,95] on PTSD development were observed in acutely trauma-exposed patients in the emergency department, in which treatment was initiated within 6 to 12 hours after the trauma. There is some evidence that low serum cortisol level is predictive of the development of post-ICU PTSD,[96] therefore stress dose hydrocortisone may offer protective effects. Kok and colleagues[97] conversely showed that exogenous administration of the glucocorticoid receptor agonist dexamethasone, compared with placebo, during cardiac surgery does not influence the prevalence of PTSD and depression. At present, pharmacologic interventions, like glucocorticoids, are not a mainstay prophylactic or intervention therapy against ICU-related PTSD.

Intranasal administration of the neuropeptide oxytocin may be a promising pharmacologic treatment to prevent PTSD.[98,99] Evidence from studies in animals and in healthy and psychiatric human populations have shown that oxytocin administration may modulate glucocorticoid and autonomic stress reactivity,[100,101] dampen anxiety, and alter neural threat processing.[102,103] However, after exposure to trauma, oxytocin administration showed detrimental effects, increasing amygdala reactivity to fearful faces and decreasing amygdala-ventrolateral prefrontal functional connectivity.[104] Moreover, other studies indicate that the effects of a single oxytocin administration may differ from the effects of repeated administration; the latter may be required to achieve clinically relevant effects regarding the prevention of PTSD.[104] Therefore, oxytocin remains investigational with respect to ICU-related PTSD.

The fragmentary nature of memories of the ICU experience and the high proportion of delusional memories that are recalled afterward make it difficult for patients to make sense of what has happened to them.[105] These altered memories may be a major precipitant of PTSD in this population.[77,82] Minimizing the occurrence of delusional memories in the ICU poses a significant clinical challenge. However, interventions focused on improving patient understanding of events occurring during critical illness have provided promising results.[93] For example, all procedures should be explained to patients and their families, and the patient should be reoriented with each physical intervention, even if the patient seems to be heavily sedated. Another possible adjunct to decrease post-ICU complications entails family integration into ICU care, as much as possible.[106]

Jones and colleagues[78] evaluated the influence of ICU diaries on symptoms of post-ICU posttraumatic stress, among both patients and their family members, after 3 months from ICU discharge. Patients in the intervention arm received their ICU diaries at 1 month following critical care discharge and the final assessment of the development of acute PTSD was made at 3 months. The incidence of new cases of PTSD was reduced in the intervention group compared with the control patients (5% vs 13%; $P = .02$). Diaries are a low-risk intervention that can probably help ICU patients to change how they think about their illness as they reread the story and build an autobiographical memory.

Families may also be helped because the diaries help to facilitate communication with the ICU patients about their treatment, and writing in the diary may allow them to express their feelings. A strong relationship has been found between high levels of PTSD-related symptoms in family members and those in ICU survivors. An ICU diary that is shared between the patient and the family may therefore be better than one that just concentrates on the patient.[78] Similarly, Garrouste-Orgeas and colleagues[107] assessed the influence of ICU diaries written by family members, nurses, and physicians on ICU survivors. At the time of ICU discharge, diaries were provided to survivors and to relatives. For both patients and relatives, levels of posttraumatic symptoms measured by the IES-R (Impact of Event Scale - Revised) were lower at 12-month follow-up, compared with prediary and postdiary controls.[107] ICU diaries have also been associated with reductions in related post-ICU psychiatric morbidities, including depressive and anxiety symptoms.[108]

Similar to diaries/journals, a single counseling session has been shown to increase both patient and family coping ability after an ICU stay.[82] Both may also prevent, reduce, or help treat PTSD.[106]

Other studies suggest that music, nature sounds, various forms of massage, and reflexology could all be used to reduce acute stress among ICU patients, including mechanically ventilated patients.[109] Because acute stress is an important precursor of long-term psychological morbidity such as PTSD, these short-term practices could also have an impact on long-term outcome. The risk of harm from such therapies is not generally high, but protocols and training for staff are needed.[109] Although several of these alternative risk factors have been identified, more work needs to be done to identify whether individual difference variables may play a role in how people cope with the stress of the ICU (**Fig. 4**).

In general, broader personality traits have been associated with greater resilience to PTSD, including extraversion and conscientiousness, whereas neuroticism and negative emotionality have been positively associated with PTSD development.[87] Social support may play an important protective role against the development of PTSD.[110] One study found that social support was significantly negatively associated with PTSD symptoms in a sample of ICU patients admitted for acute respiratory distress

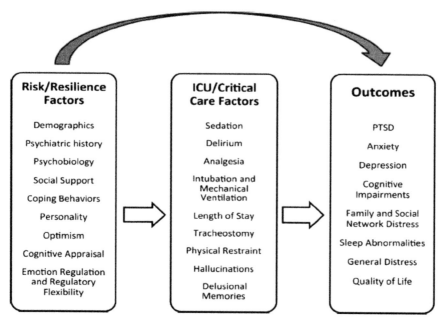

Fig. 4. Risk factors for post-ICU psychological outcome. (*From* McGiffin JN, Galatzer-Levy IR, Bonanno GA. Is the intensive care unit traumatic? What we know and don't know about the intensive care unit and posttraumatic stress responses. Rehabil Psychol 2016;61(2):120–31; with permission.)

syndrome. This association in ICU-treated individuals between social support and decreased psychological distress could represent an important topic for future research.[87,93]

REFERENCES

1. American Psychiatric Association. Diagnostic and statistical manual of mental disorders: DSM-5. Washington, DC: American Psychiatric Association; 2013.

2. Morandi A, Pandharipande P, Trabucchi M, et al. Understanding international differences in terminology for delirium and other types of acute brain dysfunction in critically ill patients. Intensive Care Med 2008;34(10):1907–15.

3. Gunther ML, Morandi A, Ely EW. Pathophysiology of delirium in the intensive care unit. Crit Care Clin 2008;24(1):45–65, viii.

4. Ely EW, Margolin R, Francis J, et al. Evaluation of delirium in critically ill patients: validation of the confusion assessment method for the intensive care unit (CAM-ICU). Crit Care Med 2001;29(7):1370–9.

5. Pandharipande P, Costabile S, Cotton B, et al. Prevalence of delirium in surgical ICU patients. Crit Care Med 2005;33(12 Suppl):A45.

6. Micek ST, Anand NJ, Laible BR, et al. Delirium as detected by the CAM-ICU predicts restraint use among mechanically ventilated medical patients. Crit Care Med 2005;33(6):1260–5.

7. Thomason JW, Shintani A, Peterson JF, et al. Intensive care unit delirium is an independent predictor of longer hospital stay: a prospective analysis of 261 non-ventilated patients. Crit Care 2005;9(4):R375–81.

8. Ely EW, Shintani A, Truman B, et al. Delirium as a predictor of mortality in mechanically ventilated patients in the intensive care unit. JAMA 2004;291(14): 1753–62.

9. Jackson JC, Hart RP, Gordon SM, et al. Six-month neuropsychological outcome of medical intensive care unit patients. Crit Care Med 2003;31(4):1226–34.

10. Milbrandt EB, Deppen S, Harrison PL, et al. Costs associated with delirium in mechanically ventilated patients. Crit Care Med 2004;32(4):955–62.

11. Lin SM, Liu CY, Wang CH, et al. The impact of delirium on the survival of mechanically ventilated patients. Crit Care Med 2004;32(11):2254–9.

12. Ely EW, Baker AM, Dunagan DP, et al. Effect on the duration of mechanical ventilation of identifying patients capable of breathing spontaneously. N Engl J Med 1996;335(25):1864–9.

13. Inouye SK, Bogardus ST Jr, Charpentier PA, et al. A multicomponent intervention to prevent delirium in hospitalized older patients. N Engl J Med 1999;340(9): 669–76.

14. Marcantonio ER, Goldman L, Mangione CM, et al. A clinical prediction rule for delirium after elective noncardiac surgery. JAMA 1994;271(2):134–9.

15. Dubois MJ, Bergeron N, Dumont M, et al. Delirium in an intensive care unit: a study of risk factors. Intensive Care Med 2001;27(8):1297–304.

16. Aldemir M, Ozen S, Kara IH, et al. Predisposing factors for delirium in the surgical intensive care unit. Crit Care 2001;5(5):265–70.

17. Brummel NE, Girard TD. Preventing delirium in the intensive care unit. Crit Care Clin 2013;29(1):51–65.

18. Barr J, Fraser GL, Puntillo K, et al. Clinical practice guidelines for the management of pain, agitation, and delirium in adult patients in the intensive care unit. Crit Care Med 2013;41(1):263–306.

19. Pandharipande P, Shintani A, Peterson J, et al. Lorazepam is an independent risk factor for transitioning to delirium in intensive care unit patients. Anesthesiology 2006;104(1):21–6.

20. Seymour CW, Pandharipande PP, Koestner T, et al. Diurnal sedative changes during intensive care: impact on liberation from mechanical ventilation and delirium. Crit Care Med 2012;40(10):2788–96.

21. Marcantonio ER, Juarez G, Goldman L, et al. The relationship of postoperative delirium with psychoactive medications. JAMA 1994;272(19):1518–22.

22. Ely EW, Gautam S, Margolin R, et al. The impact of delirium in the intensive care unit on hospital length of stay. Intensive Care Med 2001;27(12):1892–900.

23. Ouimet S, Kavanagh BP, Gottfried SB, et al. Incidence, risk factors and consequences of ICU delirium. Intensive Care Med 2007;33(1):66–73.

24. Shehabi Y, Riker RR, Bokesch PM, et al. Delirium duration and mortality in lightly sedated, mechanically ventilated intensive care patients. Crit Care Med 2010; 38(12):2311–8.

25. Pisani MA, Kong SY, Kasl SV, et al. Days of delirium are associated with 1-year mortality in an older intensive care unit population. Am J Respir Crit Care Med 2009;180(11):1092–7.

26. Klein Klouwenberg PMC, Zaal IJ, Spitoni C, et al. The attributable mortality of delirium in critically ill patients: prospective cohort study. BMJ 2014;349:g6652.

27. Salluh JI, Wang H, Schneider EB, et al. Outcome of delirium in critically ill patients: systematic review and meta-analysis. BMJ 2015;350:h2538.

28. Pandharipande PP, Girard TD, Jackson JC, et al. Long-term cognitive impairment after critical illness. N Engl J Med 2013;369(14):1306–16.

29. Hughes CG, Patel MB, Jackson JC, et al. Surgery and anesthesia exposure is not a risk factor for cognitive impairment after major noncardiac surgery and critical illness. Ann Surg 2017;265(6):1126–33.

30. Mitasova A, Kostalova M, Bednarik J, et al. Poststroke delirium incidence and outcomes: validation of the confusion assessment method for the intensive care unit (CAM-ICU). Crit Care Med 2012;40(2):484–90.

31. Naidech AM, Beaumont JL, Rosenberg NF, et al. Intracerebral hemorrhage and delirium symptoms. Length of stay, function, and quality of life in a 114-patient cohort. Am J Respir Crit Care Med 2013;188(11):1331–7.

32. Han JH, Wilson A, Graves AJ, et al. Validation of the Confusion Assessment Method for the Intensive Care Unit in older emergency department patients. Acad Emerg Med 2014;21(2):180–7.

33. van Gool WA, van de Beek D, Eikelenboom P. Systemic infection and delirium: when cytokines and acetylcholine collide. Lancet 2010;375(9716):773–5.

34. Cunningham C. Systemic inflammation and delirium: important co-factors in the progression of dementia. Biochem Soc Trans 2011;39(4):945–53.

35. Gunther ML, Morandi A, Krauskopf E, et al. The association between brain volumes, delirium duration, and cognitive outcomes in intensive care unit survivors: the VISIONS cohort magnetic resonance imaging study*. Crit Care Med 2012;40(7):2022–32.

36. Morandi A, Rogers BP, Gunther ML, et al. The relationship between delirium duration, white matter integrity, and cognitive impairment in intensive care unit survivors as determined by diffusion tensor imaging: the VISIONS prospective cohort magnetic resonance imaging study*. Crit Care Med 2012;40(7):2182–9.

37. Maldonado JR. Neuropathogenesis of delirium: review of current etiologic theories and common pathways. Am J Geriatr Psychiatry 2013;21(12):1190–222.

38. Maldonado JR. Pathoetiological model of delirium: a comprehensive understanding of the neurobiology of delirium and an evidence-based approach to prevention and treatment. Crit Care Clin 2008;24(4):789–856, ix.

39. Khan BA, Guzman O, Campbell NL, et al. Comparison and agreement between the Richmond agitation-sedation scale and the Riker sedation-agitation scale in evaluating patients' eligibility for delirium assessment in the ICU. Chest 2012;142(1):48–54.

40. Ely EW, Truman B, Shintani A, et al. Monitoring sedation status over time in ICU patients: reliability and validity of the Richmond agitation-sedation scale (RASS). JAMA 2003;289(22):2983–91.

41. Gusmao-Flores D, Salluh JI, Chalhub RA, et al. The confusion assessment method for the intensive care unit (CAM-ICU) and intensive care delirium screening checklist (ICDSC) for the diagnosis of delirium: a systematic review and meta-analysis of clinical studies. Crit Care 2012;16(4):R115.

42. Ely EW, Inouye SK, Bernard GR, et al. Delirium in mechanically ventilated patients: validity and reliability of the confusion assessment method for the intensive care unit (CAM-ICU). JAMA 2001;286(21):2703–10.

43. Smith HA, Boyd J, Fuchs DC, et al. Diagnosing delirium in critically ill children: validity and reliability of the pediatric confusion assessment method for the intensive care unit. Crit Care Med 2011;39(1):150–7.

44. Smith HA, Gangopadhyay M, Goben CM, et al. The preschool confusion assessment method for the ICU: valid and reliable delirium monitoring for critically ill infants and children. Crit Care Med 2016;44(3):592–600.

45. Meagher DJ, Trzepacz PT. Motoric subtypes of delirium. Semin Clin Neuropsychiatry 2000;5(2):75–85.

46. O'Keeffe ST, Lavan JN. Clinical significance of delirium subtypes in older people. Age Ageing 1999;28(2):115–9.
47. Ouimet S, Riker R, Bergeron N, et al. Subsyndromal delirium in the ICU: evidence for a disease spectrum. Intensive Care Med 2007;33(6):1007–13.
48. Girard TD, Pandharipande PP, Ely EW. Delirium in the intensive care unit. Crit Care 2008;12(Suppl 3):S3.
49. Brummel NE, Boehm LM, Girard TD, et al. The relationship between subsyndromal and clinical outcomes after critical illness. American Journal of Crit Care, in press.
50. Marra A, Ely EW, Pandharipande PP, et al. The ABCDEF bundle in critical care. Crit Care Clin 2017;33(2):225–43.
51. Gelinas C, Fillion L, Puntillo KA, et al. Validation of the critical-care pain observation tool in adult patients. Am J Crit Care 2006;15(4):420–7.
52. Kress JP, Pohlman AS, O'Connor MF, et al. Daily interruption of sedative infusions in critically ill patients undergoing mechanical ventilation. N Engl J Med 2000;342(20):1471–7.
53. Shehabi Y, Bellomo R, Reade MC, et al. Early intensive care sedation predicts long-term mortality in ventilated critically ill patients. Am J Respir Crit Care Med 2012;186(8):724–31.
54. Balzer F, Weiss B, Kumpf O, et al. Early deep sedation is associated with decreased in-hospital and two-year follow-up survival. Crit Care 2015;19:197.
55. Girard TD, Kress JP, Fuchs BD, et al. Efficacy and safety of a paired sedation and ventilator weaning protocol for mechanically ventilated patients in intensive care (Awakening and Breathing Controlled trial): a randomised controlled trial. Lancet 2008;371(9607):126–34.
56. Pandharipande PP, Pun BT, Herr DL, et al. Effect of sedation with dexmedetomidine vs lorazepam on acute brain dysfunction in mechanically ventilated patients: the MENDS randomized controlled trial. JAMA 2007;298(22):2644–53.
57. Riker RR, Shehabi Y, Bokesch PM, et al. Dexmedetomidine vs midazolam for sedation of critically ill patients: a randomized trial. JAMA 2009;301(5):489–99.
58. Jakob SM, Ruokonen E, Grounds RM, et al. Dexmedetomidine vs midazolam or propofol for sedation during prolonged mechanical ventilation: two randomized controlled trials. JAMA 2012;307(11):1151–60.
59. Djaiani G, Silverton N, Fedorko L, et al. Dexmedetomidine versus propofol sedation reduces delirium after cardiac surgery: a randomized controlled trial. Anesthesiology 2016;124(2):362–8.
60. Su X, Meng ZT, Wu XH, et al. Dexmedetomidine for prevention of delirium in elderly patients after non-cardiac surgery: a randomised, double-blind, placebo-controlled trial. Lancet 2016;388(10054):1893–902.
61. The Modifying the Impact of ICU-Associated Neurological Dysfunction-USA (MIND-USA) Study [Internet]. 2010 [updated June 1, 2017]. Available at: http://clinicaltrials.gov/ct2/show/NCT01211522. Accessed August 14, 2017.
62. Wang W, Li HL, Wang DX, et al. Haloperidol prophylaxis decreases delirium incidence in elderly patients after noncardiac surgery: a randomized controlled trial*. Crit Care Med 2012;40(3):731–9.
63. van den Boogaard M, Schoonhoven L, van Achterberg T, et al. Haloperidol prophylaxis in critically ill patients with a high risk for delirium. Crit Care 2013;17(1):R9.
64. Page VJ, Ely EW, Gates S, et al. Effect of intravenous haloperidol on the duration of delirium and coma in critically ill patients (Hope-ICU): a randomised, double-blind, placebo-controlled trial. Lancet Respir Med 2013;1(7):515–23.

65. Morris PE. Moving our critically ill patients: mobility barriers and benefits. Crit Care Clin 2007;23(1):1–20.
66. Herridge MS, Cheung AM, Tansey CM, et al. One-year outcomes in survivors of the acute respiratory distress syndrome. N Engl J Med 2003;348(8):683–93.
67. Herridge MS, Tansey CM, Matte A, et al. Functional disability 5 years after acute respiratory distress syndrome. N Engl J Med 2011;364(14):1293–304.
68. Sacanella E, Perez-Castejon JM, Nicolas JM, et al. Functional status and quality of life 12 months after discharge from a medical ICU in healthy elderly patients: a prospective observational study. Crit Care 2011;15(2):R105.
69. Schweickert WD, Pohlman MC, Pohlman AS, et al. Early physical and occupational therapy in mechanically ventilated, critically ill patients: a randomised controlled trial. Lancet 2009;373(9678):1874–82.
70. Davidson JE, Powers K, Hedayat KM, et al. Clinical practice guidelines for support of the family in the patient-centered intensive care unit: American College of Critical Care Medicine Task Force 2004-2005. Crit Care Med 2007;35(2):605–22.
71. Davydow DS, Desai SV, Needham DM, et al. Psychiatric morbidity in survivors of the acute respiratory distress syndrome: a systematic review. Psychosom Med 2008;70(4):512–9.
72. Unroe M, Kahn JM, Carson SS, et al. One-year trajectories of care and resource utilization for recipients of prolonged mechanical ventilation: a cohort study. Ann Intern Med 2010;153(3):167–75.
73. Jackson JC, Pandharipande PP, Girard TD, et al. Depression, post-traumatic stress disorder, and functional disability in survivors of critical illness in the BRAIN-ICU study: a longitudinal cohort study. Lancet Respir Med 2014;2(5): 369–79.
74. Patel MB, Jackson JC, Morandi A, et al. Incidence and risk factors for intensive care unit-related post-traumatic stress disorder in veterans and civilians. Am J Respir Crit Care Med 2016;193(12):1373–81.
75. Davydow DS, Gifford JM, Desai SV, et al. Posttraumatic stress disorder in general intensive care unit survivors: a systematic review. Gen Hosp Psychiatry 2008;30(5):421–34.
76. Parker AM, Sricharoenchai T, Raparla S, et al. Posttraumatic stress disorder in critical illness survivors: a metaanalysis. Crit Care Med 2015;43(5):1121–9.
77. Jones C, Backman C, Capuzzo M, et al. Precipitants of post-traumatic stress disorder following intensive care: a hypothesis generating study of diversity in care. Intensive Care Med 2007;33(6):978–85.
78. Jones C, Backman C, Capuzzo M, et al. Intensive care diaries reduce new onset post traumatic stress disorder following critical illness: a randomised, controlled trial. Crit Care 2010;14(5):R168.
79. Ehlers A, Clark DM. A cognitive model of posttraumatic stress disorder. Behav Res Ther 2000;38(4):319–45.
80. Granja C, Gomes E, Amaro A, et al. Understanding posttraumatic stress disorder-related symptoms after critical care: the early illness amnesia hypothesis. Crit Care Med 2008;36(10):2801–9.
81. Schelling G, Stoll C, Haller M, et al. Health-related quality of life and posttraumatic stress disorder in survivors of the acute respiratory distress syndrome. Crit Care Med 1998;26(4):651–9.
82. Jones C, Griffiths RD, Humphris G, et al. Memory, delusions, and the development of acute posttraumatic stress disorder-related symptoms after intensive care. Crit Care Med 2001;29(3):573–80.

83. Weinert CR, Sprenkle M. Post-ICU consequences of patient wakefulness and sedative exposure during mechanical ventilation. Intensive Care Med 2008; 34(1):82–90.

84. Davydow DS, Zatzick DF, Rivara FP, et al. Predictors of posttraumatic stress disorder and return to usual major activity in traumatically injured intensive care unit survivors. Gen Hosp Psychiatry 2009;31(5):428–35.

85. Bienvenu OJ, Gellar J, Althouse BM, et al. Post-traumatic stress disorder symptoms after acute lung injury: a 2-year prospective longitudinal study. Psychol Med 2013;43(12):2657–71.

86. Cuthbertson BH, Hull A, Strachan M, et al. Post-traumatic stress disorder after critical illness requiring general intensive care. Intensive Care Med 2004; 30(3):450–5.

87. McGiffin JN, Galatzer-Levy IR, Bonanno GA. Is the intensive care unit traumatic? What we know and don't know about the intensive care unit and posttraumatic stress responses. Rehabil Psychol 2016;61(2):120–31.

88. Girard TD, Shintani AK, Jackson JC, et al. Risk factors for posttraumatic stress disorder symptoms following critical illness requiring mechanical ventilation: a prospective cohort study. Crit Care 2007;11(1):R28.

89. Samuelson KA, Lundberg D, Fridlund B. Stressful memories and psychological distress in adult mechanically ventilated intensive care patients - a 2-month follow-up study. Acta Anaesthesiol Scand 2007;51(6):671–8.

90. Kress JP, Gehlbach B, Lacy M, et al. The long-term psychological effects of daily sedative interruption on critically ill patients. Am J Respir Crit Care Med 2003;168(12):1457–61.

91. Hauer D, Weis F, Papassotiropoulos A, et al. Relationship of a common polymorphism of the glucocorticoid receptor gene to traumatic memories and posttraumatic stress disorder in patients after intensive care therapy. Crit Care Med 2011;39(4):643–50.

92. Davydow DS, Kohen R, Hough CL, et al. A pilot investigation of the association of genetic polymorphisms regulating corticotrophin-releasing hormone with posttraumatic stress and depressive symptoms in medical-surgical intensive care unit survivors. J Crit Care 2014;29(1):101–6.

93. Long AC, Kross EK, Davydow DS, et al. Posttraumatic stress disorder among survivors of critical illness: creation of a conceptual model addressing identification, prevention, and management. Intensive Care Med 2014;40(6):820–9.

94. Delahanty DL, Gabert-Quillen C, Ostrowski SA, et al. The efficacy of initial hydrocortisone administration at preventing posttraumatic distress in adult trauma patients: a randomized trial. CNS Spectr 2013;18(2):103–11.

95. Zohar J, Yahalom H, Kozlovsky N, et al. High dose hydrocortisone immediately after trauma may alter the trajectory of PTSD: interplay between clinical and animal studies. Eur Neuropsychopharmacol 2011;21(11):796–809.

96. Schelling G, Briegel J, Roozendaal B, et al. The effect of stress doses of hydrocortisone during septic shock on posttraumatic stress disorder in survivors. Biol Psychiatry 2001;50(12):978–85.

97. Kok L, Hillegers MH, Veldhuijzen DS, et al. The effect of dexamethasone on symptoms of posttraumatic stress disorder and depression after cardiac surgery and intensive care admission: longitudinal follow-up of a randomized controlled trial. Crit Care Med 2016;44(3):512–20.

98. Olff M. Bonding after trauma: on the role of social support and the oxytocin system in traumatic stress. Eur J Psychotraumatol 2012;3.

99. Ostrowski SA, Delahanty DL. Prospects for the pharmacological prevention of post-traumatic stress in vulnerable individuals. CNS Drugs 2014;28(3):195–203.
100. Cardoso C, Kingdon D, Ellenbogen MA. A meta-analytic review of the impact of intranasal oxytocin administration on cortisol concentrations during laboratory tasks: moderation by method and mental health. Psychoneuroendocrinology 2014;49:161–70.
101. Kubzansky LD, Mendes WB, Appleton AA, et al. A heartfelt response: oxytocin effects on response to social stress in men and women. Biol Psychol 2012;90(1): 1–9.
102. Kirsch P, Esslinger C, Chen Q, et al. Oxytocin modulates neural circuitry for social cognition and fear in humans. J Neurosci 2005;25(49):11489–93.
103. Wigton R, Radua J, Allen P, et al. Neurophysiological effects of acute oxytocin administration: systematic review and meta-analysis of placebo-controlled imaging studies. J Psychiatry Neurosci 2015;40(1):E1–22.
104. van Zuiden M, Frijling JL, Nawijn L, et al. Intranasal oxytocin to prevent posttraumatic stress disorder symptoms: a randomized controlled trial in emergency department patients. Biol Psychiatry 2017;81(12):1030–40.
105. Jones C, Griffiths RD, Humphris G. Disturbed memory and amnesia related to intensive care. Memory 2000;8(2):79–94.
106. Crabtree-Buckner L, Kautz DD. Prevention of posttraumatic stress disorder in intensive care unit patients. Dimens Crit Care Nurs 2012;31(2):69–72.
107. Garrouste-Orgeas M, Coquet I, Perier A, et al. Impact of an intensive care unit diary on psychological distress in patients and relatives*. Crit Care Med 2012; 40(7):2033–40.
108. Knowles RE, Tarrier N. Evaluation of the effect of prospective patient diaries on emotional well-being in intensive care unit survivors: a randomized controlled trial. Crit Care Med 2009;37(1):184–91.
109. Wade DF, Moon Z, Windgassen SS, et al. Non-pharmacological interventions to reduce ICU-related psychological distress: a systematic review. Minerva Anestesiol 2016;82(4):465–78.
110. Brewin CR, Andrews B, Valentine JD. Meta-analysis of risk factors for posttraumatic stress disorder in trauma-exposed adults. J Consult Clin Psychol 2000; 68(5):748–66.

Management of Traumatic Brain Injury

Justin R. Davanzo, MD, Emily P. Sieg, MD, Shelly D. Timmons, MD, PhD*

KEYWORDS

- Traumatic brain injury • Neurotrauma • Secondary injury • Intracranial monitoring
- Intracranial pressure • Craniotomy • Craniectomy • Decompression

KEY POINTS

- The diagnosis of severe traumatic brain injury is based on a variety of clinical and radiographic data and encompasses a wide heterogeneity of structural and physiologic insults.
- The concept of treatment thresholds is somewhat outdated; although there are specific physiologic ranges at which secondary injury clearly takes place, treatment of an individual patient's physiology at a given point in time must take into account numerous concurrent events, including the evolution of extracerebral injuries, structural brain lesions, cerebral edema, and cerebral hypoxia/ischemia.
- The options for treatment of severe traumatic brain injury are just as varied as the presenting pathologies and may include surgery for evacuation of mass lesions or decompression of herniating or compressed cerebral tissues, drainage of cerebrospinal fluid, pharmacologic sedation and paralysis, ventilator management, hyperosmolar euvolemic therapy, and prophylaxis against seizures, thromboses, and a variety of other complications.

INTRODUCTION

According to the Centers for Disease Control and Prevention, injury remains the leading cause of death in the United States for all persons aged 1 to 44 years, is the third leading cause of death for those aged 45 to 64 years, is the fifth most common cause of death for infants less than a year of age, and ranks seventh in those 65 years and older.[1] Traumatic brain injury (TBI) comprises the cause of death for approximately one-third of people with multitrauma.[2] The public health importance of TBI, therefore, cannot be overestimated.

RELEVANT ANATOMY AND PATHOPHYSIOLOGY

Severe TBI (sTBI) has traditionally been defined as those presenting with head trauma and brain injury with a postresuscitation Glasgow Coma Scale (GCS)[3] score of 3 to 8, although other classification schema exist. Patients with sTBI, and some with

Disclosure Statement: The authors have nothing to disclose.
Department of Neurosurgery, Milton S. Hershey Medical Center, Penn State University College of Medicine, 30 Hope Drive, E.C. 110, Hershey, PA 17033, USA
* Corresponding author.
E-mail address: stimmons@mac.com

so-called moderate TBI, that is, a GCS score of 9 to 12, require intensive care, sometimes for several days to a few weeks. The pathophysiology of TBI involves the initial blow (primary injury) that may result in numerous structural pathologies as well as initiation of the chemical, electrical, and inflammatory cascade of physiologic events that comprise the secondary injury of the brain. Furthermore, secondary insults, such as hypotension, hypoxia, seizure, and other physiologic events, have a profound impact on the degree of secondary injury sustained and ultimately the functional outcome of patients. Patients with polytrauma and sTBI represent a significant challenge because of the potential for ongoing secondary insults from other organ injuries and vascular and musculoskeletal trauma.

Thus, the treatment of sTBI must begin the moment that patients are assessed by first responders. Emergency personnel and physicians in multiple specialties must be conversant with the diagnosis and management of severe TBI so as to prevent secondary insults to the degree possible, to rapidly coordinate the surgical care of structural injuries requiring surgery, and to minimize secondary cerebral injury to improve long-term outcomes after sTBI.

Structural cerebral injury occurring as part of the primary injury cannot currently be repaired, but the effects of structural injury must be mitigated. Surgical repair of a variety of structural injuries is often undertaken early (in the case of compressive lesions causing pressure on the brain) or later in the course (as in the case of evolving cerebral edema, craniofacial repairs, and treatment of cerebrospinal fluid [CSF] leak or infection). Mass lesions may be classified as extra-axial (outside the brain tissue but inside the cranium) or intra-axial (within the brain tissue). Certain intracranial hematomas require immediate surgical intervention, generally those with sufficient volume to create outright cerebral herniation or cerebral compression that is symptomatic, that is, causing coma, neurologic deficit, or intracranial hypertension.

Management of intracranial pressure (ICP) in the face of hemorrhagic lesions and cerebral edema can be challenging, depending on the space occupied in the intracranial compartment by hematomas and edematous brain tissue. The Monroe-Kellie hypothesis states that the intracranial compartment has fixed volumes of the following components: cerebral tissue, cerebral blood, and CSF. As one compartment increases in volume or a mass lesion is added to the compartment, compensation must occur to maintain a normal ICP. This compensation initially involves displacement of CSF and venous blood into the spinal canal; but once a critical volume is reached in the intracranial compartment, cerebral compliance decreases and elastance increases, resulting in larger changes in ICP with smaller changes in volume. Therefore, small reductions in CSF can have a large impact on ICP control at this stage; likewise, removing mass lesions or increasing the size of the cranial compartment via craniectomy and duraplasty can very effectively control ICP.

CLINICAL PRESENTATION

Patients with sTBI by definition present in coma. They often arrive at the hospital having been intubated in the field because of suppression of respiratory function caused by the brain injury and/or inability to protect the airway because of the depressed level of consciousness. Trauma patients with TBI must be assessed for the presence of other injuries and should be presumed to have them until proven otherwise, given their inability to report history or symptoms.

Depending on the mechanism of injury, other injuries may be rather self-evident or occult. Typical high-speed motor vehicle crash patients or a pedestrian struck by a vehicle will often present with gross signs of trauma, including abrasions, contusions, lacerations, degloving soft tissue injuries, and a variety of musculoskeletal deformities suggesting fractures, dislocations, or tendon or ligamentous injuries of the spine, thorax, pelvis, or extremities. Many of these injuries may cause sufficient internal or external blood loss resulting in hypotension and hemodynamic instability. Internal abdominal organ injuries may manifest as an acute abdomen with hypotension and abdominal distension and tympany, whereas hemopneumothorax manifests as respiratory insufficiency or cardiac arrest; cardiac or large vessel injuries may present with hypotension or cardiac arrest. Fall patients may show minimal signs of external trauma (especially for lower heights) but harbor significant internal injuries. Those presenting after assault may present with multiple missile entries and exits, stab wounds, manifestations of blunt trauma, or combinations of these. Recreational injuries may present in any number of ways, and workup requires an accounting of the activity involved and details of the mechanisms of injury.

DIAGNOSIS
Airway, Breathing, and Circulation

As with all injured patients, assessment and treatment (done simultaneously) begins with the ABCs: management of patients' *airway*, *breathing*, and *circulation* first. The next, or *D* portion of the assessment, is for *disability* (neurologic status). A GCS score is assigned both before and after resuscitation based on patients' responsiveness with respect to eye opening, motor activity, and speech (**Table 1**). As part of the motor examination, any lateralizing signs must be noted, as these can signal the location of intracranial lesions or the presence of a concurrent spinal cord injury (as can a neurologic deficit at a particular spinal level).

Glasgow Coma Scale

The GCS has been used for decades and has both high interrater reliability and prognostic value for mortality and morbidity for large populations. Prognosis relies on the postresuscitation score, and the motor examination is most sensitive. However, any given patient presenting with a specific GCS score may ultimately have a wide range of outcomes, depending on the type of structural injury, the relative degree of secondary injury burden, the development of neurologic or systemic complications,

Table 1
The Glasgow Coma Scale

GCS Component	Examination Finding	Score
Eye opening	Spontaneously	4
	To sound	3
	To pressure	2
	None	1
Verbal response	Oriented	5
	Confused	4
	Words not sentences	3
	Sounds not words	2
	None	1
Motor response	Obeys commands	6
	Localizes to pain	5
	Normal flexion	4
	Abnormal flexion	3
	Extension	2
	None	1

and a host of known and unknown genetic and epigenetic factors. Ergo, treatment is aimed at maximizing the healing milieu and minimizing detrimental events; an initial survey of traumatic findings associated with TBI must be done as rapidly as possible.

Pupils

Additional neurologic signs include the size, symmetry, and reactivity of the pupils, as abnormalities are not only helpful in determining the presence of cerebral herniation requiring emergency interventions but are also associated with other forms of trauma, including blunt vascular injury (Horner syndrome), direct trauma to the globe, or direct injury of the third nerve (as opposed to compression caused by cerebral herniation). Pinpoint pupils may signify a brainstem injury. Other factors affecting the level of consciousness, such as the presence of certain intoxicants, can also affect the pupillary examination. The absence of brainstem reflexes, such as corneal and gag reflexes, after adequate establishment of perfusion and oxygenation from resuscitation and restoration of normothermia, portends a poor prognosis but is sometimes reversible with ongoing stabilization.

Cranium

After the rapid neurologic examination and GCS score are obtained, signs of trauma to the head and neck must be identified. External signs of head trauma must be carefully sought and documented, sometimes requiring clipping of hair to determine the nature and extent of scalp abrasions, contusions, and lacerations and the presence of open depressed skull fractures within lacerations. The presence of mastoid ecchymoses (Battle's sign) or bilateral periorbital ecchymoses (raccoon eyes) are often associated with basilar skull fractures. The calvarium should be palpated for deformities signifying closed skull fractures.

Eyes

Early survey including pupillary examination and assessment of corneal reflexes and the presence of periorbital ecchymoses has been mentioned. Periorbital edema may make the ocular examination more difficult; head elevation, application of iced-saline-soaked gauze pads, and the use of instruments to evert the eyelids may aid the examination. Extraocular movements should be assessed as soon as patients are able to follow commands, as cranial nerve palsies may be due to impingement in the orbit, compression within the cranium, or primary damage to the nuclei. Gaze deviation may signal the presence of nonconvulsive seizure activity/status epilepticus. The presence of important signs should be noted. For example, hyphema (typically an ophthalmologic emergency) or subconjunctival hemorrhage indicate direct trauma to the globe and conjunctival petechiae may indicate hypoxemia. For those with the most devastating of injuries resulting in brain death, the presence of oculocephalic and oculovestibular reflexes needs to be assessed.

Ears and Nose

The presence of hemotympanum or external auditory canal hemorrhage on otoscopic evaluation should be investigated for cause and associated injuries (eg, skull fracture, ruptured tympanic membrane, or trauma to the ossicles and other structures of the ear). The presence of CSF otorrhea or rhinorrhea signifies skull base fracture and dural laceration and is a risk factor for later development of meningitis. Although most skull base fracture-associated CSF leaks resolve spontaneously and do not require any treatment (including lumbar drainage or administration of antibiotics), some CSF leaks may require later lumbar drainage; others may require immediate or delayed open or endoscopic surgical repair, especially those associated with frontal sinus fractures. Except for transoral gunshot wounds, antibiotics are generally reserved for perioperative surgical patients (as per standard practice for craniotomy), so as to avoid selection of resistant organisms should infection occur. Epistaxis must be controlled, especially if arterial; this may require careful packing or interventional embolization.

Face

Concomitant facial fractures and soft tissue injuries are common and may impact surgical decision-making, so a thorough assessment of these injuries is mandatory, including imaging when needed and careful repair and control of active bleeding. Cranial integrity in multiple fractures relies on craniofacial bone structural integrity; however, fracture repair is often delayed because of the presence of brain edema, so surgical approaches must be coordinated among specialists.

Neck

Coincident blunt vascular injury (BVI) may occur and should be suspected in the following clinical scenarios[4]:

- Neurologic deficit unexplained by brain computed tomography (CT)
- Monoparesis in alert patients without brachial plexus injury suspected
- Lucid interval followed by neurologic deterioration
- Isolated dysphasia
- Unilateral headache after trauma
- Arterial epistaxis
- Horner syndrome (ptosis, miosis, anhidrosis)
- Neck hematoma, ecchymosis, or crepitus

Risk factors for blunt cerebrovascular injury include[5]

- Cervical hyperextension injury, especially with rotation
- GCS of 8 or less
- Seatbelt injury to the neck, hanging, or strangulation mechanism
- Skull base fracture, especially through the foramen lacerum or carotid canal
- Facial fractures, especially Le Fort II and III
- Cervical spine fracture
- Other vascular injuries, for example, thoracic aorta

Maintaining a high index of suspicion and evaluating for blunt vascular injury (BVI) in appropriate cases is important, as the consequences of dissection, thromboembolism, and occlusion are avoidable secondary insults to the brain resulting in potentially large territories of ischemia, which can not only add to the neurologic deficit burden but may also be fatal.[6,7]

Secondary Surveys

As soon as patients are testable, more detailed assessments should be done, including tests of all cranial nerve functionality, sensory and motor abilities (including tremor and coordination), speech (for dysarthria, expressive and receptive dysphasia), and cognition (multiple domains, especially awareness and memory early on).

DIAGNOSTIC PROCEDURES

Systemic causes of a depressed level of consciousness must be ruled out, including hypoxia, hypoperfusion, hypoglycemia or hyperglycemia or the presence of intoxicants. Arterial blood gases, serum electrolytes and glucose, serum alcohol level, and urine toxicology tests are, therefore, commonly needed emergently to gauge the impact of physiologic derangements on the neurologic examination.

Neuroimaging

Once patients have been adequately hemodynamically stabilized, the mainstay of diagnosis for sTBI is CT of the brain and skull. This imaging may be augmented by CT angiography for potential blunt craniocervical vascular injury and CT of the face (to fully evaluate craniofacial fractures and degree of pneumocephalus) and should always also include high-quality, thin-cut, 3-dimensional reconstructed views of the cervical spine, if available, in order to diagnose any comorbid cervical column injuries (common). MRI of the brain is not typically used in the workup of acute trauma because of the safety of the scanner environment, the length of time to obtain the study, and the lack of meaningful additional information to guide emergency management. Diagnostic cerebral angiography is not used in the diagnosis of brain injury itself but may be needed to assess blunt vascular injuries more fully in the hours or days after presentation. Advanced neuroimaging with PET or single-photon emission CT is sometimes used in the intensive care phases of sTBI management in research centers or high-acuity centers with advanced imaging and other treatment modalities available. The timing and number of follow-up CT scans depends on patients' presenting clinical and radiographic findings, presence of antithrombotic drugs or coagulopathy, trends in neuromonitoring values, age, and ability to obtain adequate serial neurologic examinations.

Neuromonitoring

After initial stabilization and treatment of patients with sTBI, consideration is given to the use of invasive and noninvasive neuromonitoring techniques. Such monitoring devices may be intraparenchymal (fiber-optic catheters inserted through the lumen of a bolt secured to the skull) or intraventricular. These catheters may be used to measure continuous ICP; from that value, the cerebral perfusion pressure (CPP) may be calculated as the difference between mean arterial pressure and ICP. The advantages of parenchymal catheters include ease of placement and ultralow complications rates.

Numerous studies have demonstrated improvements in mortality and outcome with ICP monitoring and goal-directed treatment,[8-11] although rigorous scientific conclusions have been somewhat inhibited by their retrospective nature or other limitations in study design.[12] Although one prospective controlled trial[13] at 6 hospitals in South America randomizing patients with sTBI to either ICP monitor-guided treatment or treatment guided by frequent clinical reexamination and radiographic studies showed no statistically significant difference in 6-month outcome (as assessed by the Glasgow Outcome Scale-Extended), this study is not an indictment of the use of ICP monitoring; rather, it highlights that primary use of numerical electronic ICP values or signs of intracranial hypertension on examination or radiographic studies may be equally as important in driving ICP-related decision-making. Practically speaking, such decisions are made on a daily basis through the synthesis of numerical ICP data, clinical examination changes, and radiographic imaging evolution.

External ventricular drainage catheters may be used in a therapeutic manner as well as diagnosticly. There are 2 forms available; one is a simple ventricular catheter and a fluid-coupled transducer to measure ICP and monitor the ICP waveform. The disadvantage of this method is that during periods when the catheter is open to drainage for therapeutic purposes (to remove CSF volume and, therefore, decrease ICP), an accurate reading cannot be obtained. Thus, a second technology has been developed that contains a fiber-optic transducer at the tip of the catheter that can read ICP continually, even when the system is open to drain CSF. Disadvantages of EVD in general include higher infection and hemorrhage rates than for parenchymal monitors.

In addition to ICP monitoring, there are multiple other advanced neuromonitoring options for patients with sTBI. These options include parenchymal catheters to measure brain tissue oxygen (pB_tO_2)[14] and brain temperature and cerebral microdialysis to monitor extracellular glutamate,[15] lactate, and pyruvate (among other molecules) to assess for excitotoxicity and tissue ischemia.[16,17] Additionally, intravenous jugular bulb catheters to assess jugular venous saturation of oxygen ($S_{jv}O_2$) as an estimation of cerebral extraction of oxygen are sometimes used.[18–20] Parenchymal pB_tO_2 monitoring techniques tend to be used in patients with worse injuries requiring more intensive care interventions, and the use of the technique has been associated with improvement in outcomes.[21–26] Microdialysis techniques tend to be used only in highly specialized centers or research settings, but preliminary work suggests that using data derived from microdialysis techniques may help predict outcomes (both mortality and functional outcome at 6 months). The use of $S_{jv}O_2$ monitoring in sTBI requires a fair amount of troubleshooting and interpretation. Any maneuver or physiologic event that results in decreased oxygen delivery to the brain or increased oxygen extraction by the brain will result in low $S_{jv}O_2$, provided the device is reading the venous saturation properly, so the values cannot be interpreted in isolation. The technique must be used in conjunction with other assessments (systemic hypoxia, ventilator settings, pB_tO_2 measurements, and so forth) to put the $S_{jv}O_2$ values into context to drive clinical decision-making. That being said, some studies have shown improvements in outcome when the technique is used to guide treatment of jugular venous desaturations.[18,19] Parenchymal probes to assess regional cerebral blood flow (CBF) are also available,[27] though not yet in common usage; however, as techniques become more reliable and more data become available, the addition of direct measurements of blood flow in the injured brain will likely prove to be a valuable adjunct in the intensive care management of sTBI. Finally, the use of electroencephalography (EEG), particularly continuous EEG, in comatose intensive care unit (ICU) patients with TBI plays an important role in diagnosing subclinical seizures so that they can be treated in a timely fashion to prevent secondary injury.[28,29]

MANAGEMENT OPTIONS AND OUTCOMES
Treatment Thresholds

The concept of treatment thresholds has been an important part of decision-making for decades; however, understanding the physiology behind these thresholds and acting accordingly is more important than blind adherence to maintaining a particular set of numeric values.

Hypotension has long been known to have an adverse effect on patient mortality after TBI (mortality being 35% in those admitted with TBI and systolic blood pressure [SBP] of less than 85 mm Hg vs 6% without hypotension in a seminal study from the 1980s).[30] This concept was confirmed in a Traumatic Coma Data Bank study demonstrating a doubling of mortality (from 27% to 55%) in patients with sTBI experiencing early hypotension (any measurement of SBP <90 mm Hg).[31] Avoiding any SBP less than 90 mm Hg requires a higher average SBP than 90 mm Hg, and for decades maintenance of SBP well greater than 90 to 100 mm Hg has been a mainstay of therapy (as long as autoregulatory collapse does not cause major elevations in ICP). In young healthy patients, permissive hypertension can sometimes be used. Pain or dysautonomia must be considered for those with persistent hypertension and no premorbid hypertension diagnosis. Age is a factor in determining appropriate blood pressure thresholds, and recent data suggests that for patients 50 to 69 years of age, SBP should be maintained at greater than 100 mm Hg and greater than 110 mm Hg for patients 15 to 49 years of age or greater than 70 years of age.[32] In general, the strict avoidance of hypotension and concomitant hypoperfusion of the brain is a critical aspect of sTBI management. Hypoxia is also to be avoided, as any episode of hypoxia (defined as Pao_2 $\leq$60 mm Hg or apnea or cyanosis in the field) is independently associated with a poor outcome after sTBI.[33]

ICP has variably been considered to be normal at less than 20 or 25 mm Hg in sTBI studies. Traditionally, ICP target ranges of less than 20 mm Hg have been used; but slightly higher values are tolerable as long as CPP is adequate (60–70 mm Hg or greater), ICP waveforms are not pathologic, and/or significantly higher or sustained elevations are not occurring. In decades past, aggressive attempts to artificially elevate the CPP to sustained levels higher than 70 mm Hg using fluid and pressors led to systemic complications, most notably adult respiratory distress syndrome[20,34], so global application of that technique has largely been abandoned for nearly 2 decades. However, a specific patient may require higher CPP if, for example, there are consistent pressure-dependent examination changes or neuromonitoring parameters suggest cerebral ischemia.

Surgical Management

Rapid evacuation of mass lesions causing neurologic compromise most commonly occurs shortly after arrival to the hospital. Although each patient must be considered individually for his or her surgical indications, size and volume criteria as well as guidelines based on midline shift, appearance of cisterns, and other markers of mass effect have been published.[35–39] Occasionally, patients are managed nonoperatively initially, but expansion of mass lesions in the first hours or days after admission will prompt surgical evacuation. This decision may be based on uncontrollable ICP, new or worsening neurologic deficit, and/or new or worsening findings on CT.

When patients are taken for craniotomy and evacuation of mass lesions, the decision must be made whether or not to replace the bone flap. This decision is usually made based on a combination of factors, including but not limited to the occurrence of hypotension or hypoxia, the presence of a major vascular injury, the degree of cerebral edema on CT scan (including midline shift out of proportion to extra-axial hematoma thickness and compressed or absent cisterns), the degree of hemorrhage and hemispheric swelling seen at surgery, the degree of observed intraoperative coagulability, the presence of extracranial injuries that are expected to produce ongoing problems with hypotension or hypoxia, and others. When the bone flap is left out, it must comprise a large fronto temporoparietal craniotomy with squamous temporal craniectomy to the middle fossa floor, and duraplasty of some form must be performed to avoid hemispheric compression.

Delayed decompressive craniotomy/craniectomy may be done in cases of medically refractory intracranial hypertension. Two randomized controlled clinical trials of surgical decompression have been performed,[40,41] with variable results due to differences in methodological considerations. However, many prior studies have demonstrated the effectiveness of this technique in controlling ICP, and the practice of decompressive surgery in these patients is commonplace. The potential for meaningful recovery based on patient values is a critical part of decision-making, so careful patient selection is most important.

Medical Management

Medical management of TBI centers on several principles, namely, reduction of cerebral edema and ICP, avoidance of tissue hypoxia and ischemia, neuroprotection via mitigation of inflammation and reduction in metabolic demand, correction of coagulopathies and avoidance of hemorrhagic progression, and prevention of systemic complications (primarily pulmonary, infectious, nutritional, thromboembolic, musculoskeletal, and neurologic, such as seizure). The critical care management of sTBI involves meticulous attention to the maintenance of adequate CBF for oxygen and glucose delivery, which is practically managed by keeping ICP low and CPP adequate. Because, to date, numerous clinical trials of neuroprotective agents for sTBI have failed,[42] clinical care must rely on providing the best environment for healing to occur while avoiding complications.

Treatments aimed at controlling ICP include sedation and neuromuscular paralysis. Ideal sedative agents would have neuroprotective effects on the brain and not aggravate the neurochemical cascades leading to excitotoxicity and secondary injury. Any agent used for this purpose should be short acting to allow for neurologic assessment, should not increase ICP, and should not decrease cerebral perfusion. Unfortunately, no one agent meets these criteria. Propofol[43] and narcotics are the most commonly used agents for sedation in sTBI, with benzodiazepines a less ideal alternative. However, caution with high doses of propofol is warranted; adequate intravascular volume should be ensured in an effort to avoid the rare complication of propofol infusion syndrome,[44] which is characterized by cardiovascular collapse, renal failure, metabolic acidosis, and rhabdomyolysis. In difficult-to-control intracranial hypertension, barbiturate coma may be used; but it is not used prophylactically.[45–47] Barbiturate therapy also reduces cerebral metabolism. Patients may be responders or nonresponders; before initiating a barbiturate coma, test doses may be given to ensure that the desired effect on ICP is present, because of the risk of morbidity associated with barbiturate coma (infection, hypotension). Any patient being considered for a barbiturate coma should have confirmation of adequate intravascular volume before initiation, should be hemodynamically stable without hypotension, and should undergo continuous EEG to monitor for adequate effect (burst suppression). Short-acting neuromuscular paralytics (intermittent doses or low-dose continuous infusions) may rarely be required to help control ICP, typically in difficult-to-ventilate patients.

The use of osmotic agents to reduce cerebral edema is also commonly used, namely, mannitol for the acute reduction of increased ICP, and hypertonic saline (HTS) for multiple effects. Mannitol has multiple mechanisms of action in addition to reduction of interstitial edema via osmotic gradients, including increasing CBF and decreasing blood viscosity via hemodilution and alterations in red blood cell viscosity (potentially increasing oxygen delivery) as well as reducing ICP via reductions in blood volume from arteriolar constriction and inhibition of CSF production.[48,49] HTS may also decrease ICP, in addition to serving as a microresuscitation fluid for improved microcirculatory CBF and as a mitigator of inflammation.[50] The two therapies are not necessarily mutually exclusive and may be used at different time points or even simultaneously during the management of a single patient. Further research is needed to define optimal hyperosmolar euvolemic therapeutic laboratory values and physiologic parameters to guide therapy as well as modes of delivery, that is, rapid bolus of very concentrated formulae, slower boluses or self-limited drips, or continuous drips, all of which are in clinical usage for different situations.

Although hypothermia has shown significant promise in preclinical research and early clinical studies,[51,52] it has not borne out in large clinical trials as a viable therapeutic alternative due in part to methodological considerations, that is, time to target temperature not being achieved, possibly suboptimal rewarming rates, and the like.[53–55] However, some centers with expertise in its use do use the technique in select patients. Furthermore, certain subsets of patients may benefit, including those with evacuated subdural hematoma; ongoing research is being done in this area (the Hypothermia for Patients requiring Evacuation of Subdural Hematoma: A Multicenter, Randomized Clinical [HOPES] Trial). What is clear is the detrimental effect of hyperthermia and elevated core brain temperature[50]; therefore, active attempts to keep patients with sTBI euthermic should be used, at a minimum.

Although prolonged, prophylactic hyperventilation is not recommended in patients with sTBI because of the potential for harm,[56] hyperventilation is still an acceptable temporizing measure in the setting of elevated ICP.[12] Hyperventilation to reduce the systemic Pco_2 results in cerebral vasoconstriction (via pH changes in the blood) and a reduction in CBF and volume leading to acute decreases in ICP. Hyperemic patients may respond particularly well to this intervention. However, careful use is essential so as to avoid cerebral tissue ischemia. Oxygenation monitoring (pB_tO_2 or $S_{jv}O_2$) is a useful adjunct when using hyperventilation.

Corticosteroids are not used in the treatment of sTBI. The Corticosteroid Randomisation After Significant Head Injury (CRASH) trial[57,58] demonstrated deleterious effects in patients with sTBI and was halted early. This study of 10,008 patients, 3966 of whom had sTBI, led to the only current evidence-based level I recommendation in sTBI, namely, that the use of steroids is not recommended to improve outcomes or control ICP in sTBI. In addition, high-dose methylprednisolone is associated with increased mortality in sTBI patients and is, therefore, contraindicated.[12]

Early nutritional replacement to meet the increased metabolic needs of coma is critical in the management of sTBI and may reduce cerebral inflammation. Early nutritional replacement (within 5 days) has been demonstrated to reduce 2-week mortality after sTBI[59] and reduce the incidence of ventilator-associated pneumonias (VAPs).[58] Certainly, the critical care and trauma literature on early nutritional replacement for the avoidance of the systemic inflammatory response[60] and infectious complications[61] also applies to patients with sTBI. Transpyloric feeding is favored over gastric feeding because of the decreased incidence of VAPs.[62]

Strict glycemic control has been espoused as a mechanism to reduce the complications of hyperglycemia in critical care patients; however, in sTBI hypoglycemia may be detrimental to the injured brain, because cerebral metabolism relies on a steady supply of glucose for oxidative metabolism. No differences in mortality have been shown with various glycemic control protocols in sTBI, although there has been some evidence of improved outcome[63] when hyperglycemia is avoided. However, studies have also shown increased frequency of hypoglycemic episodes[64,65] in the more strictly controlled groups. In general, euglycemia is targeted in critical care patients with sTBI, with great care taken to avoid hypoglycemic episodes.

Coagulopathy is common in sTBI, both from acute blood loss from polytrauma and resuscitation-related hemodilution as well as release of tissue factor and other proteins from damaged brain tissue.[66] Standard coagulation panels, including partial thromboplastin time, prothrombin time, and the international normalized ratio, may need to be performed serially within the first 72 hours of injury or longer. Full disseminated intravascular coagulation panels should be done for uncorrectable coagulopathies as evidenced by abnormal laboratory values or excessive and protracted bleeding at surgery or from injuries. Studies of platelet function, such as thromboelastography, are also sometimes required, particularly for patients with major blood loss, patients on antiplatelet medications, or those with chronic alcohol abuse.

Correction of coagulopathy (including those on anticoagulants for comorbidities) is particularly important for those patients undergoing cranial surgery, intracranial monitor placement, and for those harboring significant intracranial hemorrhage, in general (**Table 2**). Administration of platelets for patients on antiplatelet therapy is reserved for surgical patients, as there is no strong evidence that administration of platelets in these patients is effective at improving outcomes or reducing lesion progression.[67,68]

Infection prevention in patients with sTBI is difficult, and a significant proportion of patients admitted to the ICU with sTBI will have some form of infection. Prolonged mechanical ventilation increases the risk of pneumonia, as does prolonged immobilization. Although oral care with povidone-iodine has been promulgated as a means of reducing VAP risk for orally intubated patients over the last several years, there is at least some evidence that it may contribute to increased infectious risk as well as the development of adult respiratory distress syndrome.[69] Early tracheostomy may afford some degree of protection from VAP in patients with sTBI in that mechanical ventilation days can be reduced,[70] although actual VAP incidence and mortality rates have not been shown to be directly affected.[70,71] Again, the benefits of early tracheostomy as seen in general trauma patients apply as well to patients wutg sTBI, as long as the procedure does not lead to deleterious effects on ICP, brain edema, and so forth, which have largely been reduced with rapid surgical technique and minimally invasive tracheostomy techniques that can be used in the ICU. In addition to reduced ICU length of stay, these benefits include avoidance of vocal cord injury and stenosis, improved pulmonary toilet, reduced work of spontaneous breathing, and enhanced ability to wean mechanical ventilation (ability to go on and off of the ventilator). Surgical complications are unusual and include infection and hemorrhage as well as tracheal stenosis. For patients with sTBI whose return to consciousness is generally expected to be greater than 7 days, consideration for tracheostomy between days 3 and 7 should be given.

The potential for central nervous system infection related to surgery, monitoring procedures (especially EVD), or the primary injury (especially for penetrating injuries, open depressed skull fractures, and dural laceration with CSF leak) requires extra vigilance. Two meta-analyses[72,73] have concluded that the use of antibiotic-impregnated catheters significantly reduced catheter-related infections; however, when considering only studies with adequate allocation concealment, this difference was not seen in one of these analyses.[72]

Table 2 Structural intracranial injuries		
Extra-Axial Hematomas	**Intra-Axial Hematomas**	**Primary Brain Injuries**
Epidural hematoma	Intraparenchymal hemorrhage Contusion Hematoma	Intraparenchymal hemorrhage Contusion Hematoma
Subdural hematoma	Intraventricular hemorrhage[b]	Cerebral laceration
Subarachnoid hemorrhage[a]		Diffuse axonal injury

[a] Although traumatic subarachnoid hemorrhage (tSAH) is technically a form of extra-axial hemorrhage, the presence of diffuse tSAH portends a poor prognosis, as it can be a marker of structural damage to the underlying cerebral tissue.
[b] Although intraventricular hemorrhage is often classified as intra-axial because of the deep location within the ventricles of the brain, it is technically not within the substance of the brain, and the ventricular space and CSF are in communication with the subarachnoid space.

Venous thromboembolism (VTE) prophylaxis is particularly important in patients in a prolonged coma and its resultant immobility. Clinical questions of timing, choice of agent, and duration of therapy persist. Expectations for intracranial monitor or ventricular catheter insertions and removals and cranial surgeries impact the timing and choice of agent. Surgical staving of cerebral arteriolar and venular bleeding relies on the use of careful bipolar cautery to minimize brain tissue trauma, and adequate clotting is required for cautery to be effective. Surgery on patients who already have significant tissue trauma with friable brain tissue can be adversely affected by the presence of anticoagulants, in particular low-molecular-weight heparin (LMWH). LMWH used early has also been shown to significantly increase hemorrhagic progression on imaging after blunt TBI, with a proportion of those patients requiring surgery for the hemorrhagic progression.[74] Another study showed no difference in radiographic progression but suffered from the grouping of subcutaneous heparin and LMWH together as "chemoprophylaxis."[75] An examination of VTE rates in patients with sTBI treated with early or late LMWH (enoxaparin) prophylaxis showed no difference in VTE rate.[76] Most studies on this subject are limited by their retrospective nature. The utilization of a protocol for initiation of chemoprophylaxis alone may be sufficient to improve VTE rates.[77] The protocol used by the senior author is demonstrated in **Fig. 1**.

Posttraumatic seizures (PTSs) are classified into 3 categories: immediate, early (within 7 days of injury), or late (after 7 days). Posttraumatic epilepsy is defined as recurrent seizures occurring in the late seizure period. The incidence of clinical PTSs may be as high as 12%, with the rate of subclinical seizures detected on EEG

For Severe Traumatic Patients with Brain Injury Expected Prolonged Coma

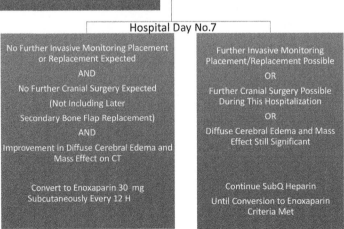

Fig. 1. Senior author's protocol for VTE prophylaxis in patients with sTBI. SubQ, subcutaneous.

being even higher.[28,78] To date, the largest randomized controlled clinical trials have shown that phenytoin significantly reduces the incidence of early but not late seizures,[79] with no differences in 12-month neuropsychologic testing outcomes.[80] Valproic acid has similar efficacy for the prevention of early PTS but not late PTS but is associated with higher mortality.[81] Phenytoin is, therefore, indicated for prevention of early PTS. Strong evidence for the use of levetiracetam in the prevention of early PTS in patients with sTBI is so far lacking. Late PTS is treated with a broader array of antiepileptic drugs (AEDs), congruent with the treatment of new-onset epilepsy from other causes, until further evidence is forthcoming. No anticonvulsant is free from side effects. Phenytoin may be associated with excessive sleepiness and if levels become too high, ataxia and imbalance. Levetiracetam has been independently associated with mood and behavioral side effects (depression, nervousness, agitation, anger, and aggression) and other adverse effects, such as upset stomach and sleep disturbance.[82] A thorough familiarity with the medication kinetics and adverse effect profiles for any AED under consideration for the prevention of early PTS or treatment of late PTS is of critical importance, as many of the adverse effects mimic the sequelae, signs, and symptoms of TBI (eg, confusion, depression, anxiety, somnolence, anger and aggression, sleep disturbance, ataxia, and more). Age and prior neuropsychiatric disease also play roles in AED selection.

SUMMARY

The management of patients with sTBIs requires meticulous attention to a variety of details and involves team members from a variety of specialties. A thorough understanding of the pathophysiology of cerebral edema and secondary injury cascades is a critical foundation for determining therapeutic decisions, particularly in areas where evidence is lacking.

REFERENCES

1. Centers for Disease Control and Prevention, National Center for Injury Prevention and Control. Web-based Injury Statistics Query and Reporting System (WISQARS). 2005. Available at: www.cdc.gov/injury/wisqars. Accessed July 23, 2017.
2. National Vital Statistics System (NVSS) 2006-2010. Data source is maintained by the CDC National Center for Health Statistics. 2010.
3. Teasdale G, Jennett B. Assessment of coma and impaired consciousness. A practical scale. Lancet 1974;2(7872):81–4.
4. Watridge CB, Muhlbauer MS, Lowery RD. Traumatic carotid artery dissection: diagnosis and treatment. J Neurosurg 1989;71(6):854–7.
5. Biffl WL, Moore EE, Ryu RK, et al. The unrecognized epidemic of blunt carotid arterial injuries: early diagnosis improves neurologic outcome. Ann Surg 1998; 228(4):462–70.
6. Miller PR, Fabian TC, Bee TK, et al. Blunt cerebrovascular injuries: diagnosis and treatment. J Trauma 2001;51(2):279–85 [discussion: 285–6].
7. Miller PR, Fabian TC, Croce MA, et al. Prospective screening for blunt cerebrovascular injuries: analysis of diagnostic modalities and outcomes. Ann Surg 2002;236(3):386–93 [discussion: 393–5].
8. Farahvar A, Gerber LM, Chiu YL, et al. Increased mortality in patients with severe traumatic brain injury treated without intracranial pressure monitoring. J Neurosurg 2012;117(4):729–34.

9. Alali AS, Fowler RA, Mainprize TG, et al. Intracranial pressure monitoring in severe traumatic brain injury: results from the American College of Surgeons Trauma Quality Improvement Program. J Neurotrauma 2013;30(20):1737–46.

10. Gerber LM, Chiu YL, Carney N, et al. Marked reduction in mortality in patients with severe traumatic brain injury. J Neurosurg 2013;119(6):1583–90.

11. Talving P, Karamanos E, Teixeira PG, et al. Intracranial pressure monitoring in severe head injury: compliance with brain trauma foundation guidelines and effect on outcomes: a prospective study. J Neurosurg 2013;119(5):1248–54.

12. Carney N, Totten AM, O'Reilly C, et al. Guidelines for the management of severe traumatic brain injury, fourth edition. Neurosurgery 2017;80(1):6–15.

13. Chesnut RM, Temkin N, Carney N, et al. A trial of intracranial-pressure monitoring in traumatic brain injury. N Engl J Med 2012;367(26):2471–81.

14. Martini RP, Deem S, Yanez ND, et al. Management guided by brain tissue oxygen monitoring and outcome following severe traumatic brain injury. J Neurosurg 2009;111(4):644–9.

15. Chamoun R, Suki D, Gopinath SP, et al. Role of extracellular glutamate measured by cerebral microdialysis in severe traumatic brain injury. J Neurosurg 2010; 113(3):564–70.

16. De Fazio M, Rammo R, O'Phelan K, et al. Alterations in cerebral oxidative metabolism following traumatic brain injury. Neurocrit Care 2011;14(1):91–6.

17. Sanchez JJ, Bidot CJ, O'Phelan K, et al. Neuromonitoring with microdialysis in severe traumatic brain injury patients. Acta Neurochir Suppl 2013;118:223–7.

18. Robertson C. Desaturation episodes after severe head injury: influence on outcome. Acta Neurochir Suppl (Wien) 1993;59:98–101.

19. Robertson CS, Gopinath SP, Goodman JC, et al. SjvO2 monitoring in head-injured patients. J Neurotrauma 1995;12(5):891–6.

20. Robertson CS, Valadka AB, Hannay HJ, et al. Prevention of secondary ischemic insults after severe head injury. Crit Care Med 1999;27(10):2086–95.

21. Bardt TF, Unterberg AW, Härtl R, et al. Monitoring of brain tissue PO2 in traumatic brain injury: effect of cerebral hypoxia on outcome. Acta Neurochir Suppl 1998; 71:153–6.

22. Valadka AB, Gopinath SP, Contant CF, et al. Relationship of brain tissue PO2 to outcome after severe head injury. Crit Care Med 1998;26(9):1576–81.

23. van den Brink WA, van Santbrink H, Steyerberg EW, et al. Brain oxygen tension in severe head injury. Neurosurgery 2000;46(4):868–76 [discussion: 876–8].

24. Stiefel MF, Udoetuk JD, Spiotta AM, et al. Conventional neurocritical care and cerebral oxygenation after traumatic brain injury. J Neurosurg 2006;105(4):568–75.

25. Chang JJ, Youn TS, Benson D, et al. Physiologic and functional outcome correlates of brain tissue hypoxia in traumatic brain injury. Crit Care Med 2009;37(1): 283–90.

26. Eriksson EA, Barletta JF, Figueroa BE, et al. The first 72 hours of brain tissue oxygenation predicts patient survival with traumatic brain injury. J Trauma Acute Care Surg 2012;72(5):1345–9.

27. Vajkoczy P, Roth H, Horn P, et al. Continuous monitoring of regional cerebral blood flow: experimental and clinical validation of a novel thermal diffusion microprobe. J Neurosurg 2000;93(2):265–74.

28. Vespa PM, Nuwer MR, Nenov V, et al. Increased incidence and impact of nonconvulsive and convulsive seizures after traumatic brain injury as detected by continuous electroencephalographic monitoring. J Neurosurg 1999;91(5):750–60.

29. Vespa P. Continuous EEG monitoring for the detection of seizures in traumatic brain injury, infarction, and intracerebral hemorrhage: "to detect and protect". J Clin Neurophysiol 2005;22(2):99–106.

30. Klauber MR, Marshall LF, Luerssen TG, et al. Determinants of head injury mortality: importance of the low risk patient. Neurosurgery 1989;24(1):31–6.

31. Chesnut RM, Marshall SB, Piek J, et al. Early and late systemic hypotension as a frequent and fundamental source of cerebral ischemia following severe brain injury in the Traumatic Coma Data Bank. Acta Neurochir Suppl (Wien) 1993;59: 121–5.

32. Berry C, Ley EJ, Bukur M, et al. Redefining hypotension in traumatic brain injury. Injury 2012;43(11):1833–7.

33. Chesnut RM, Marshall LF, Klauber MR, et al. The role of secondary brain injury in determining outcome from severe head injury. J Trauma 1993;34(2):216–22.

34. Contant CF, Valadka AB, Gopinath SP, et al. Adult respiratory distress syndrome: a complication of induced hypertension after severe head injury. J Neurosurg 2001;95(4):560–8.

35. Bullock MR, Chesnut R, Ghajar J, et al. Surgical management of acute subdural hematomas. Neurosurgery 2006;58(3 Suppl):S16–24 [discussion: Si–iv].

36. Bullock MR, Chesnut R, Ghajar J, et al. Surgical management of acute epidural hematomas. Neurosurgery 2006;58(3 Suppl):S7–15 [discussion: Si–iv].

37. Bullock MR, Chesnut R, Ghajar J, et al. Surgical management of traumatic parenchymal lesions. Neurosurgery 2006;58(3 Suppl):S25–46 [discussion: Si–iv].

38. Bullock MR, Chesnut R, Ghajar J, et al. Surgical management of posterior fossa mass lesions. Neurosurgery 2006;58(3 Suppl):S47–55 [discussion: Si–iv].

39. Bullock MR, Chesnut R, Ghajar J, et al. Surgical management of depressed cranial fractures. Neurosurgery 2006;58(3 Suppl):S56–60 [discussion: Si–iv].

40. Cooper DJ, Rosenfeld JV, Murray L, et al. Decompressive craniectomy in diffuse traumatic brain injury. N Engl J Med 2011;364(16):1493–502.

41. Hutchinson PJ, Kolias AG, Timofeev IS, et al. Trial of decompressive craniectomy for traumatic intracranial hypertension. N Engl J Med 2016;375(12):1119–30.

42. Maas AI, Steyerberg EW, Murray GD, et al. Why have recent trials of neuroprotective agents in head injury failed to show convincing efficacy? A pragmatic analysis and theoretical considerations. Neurosurgery 1999;44(6):1286–98.

43. Kelly DF, Goodale DB, Williams J, et al. Propofol in the treatment of moderate and severe head injury: a randomized, prospective double-blinded pilot trial. J Neurosurg 1999;90(6):1042–52.

44. Kang TM. Propofol infusion syndrome in critically ill patients. Ann Pharmacother 2002;36(9):1453–6.

45. Ward JD, Becker DP, Miller JD, et al. Failure of prophylactic barbiturate coma in the treatment of severe head injury. J Neurosurg 1985;62(3):383–8.

46. Eisenberg HM, Frankowski RF, Contant CF, et al. High-dose barbiturate control of elevated intracranial pressure in patients with severe head injury. J Neurosurg 1988;69(1):15–23.

47. Roberts I, Sydenham E. Barbiturates for acute traumatic brain injury. Cochrane Database Syst Rev 2012;(12):CD000033.

48. Nissenson AR, Weston RE, Kleeman CR. Mannitol. West J Med 1979;131(4): 277–84.

49. Winkler SR, Munoz-Ruiz L. Mechanism of action of mannitol. Surg Neurol 1995; 43(1):59.

50. Timmons SD. Current trends in neurotrauma care. Crit Care Med 2010;38(9 Suppl):S431–44.

51. Clifton GL, Allen S, Barrodale P, et al. A phase II study of moderate hypothermia in severe brain injury. J Neurotrauma 1993;10(3):263–71 [discussion: 273].

52. Marion DW, Penrod LE, Kelsey SF, et al. Treatment of traumatic brain injury with moderate hypothermia. N Engl J Med 1997;336(8):540–6.

53. Clifton GL, Valadka A, Zygun D, et al. Very early hypothermia induction in patients with severe brain injury (the National Acute Brain Injury Study: Hypothermia II): a randomised trial. Lancet Neurol 2011;10(2):131–9.

54. Clifton GL, Coffey CS, Fourwinds S, et al. Early induction of hypothermia for evacuated intracranial hematomas: a post hoc analysis of two clinical trials. J Neurosurg 2012;117(4):714–20.

55. Adelson PD, Wisniewski SR, Beca J, et al. Comparison of hypothermia and normothermia after severe traumatic brain injury in children (Cool Kids): a phase 3, randomised controlled trial. Lancet Neurol 2013;12(6):546–53.

56. Muizelaar JP, Marmarou A, Ward JD, et al. Adverse effects of prolonged hyperventilation in patients with severe head injury: a randomized clinical trial. J Neurosurg 1991;75(5):731–9.

57. Edwards P, Arango M, Balica L, et al. Final results of MRC CRASH, a randomised placebo-controlled trial of intravenous corticosteroid in adults with head injury-outcomes at 6 months. Lancet 2005;365(9475):1957–9.

58. Roberts I, Yates D, Sandercock P, et al. Effect of intravenous corticosteroids on death within 14 days in 10008 adults with clinically significant head injury (MRC CRASH trial): randomised placebo-controlled trial. Lancet 2004; 364(9442):1321–8.

59. Härtl R, Gerber LM, Ni Q, et al. Effect of early nutrition on deaths due to severe traumatic brain injury. J Neurosurg 2008;109(1):50–6.

60. Kudsk KA. Effect of route and type of nutrition on intestine-derived inflammatory responses. Am J Surg 2003;185(1):16–21.

61. Kudsk KA. Early enteral nutrition in surgical patients. Nutrition 1998;14(6):541–4.

62. Taylor SJ, Fettes SB, Jewkes C, et al. Prospective, randomized, controlled trial to determine the effect of early enhanced enteral nutrition on clinical outcome in mechanically ventilated patients suffering head injury. Crit Care Med 1999; 27(11):2525–31.

63. Yang M, Guo Q, Zhang X, et al. Intensive insulin therapy on infection rate, days in NICU, in-hospital mortality and neurological outcome in severe traumatic brain injury patients: a randomized controlled trial. Int J Nurs Stud 2009;46(6):753–8.

64. Bilotta F, Caramia R, Cernak I, et al. Intensive insulin therapy after severe traumatic brain injury: a randomized clinical trial. Neurocrit Care 2008;9(2):159–66.

65. Coester A, Neumann CR, Schmidt MI. Intensive insulin therapy in severe traumatic brain injury: a randomized trial. J Trauma 2010;68(4):904–11.

66. Zhang J, Jiang R, Liu L, et al. Traumatic brain injury-associated coagulopathy. J Neurotrauma 2012;29(17):2597–605.

67. Joseph B, Pandit V, Sadoun M, et al. A prospective evaluation of platelet function in patients on antiplatelet therapy with traumatic intracranial hemorrhage. J Trauma Acute Care Surg 2013;75(6):990–4.

68. Baharoglu MI, Cordonnier C, Al-Shahi Salman R, et al. Platelet transfusion versus standard care after acute stroke due to spontaneous cerebral haemorrhage associated with antiplatelet therapy (PATCH): a randomised, open-label, phase 3 trial. Lancet 2016;387(10038):2605–13.

69. Seguin P, Laviolle B, Dahyot-Fizelier C, et al. Effect of oropharyngeal povidone-iodine preventive oral care on ventilator-associated pneumonia in severely

brain-injured or cerebral hemorrhage patients: a multicenter, randomized controlled trial. Crit Care Med 2014;42(1):1–8.

70. Bouderka MA, Fakhir B, Bouaggad A, et al. Early tracheostomy versus prolonged endotracheal intubation in severe head injury. J Trauma 2004;57(2):251–4.

71. Sugerman HJ, Wolfe L, Pasquale MD, et al. Multicenter, randomized, prospective trial of early tracheostomy. J Trauma 1997;43(5):741–7.

72. Ratilal B, Costa J, Sampaio C. Antibiotic prophylaxis for surgical introduction of intracranial ventricular shunts: a systematic review. J Neurosurg Pediatr 2008; 1(1):48–56.

73. Wang X, Dong Y, Qi XQ, et al. Clinical review: efficacy of antimicrobial-impregnated catheters in external ventricular drainage - a systematic review and meta-analysis. Crit Care 2013;17(4):234.

74. Kwiatt ME, Patel MS, Ross SE, et al. Is low-molecular-weight heparin safe for venous thromboembolism prophylaxis in patients with traumatic brain injury? A Western Trauma Association multicenter study. J Trauma Acute Care Surg 2012;73(3):625–8.

75. Scudday T, Brasel K, Webb T, et al. Safety and efficacy of prophylactic anticoagulation in patients with traumatic brain injury. J Am Coll Surg 2011;213(1): 148–53 [discussion: 153–4].

76. Daley MJ, Ali S, Brown CV. Late venous thromboembolism prophylaxis after craniotomy in acute traumatic brain injury. Am Surg 2015;81(2):207–11.

77. Farooqui A, Hiser B, Barnes SL, et al. Safety and efficacy of early thromboembolism chemoprophylaxis after intracranial hemorrhage from traumatic brain injury. J Neurosurg 2013;119(6):1576–82.

78. Torbic H, Forni AA, Anger KE, et al. Use of antiepileptics for seizure prophylaxis after traumatic brain injury. Am J Health Syst Pharm 2013;70(9):759–66.

79. Temkin NR, Dikmen SS, Wilensky AJ, et al. A randomized, double-blind study of phenytoin for the prevention of post-traumatic seizures. N Engl J Med 1990; 323(8):497–502.

80. Dikmen SS, Temkin NR, Miller B, et al. Neurobehavioral effects of phenytoin prophylaxis of posttraumatic seizures. JAMA 1991;265(10):1271–7.

81. Temkin NR, Dikmen SS, Anderson GD, et al. Valproate therapy for prevention of posttraumatic seizures: a randomized trial. J Neurosurg 1999;91(4):593–600.

82. Kowski AB, Weissinger F, Gaus V, et al. Specific adverse effects of antiepileptic drugs–A true-to-life monotherapy study. Epilepsy Behav 2016;54:150–7.

Brain Death

Mack Drake, DO[a],*, Andrew Bernard, MD[a], Eugene Hessel, MD[b,c]

KEYWORDS

- Brain death • Organ donor • Brain injury • Critical care • Confirmatory testing
- Ancillary testing • Clinical examination

KEY POINTS

- Critical care both improves outcome in survivors and improves organ graft function in those who do not survive but become brain dead organ donors.
- Brain death determination technique varies among hospitals and clinicians.
- Mimickers of brain death must be carefully considered and factors that confound the brain death examination must be absent.
- Published guidelines provide structure and process to the brain death determination process.
- Ethical controversies remain, therefore clinicians who care for neurologically injured patients should continue to engage in dialogue and research.

BRAIN DEATH IN CONTEXT

Critical care physicians are frequently called on to diagnose and manage brain death. Although the medical and legal concepts of brain death are generally accepted, establishing the diagnosis is not simple and must be performed accurately. The details of how to diagnose brain death have been codified in guidelines by panels of experts[1–4]; however, precision in the brain death examination varies, and skepticism has been expressed in the lay literature about the accuracy of brain death determination.[5] Thus, it is imperative that clinicians perform brain death determination accurately

Disclosure: Drs M. Drake, A. Bernard and E. Hessel receive stipends from Kentucky Organ Donor Affiliates to provide organ donor critical care. Dr A. Bernard receives salary support as institutional liaison for UK Healthcare to Kentucky Organ Donor Affiliates. Dr A. Bernard serves as a board member benefits for Kentucky Organ Donor Affiliates (includes travel, lodging, meals, continuing education).

[a] Section on Trauma and Acute Care Surgery, Division of General Surgery, Department of Surgery, University of Kentucky College of Medicine, C224, 800 Rose Street, Lexington, KY 40536-0298, USA; [b] Department of Anesthesiology, University of Kentucky College of Medicine, 800 Rose Street, Lexington, KY 40536-0298, USA; [c] Department of Surgery, University of Kentucky College of Medicine, 800 Rose Street, Lexington, KY 40536-0298, USA
* Corresponding author. Division of General Surgery, UKCOM, C224, 800 Rose Street, Lexington, KY 40536.
E-mail address: mack.drake@uky.edu

Surg Clin N Am 97 (2017) 1255–1273
http://dx.doi.org/10.1016/j.suc.2017.07.001
0039-6109/17/© 2017 Elsevier Inc. All rights reserved.

and beyond reproach. In this article, we describe the critical components of brain death examination and briefly review the management of patients with impending and established brain death.

The most common causes of brain death in adults are traumatic brain injury and spontaneous subarachnoid hemorrhage. In children, the most common cause is non-accidental trauma.[6] Surgeons are keenly aware of the prevalence of end-stage chronic organ failure and the importance of organ transplantation and therefore tend to be diligent and timely in brain death evaluations and support of potential organ donors.

In caring for patients with severe neurologic injury, clinicians must first remember that most will recover. Half of patients who present with a Glasgow Coma Scale score of 3 will survive.[7] Clinicians should not make hasty judgments but should provide optimal physiologic support and careful neurologic examination. Principles of optimal care for neurologic injury are the same as for the potential organ donor, so good critical care is always the first priority.

Today, the medical community is generally comfortable with the general concept of brain death, but testing for and determination of brain death still draws occasional uncertainty and disagreement among providers; there is significant variability across hospitals.[8] Guidelines are available and any clinician performing brain death examination or supervising intensive care units should review and implement practice standards accordingly. The American Academy of Neurology (AAN) is considered the authoritative body on brain death testing in the United States. The AAN first promulgated its guideline, the American Academy of Neurologic Practice Parameters (AANPP), for diagnosis of brain death in adults in 1995[1] and an updated version in 2010.[2] The update is more prescriptive and definitive. The Society of Critical Care Medicine, American Academy of Pediatrics, and the Child Neurology Society updated their guidelines for determination of brain death in infants and children in 2011.[3,4]

Brain death testing has become more consistent across major neurologic centers but still lacks uniformity across the United States.[8] Variability is greater in smaller hospitals in which specialized neurologic and critical care expertise may be lacking.[9] Two areas of major concordance today between the guidelines and actual practice that had not existed previously are the use of apnea testing and the use of ancillary tests. Major areas of continued practice variability are the exclusion of confounders of brain death determination and the precise components and technique of clinical examination. In a recent survey, only 56% of surveyed hospitals excluded hypotension and only 79% excluded hypothermia.[8] These confounders of the examination and others, like acid-base disorders, electrolyte abnormalities, and intoxication, could reduce the examination's diagnostic accuracy. Failure to fully implement the 2010 AANPP guidelines may be due to overconfidence by providers or institutions or a lack of regulatory oversight, such as by hospital policy or leadership.

HISTORY

Mollaret and Goulon[10] from the Hospital Claude Bernard in Paris first described irreversible coma ("le coma depasse") in 1959. In 1968, Harvard Medical School convened an ad hoc committee to examine the concept of brain death from a clinical and ethical perspective. Led by renowned ethicist Henry Beecher, the committee published what it felt to be its unbiased and relatively simple assessment in *JAMA* that same year.[11] Three years later, Mohandas and Chou[12] expanded on this work by emphasizing the role of the brainstem in brain damage in 1971. A 1976 Conference of Royal Medical Colleges in the United Kingdom described loss of brain stem function as a part of brain death.[13] The Uniform Brain Death Act of 1978 attempted to clarify ambiguity regarding the definition of brain death and was then later replaced by the Uniform Determination of Death Act (UDDA) of 1980, which also included the definition of cardiorespiratory death. Most state laws governing brain death determination are now based on the UDDA legal standards. In 1981, a US President's Commission examined brain death determination, including confirmatory tests and waiting periods for anoxic deaths, and concluded that providers had in the past wrongly diagnosed brain death in some individuals who suffered from drug intoxication or other confounders. The AAN put forth the first evidence-based practice guidelines in its 1995 and 2010 publications.[2]

BRAIN DEATH POLICIES

Every hospital caring for patients with severe neurologic injury should have a policy for determining brain death. This policy should specify what specialties and professional roles (eg, attending, resident) might determine brain death, how they will be trained, whether credentialing for brain death determination will be required, and the precise criteria and parameters for the process. These should all be in accordance with or at least in consideration of the AAN guidelines.

A recent survey found that almost half of US hospitals require training for those determining brain death.[8] Forty-nine percent of those surveyed require that a neurologist or neurosurgeon be involved, but this is not a mandate in the AAN guideline. Although the AAN advocates the involvement of a neurologist, the guideline goes on to say, "neurosurgeons and intensive care specialists may have specialized expertise. It seems reasonable to require that all physicians making a determination of brain death be intimately familiar with brain death criteria and have demonstrated competence in this complex examination."[2]

Professional credentials, training, and even components and thresholds of the examination itself differ among countries, states, and individual hospitals. Intensivists and hospital leaders should maintain a high standard for who may perform brain death determination. Not all provider groups will maintain the same knowledge, experience, and skill set. Few hospitals require credentialing to perform brain death testing but such a practice merits consideration.

There is little evidence showing that 2 clinical examinations are superior to 1, although many hospitals and state statutes require 2.[9] A second test can delay the process of brain death determination and complicate the organ donation process.[14] Mandatory waiting periods and multiple examinations are very important for some clinical scenarios, such as in very young children and after cardiac arrest.

Many hospital brain death policies lack sufficient detail with regard to parameters necessary for allowing the clinical determination of brain death. Examples include thresholds for temperature, blood pressure, serum levels for confounding drugs, and details surrounding the performance of apnea testing.[8] Specificity is most lacking outside major neurologic specialty centers. Variability in hospital policy with regard to determining brain death should be considered avoidable risk.

NEUROIMAGING IN BRAIN DEATH

Determination of brain death begins with identifying a cause. Cause is determined by history, clinical examination, and neuroimaging studies. Clinicians should take pause when the circumstances are unclear or when imaging appears normal. Computerized tomography (CT) findings after neurologic injury include hemorrhage, edema, mass lesions, or ischemia, but imaging may be normal in the first 24 to 48 hours or longer in situations of hypoxic injury and central nervous system (CNS) infection. In the case of hypoxic injury, as seen with hanging or following severe shock and cardiac arrest, a waiting period of up to 24 hours followed by an interval clinical examination is necessary. Therapeutic hypothermia following cardiac arrest should be considered a confounder preventing clinical diagnosis of brain death until normothermia is restored.

Even when circumstances of the neurologic injury are clear and imaging is abnormal, a regimented, detailed and precise clinical examination is fundamental. Some neurologic findings are reversible. For example, numerous cases have been reported of transtentorial herniation being reversed with aggressive critical care maneuvers, even to favorable outcomes.[15,16] So the clinician must approach severe neurologic injury without bias or supposition. Abnormal imaging supports the brain death diagnosis but is only one part of a complete evaluation.

CLINICAL CRITERIA

After establishment of cause, review of neuroimaging and assurance that other prerequisites have been met, brain death determination may proceed. The process involves neurologic tests, consideration of confounders, resolution of any misleading or conflicting evidence, and if necessary, performance of confirmatory tests. Normothermia, hemodynamic stability, correction of extreme electrolyte disturbances, and confirmation of absence of neuromuscular blockade are essential before examination (**Box 1**). Neurologic testing is based on 3 fundamental findings: (1) coma, (2) absence of brainstem reflexes, and (3) apnea. Assess coma by inducing a pain stimulus to all 4 extremities (eg, nail beds), trunk (eg, sternum), and head (eg, supraorbital nerve or temporomandibular joint). The latter is important to avoid a false-positive test in the event of occult spinal cord injury. Seven brainstem reflexes must be assessed (**Box 2**). (1) Pupils should be fixed at "mid-position"; that is, between constricted and dilated, usually approximately 4 mm, and nonreactive to bright light. Pupillary dilation alone is not a sign of brain death and this examination finding should not withhold resuscitation of what may be a salvageable patient.[17] (2) Oculocephalic reflexes (doll's

---

Box 1
Prerequisites for brain death examination

1. Cause of irreversible brain death established

2. Supported by neuroimaging

3. Observed for at least 4 hours
   a. In cases of anoxic brain injury or following cardiac arrest observed for 24 hours
   b. If treated with hypothermia observe for 24 hours after resumed to normothermia

4. Normothermic. Adults $\geq 36°C$; children (<15 years old) $\geq 35°C$

5. Adequate systolic arterial pressure (with or without vasopressor support). Adults ≥ 100 mm Hg; children (<15 years old) above 2 SD below norm for age

6. No evidence of neuromuscular blockade (normal twitch to peripheral nerve stimulation)

7. Confounding factors ruled out
   a. Shock or severe hypotension
   b. Significant levels of central nervous system depressants (pentobarbital >10 µg/mL)
   c. Hyperosmolar coma, hepatic encephalopathy
   d. Extreme abnormalities of glucose, sodium, and pH

Box 2
Steps in the determination of death by neurologic criteria

1. Meets all prerequisites (see **Box 1**)

2. The clinical neurologic examination
   a. Establishment of irreversible coma
      Lack of motor responses to noxious stimuli including those applied above the neck (Glasgow Coma Score = 3)
   b. Absence of brainstem reflexes
      i. Absent pupillary response to light
      ii. Absent oculocephalic reflex (dolls eyes)
      iii. Absent of oculovestibular reflex (cold calorics)
      iv. Absence of corneal reflex
      v. Absence of facial muscle movement to noxious stimulus
      vi. Absence of pharyngeal reflex (gag)
      vii. Absence of tracheal reflex (cough)
   c. Apnea (**Box 3**)

3. In certain circumstances, ancillary testing (**Boxes 4** and **5**)

---

eyes) are tested by rapidly turning the head but this can be difficult to perform after injury and is prohibited in patients with spinal cord injury. (3) Vestibulo-ocular reflex (cold caloric responses) should be absent when irrigating the auditory canal with cold water with the head turned at 30°. Occlusion of the meatus or auditory canal can confound this test. (4) Corneal reflexes should be absent when stimulated with a swab. (5) A gag reflex should be absent on stimulation of the posterior pharynx. (6) A cough reflex should be absent with endotracheal suctioning. Cough reflex should not be tested with manipulation of the endotracheal tube alone. (7) Facial muscle movement should be absent in response to deep pressure on the temporomandibular condyles and supraorbital ridges.

APNEA TESTING

After establishing coma and absence of the 7 brainstem reflexes, confirmation of apnea is the third and final step in determining brain death. Various methods exist but all of them rely on a period of observing the patient during cessation of mechanical ventilation.[18] Essential steps are shown in **Box 3**. Before apnea testing, the patient must be preoxygenated for at least 10 minutes with 5 or more cm H_2O of positive end-expiratory pressure (PEEP) to wash out respiratory nitrogen and facilitate oxygen transport. This critical step reduces the risk of hypoxemia during testing, which is a common reason for arrhythmias and hypotension during apnea testing.[19] Minute ventilation is also adjusted, usually decreased, before commencing the period of apnea testing so that the examination begins with $Paco_2$ in the normal range. An arterial blood gas (ABG) is obtained after preoxygenation and before commencement of apnea testing to document baseline $Paco_2$ and pH. Mechanical ventilation is then discontinued. The traditional technique is to disconnect the ventilator circuit, pass oxygen tubing down the endotracheal tube to the carina, and instill 5 to 10 L/min oxygen. Alternatively, a T-piece may be used through which oxygen is insufflated at 5 to 10 L/min and on which the exhaust end is covered with a PEEP valve set at 5 to 10 cm H_2O. Addition of the PEEP valve may reduce hypoxia during apnea.[20,21] The patient is observed for any respiratory effort for at least 8 to 10 minutes and until the $Paco_2$ is expected to rise to $\geq$60 mm Hg. Carbon dioxide rises at a rate of about

---

Box 3
Apnea testing

1. Prerequisites
   a. Patient must have met all of the prerequisites for preforming a clinical examination for brain death
   b. First 2 components of the clinical examination (deep coma and absence of brain stem reflexes) must be compatible with diagnosis of brain death

2. Conduct
   a. Place on 100% Fio_2 and a low rate (~6 BPM) and 5 cm positive end-expiratory pressure (PEEP) for at least 10 minutes
   b. Then obtain baseline arterial blood gas (ABG) and ensure satisfactory parameters:
      i. Pao_2 >200
      ii. $Paco_2$ ~40
      iii. Treat severe base deficit (>6) with bicarbonate
   c. Take patient off ventilator and
      i. Insufflate oxygen at 10 L/min via a small catheter (small compared with ID of ETT) threaded into the trachea through the ETT, or better,
      ii. Attach a T-piece supplied with oxygen at 5 to 10 L/min to the ETT with a PEEP valve set at 5 to 10 cm H_2O at end of exhaust tube of T-piece
   d. Observe chest and abdomen for any respiratory activity for ≥10 minutes
   e. Must maintain SpO_2 >85%, mean arterial pressure >60, and systolic arterial pressure >90 (otherwise MUST abort and perform ancillary test)
   f. Obtain ABG after 10 minutes (to ensure that $Paco_2$ ≥60)
   g. Resume ventilation

3. Abort if become hypoxic (SpO_2 <85) or hypotensive (systolic pressure <90) and obtain an ancillary test

4. Interpretation
   a. Confirms brain death
      i. Considered a positive test if no respiratory activity despite a $Paco_2$ of ≥60 mm Hg
   b. Uninterpretable if test aborted. Must be followed with ancillary test
   c. May be unreliable if positive in presence of (and hence an ancillary test may be indicated):
      i. High levels central nervous system (CNS) depressants
      ii. Severe neuromuscular disease
      iii. High spinal cord injury
      iv. Preexisting carbon dioxide retainer
         1. If known, require $Paco_2$ 20 mm above usual premorbid baseline
         2. If unknown but suspected obtain ancillary test

---

3 mm Hg per minute. An ABG is then drawn and ventilation is resumed. Absence of respiratory effort while $Paco_2$ has risen to the target threshold constitutes a positive apnea test that is consistent with brain death. The apnea test must be aborted if the patient becomes hypoxic or hemodynamically unstable. If the $Paco_2$ did not reach 60 mm Hg at the completion of the test, it must be repeated with a longer period of apnea to produce the desired level of CO_2. Variations in apnea testing include how the test is performed (continuous positive airway pressure, oxygen tubing blow-by, T-piece) and how the results are interpreted. For example, patients who are CO_2 retainers have a higher baseline $Paco_2$ so in these patients, apnea testing should be based on a rise in $Paco_2$ of 20 mm Hg above their normal premorbid baseline. If a patient's baseline value is not known but the patient has severe chronic obstructive pulmonary disease and is suspected of being a CO_2 retainer, the apnea test must be interpreted with some skepticism and consideration given to performance of an ancillary test.

Box 4
Indications for ancillary testing

- Portions of clinical examination cannot be performed because of anatomic limitations or injuries
- Apnea test had to be aborted due to hypotension or hypoxia
- Limitations to interpreting a positive apnea test because of high levels of CNS depressants, severe neuromuscular disease, high spinal cord injury, or suspected preexisting carbon dioxide retainer
- Possible high levels of CNS depressants, for example, barbiturates
- Less than 24 hours since cardiac arrest, hypoxic brain damage or recovery from hypothermia therapy
- Disturbing residual movements/possible spinal reflexes
- Physician or family discomfort with diagnosis of brain death

---

MISLEADING MOTOR MOVEMENTS

Muscle movements in brain dead patients can confuse and cause uncertainty among clinicians, staff, and families. The exact physiologic basis for such movements is not known.[18] These movements arise from the spinal cord and include spontaneous twitches, movements of the limbs, including arm raises, head turning, toe twitching, positive Babinski, triple flexion response (hip and leg flexion and foot dorsiflexion), respiratorylike movements that can trigger the ventilator and confuse apnea testing, and even contraction of the abdominal muscles during organ retrieval or appearance of a brief attempt to sit up in the bed.[18] Saposnik and colleagues[22] observed 107 brain dead patients over a 5-year study period and almost half had spontaneous and reflexive movements, most commonly "undulating toe reflex" and the "triple flexion response." A follow-up review of 131 published reports concluded that such movements are present in 40% to 50% of brain dead patients and that these phenomena should not preclude diagnosis of death or eligibility for organ donation.[23] Any question regarding the relevance of such movements by the examining clinician should be

---

Box 5
Ancillary testing

1. Whole brain blood flow
   - 4-vessel contrast intra-arterial cerebral angiogram
   - Nuclear perfusion scan (single-photon emission computed tomography with Technetium 99m hexamethylpropyleneamine oxime)
   - Computed tomography angiography
   - Magnetic resonance angiography
   - Transcranial Doppler

2. Electrical activity in brain
   - Electroencephalogram
   - BIS
   - SSEP

3. Other imaging
   - MRI
   - PET

allayed by a complete clinical examination that is consistent with brain death followed by an ancillary test.[22–24] Proper terminology and careful explanation is important for both families and staff. Jain and Degeorgia[25] suggest referring to movements provoked by stimulus and brain death–associated reflexes and spontaneous movements as "brain death–associated automatisms." This nomenclature does not address specific pathophysiology of each movement, but does help ensure that they are categorized according to inciting action and avoids usage of the term "spontaneous motor movements."

CONDITIONS THAT MIMIC BRAIN DEATH

Three conditions may mimic brain death: locked-in syndrome, hypothermia, and drug intoxication. Locked-in syndrome results from an injury at the level of the pons with preservation of portions of the midbrain. The patient cannot move his or her limbs, grimace, or swallow but consciousness is preserved, as are blinking and vertical gaze. Locked-in syndrome most commonly results from basilar artery embolic stroke.[26] A similar clinical picture can occur with Guillan-Barre in which cranial and peripheral nerves are lost. In this specific syndrome, recovery is quite possible, which raises the alarming notion that these patients could be mistaken as brain dead.[27] The locked-in and Guillan-Barre syndromes are examples of cases in which the involvement of a consultant in the field of neuroscience with specific expertise in these disorders would be valuable to avoid errors in diagnosis. Hypothermia is a well-known mimicker of brain death. Cranial nerve reflexes disappear at approximately 28° Celsius but can then be recovered with rewarming.[28]

Drug intoxication can mimic brain death. Brain stem reflexes are normally preserved with intoxication so a complete examination is essential. Autopsy reports of brain death determined clinically in the context of sedative or toxic levels of pentobarbital raise the frightening specter of this error in clinical practice.[29] Critically ill or injured patients have altered drug clearance and may require more than 72 hours for pentobarbital or other drugs to be eliminated. Pentobarbital's lower limit of therapeutic range is 10 mg/L but there is no clinical consensus on the minimum concentration threshold for pentobarbital or any other barbiturates when determining brain death.[30] It is prudent to obtain a quantitative drug level before determining brain death in cases of drug intoxication. No specific waiting period has been reported in drug-intoxicated patients but the investigators recommend waiting 4 half-lives of whatever drug is present.

Urine drug screens cannot be considered inclusive of the effects of all drugs because not every drug or metabolite is routinely measured with standard screening assays. Particularly elusive are lithium, fentanyl, and cyanide. Drug ingestion should be particularly considered in cases in which neuroimaging is inconsistent with clinical examination.[31] Unless there is irrefutable evidence that drug effects have subsided, clinicians are wise to either prolong the period of delay in performing clinical brain death examination or proceed with ancillary testing.[18] At the time of this writing, there exists significant controversy regarding the management of clinically brain dead patients who also have drug/substance intoxication. Mandatory ancillary testing in intoxication situations is being debated. Even at the US federal level there is ongoing discussion regarding regulation over clinical criteria for brain death and specifics regarding these controversial circumstances.

ANCILLARY TESTING

Brain death is primarily a clinical diagnosis. After clinical confirmation of brain death as described previously, including confirmation of apnea, death may be declared. In adults, ancillary tests are not required except when the examination is not reliable or when mandated by institutional guidelines. Some advocate routine use of ancillary tests in conjunction with the clinical examination for the determination of brain death,[32] whereas others argue that confirmatory tests are unnecessary and if determination of brain death cannot be made based on clinical examination, then brain death should not be determined at all.[2,4] Ancillary tests may be indicated when elements of the clinical examination cannot be performed (eg, facial trauma, preexisting cranial nerve deficits), motor movements are present, or when the apnea testing cannot be completed due to hypoxia or hypotension or when confounding factors are present (see **Box 4**). Ancillary testing has been used to assist families with understanding the finality of brain death, but this practice should be avoided.[33]

Ancillary testing must not replace a thorough clinical examination. Ancillary tests should not be performed until all prerequisites for the clinical examination have been met and all evaluable components of the clinical examination including the apnea test are consistent with brain death. At many centers, ancillary tests are routinely used when declaring brain death in children, although they are not required in all infants and children by the most recent pediatric guidelines.[3] When ancillary testing is used, the time of death is best recorded as the time the testing results are finalized or reported. In clinical cases, time of death is reported as the time the $Paco_2$ reaches its maximum value, thus representing an apnea test confirmatory of brain death.

MECHANISTIC BASIS FOR ANCILLARY TESTING

Ancillary tests are based on either absence of cerebral blood flow or lack of electrical activity (see **Box 5**). To understand the mechanism by which confirmatory tests determine brain death, one must consider brain death physiology. Palmer and Bader[34] suggest hypothetical mechanisms for brain death. First, intracranial pressure exceeds mean arterial pressure (ICP > MAP) resulting in brain and brainstem death due to lack of blood flow. This first hypothesis is the one on which most ancillary tests are based. Second, ICP does not exceed MAP, therefore the cerebral blood flow is preserved but intrinsic pathology is present that causes neuronal and axonal injury, ultimately resulting in brain death. This second mechanistic hypothesis would make any confirmatory test based on blood flow falsely negative.[35–37] In the final and least common mechanistic hypothesis, direct catastrophic brainstem or cerebral pathology may exist.[34]

TYPES OF ANCILLARY TESTING

The 3 most commonly performed ancillary tests are cerebral scintigraphy (hexamethylpropyleneamine oxime [HMPAO]), cerebral angiography, and electroencephalogram (EEG). Other potential confirmatory tests include transcranial Doppler study (TCD), CT angiography, and magnetic resonance angiography (MRA). Conventional MRI and CT lack the sensitivity and specificity required to act as an ancillary test for brain death. The Canadian Guidelines[38] and the Australian-New Zealand Intensive Care Society (ANZICS) Guideline[39] do not include EEG or TCD. The American pediatric guidelines[3] do not include TCD. However, the American adult guidelines[2] accept all 4 studies but prefer EEG, cerebral angiography, and nuclear scan. The Canadian Forum on Determining Brain Death[38] recommends that demonstration of absence of intracerebral flow be the standard ancillary test.[40] Ancillary tests based on assessing blood flow are based on the hypothesis that if blood flow to the entire brain is absent for a substantial period, there can be no brain function. Therefore, the absence of flow is compatible with the clinical diagnosis of brain death. On the other hand, some persistent blood flow does not rule out clinical brain death. Tests of electrical activity (eg, EEG) assume that the absence of electrical activity indicates absence of brain function. Each ancillary test carries its own potential pitfalls (see **Box 4**) and each its own reportable rates of specificity and sensitivity. Most require transport of the critically ill patient out of the care area.

CEREBRAL ANGIOGRAPHY

Cerebral angiography is the test by which most other ancillary tests are referenced. However, angiography is invasive, requires prolonged travel to the angiography suite, is not readily available and interpretable at many centers, and is relatively expensive. Proper technique for cerebral angiography is specified in the AANPP guideline and includes high-pressure injection into the aortic arch, contrast medium should reach both anterior and posterior circulations, no intracerebral filling at the level of entry of the carotid or vertebral artery to the skull. The external carotid circulation should be visualized as a positive control. Filling of the superior longitudinal sinus may be delayed and does not affect accuracy.[2] No false-positive cases have been reported in the literature using cerebral angiography. False negatives (cerebral flow in the face of apparent brain death) have been reported, usually when ICP was not elevated.[40]

CEREBRAL SCINTIGRAPHY

Scintigraphy, often called nuclear flow testing or SPECT (single-photon emission CT), uses a gamma-emitting radioactive tracer instilled into the venous system and detected by a radio counter in nuclear medicine. Reliability is comparable to cerebral angiography.[41] The tracer is technetium 99m-HMPAO (Tc99-HMPAO). Nuclear scintigraphy requires instrumentation, a radiologist with expertise to interpret the test, and the relatively expensive radioisotope that must be reconstituted by a specialty pharmacy. Technical specifics include injecting the isotope within 30 minutes of reconstitution, collection of images from anterior and both lateral planar views immediately, between 30 to 60 minutes later, and at 2 hours after injection, liver uptake as a positive control, no radionuclide localization in the middle cerebral artery, anterior cerebral artery, or basilar artery territories of the cerebral hemispheres (hollow skull phenomenon), and no tracer in superior sagittal sinus. Minimal tracer can come from the scalp.[2,42,43]

If perfusion is identified on HMPAO SPECT, brain death cannot be determined. If a repeat test is planned, most radiologists recommend waiting 24 to 48 hours.[40] Proposed explanations for blood flow on scintigraphy in the circumstance of clinical brain death include the temporal relationship between actual cessation of flow and clinical diagnosis, as well as a potential rostrocaudal necrosis of neuraxial tissue that makes lower brain blood flow the last to dissipate.[40]

ELECTROENCEPHALOGRAPHY

EEG in brain dead patients seeks to establish a lack of reactivity to intense somatosensory or audiovisual stimuli. Techniques for reliable testing are demanding and specific and include a minimum of 8 scalp electrodes, a check of the entire recording system, a distance between electrodes of least 10 cm, and sensitivity increased to at least 2 μV for 30 minutes.[2] EEG is the most technically cumbersome to perform and interpret, time-consuming, and least often used ancillary test.

TRANSCRANIAL DOPPLER ULTRASONOGRAPHY

Transcranial doppler ultrasonography (TCD) is noninvasive, bedside, and relatively quick to perform and interpret, but there is little consensus on the usefulness of TCD as an ancillary test, as it does not necessarily quantify cerebral blood flow. TCD is very technician and interpreter-dependent. It requires visualization of each hemisphere (both internal carotid arteries and the basilar artery) and demonstration of an abnormal flow pattern. TCD is useful only if a reliable signal is found. Up to 20% of patients are poor candidates for TCD secondary to increased thickness of cranial vaults or other technical limitations.[44]

Abnormalities consistent with brain death include either reverberating flow or small systolic peaks in early systole. Complete absence of flow is not reliable, as it may result from inadequate transtemporal windows. Reliability is augmented if the patient has had prior TCD studies by the same TCD team with the previous studies noting normal flow in all 3 vessels. Technical details are critically important. Many reports in the literature of both false positives and negatives make the utility of TCD as an ancillary test in brain death questionable.[2,45]

COMPUTED TOMOGRAPHY ANGIOGRAPHY

Computed tomography angiography (CTA) was first reported as an ancillary test in the diagnosis of brain death in 1998 as having 100% specificity.[46] It is used widely in Europe as an ancillary test to determine cessation of cerebral blood flow but has not yet been adopted in the United States.[47] CTA is readily available, relatively inexpensive, easy to acquire, minimally invasive, and fast, but requires precision performance. Diagnostic criteria are lack of intracranial arterial contrast opacification, defined as vertebrobasilar circulation within the dura and within the internal carotids above the clinoid. Some investigators suggest interpretation should specifically reference lack of filling of the cortical middle cerebral artery branches and cerebral veins.[48,49] CTA was compared with nuclear perfusion study in 2010 among 25 clinically brain dead patients with no false negatives, but the investigators found 3 patients without flow on nuclear perfusion who showed minimal flow on CTA, all of whom had open skull defects, suggesting that CTA is even more sensitive than HMPAO SPECT for detecting blood flow just above the skull base.[50]

Nonangiographic CT perfusion scans, such as Xenon CT, are more difficult to interpret and less available. Critics cite incomplete quantitative measurement of cerebral blood flow. Xenon CT shows some promise, but at this point is limited to large academic centers and should not be considered the standard of care.

MAGNETIC RESONANCE ANGIOGRAPHY

Determination of brain death by MRA should be based on the same criteria as CTA. Although likely a reliable test for cerebral blood flow, MRA has not yet been proven as an ancillary test in brain death. Like any MRI, the patient must be transported to the radiology suite, examination time is longer than CT or HMAO-SPECT, and the patient and monitors must be MRI-compatible.[2]

Regardless of the test used, radiologists and others who interpret the tests hold a precarious position in brain death determination. They rarely perform clinical examination of the patient, but the radiologic study is often used as the final examination determining brain death. The time of death is often recorded as the time the report is finalized. It is recommended that radiologists refer strictly to brain blood flow testing and avoid the terminology "consistent with brain death" when referencing their assessment that cerebral blood flow is absent.[51] This practice will allow the radiologist to maintain the appropriate relationship with respect to the process of brain death determination.

DOCUMENTATION OF BRAIN DEATH

The authors endorse the use of the checklists provided in both adult and pediatric published guidelines.[2,3] We include these in the documentation of brain death examination in the electronic health record at our institution and believe it serves to remind the examiner to perform a complete examination and documents the examination accurately in the medical record. If all requirements are not met, the electronic record should not accept the note.

CRITICAL CARE OF THE BRAIN DEAD PATIENT

Cerebral ischemia progresses from rostral to caudal as brain death ensues and physiologic changes occur simultaneously. First, cerebral ischemia results in vagal activation with bradycardia and possibly hypotension. Next, the pons becomes ischemic, stimulating the Cushing response of sympathetic stimulation with parasympathetic modulation resulting in moderate hypertension and bradycardia. With uncal herniation, the upper medulla becomes ischemic. A "sympathetic storm" is caused by sympathetic stimulation without parasympathetic modulation. Severe hypertension and tachycardia occur, which may in turn be responsible for the myocardial dysfunction often encountered in brain death as well as neurogenic pulmonary edema.

Finally, herniation of the cerebellar tonsils, also called coning, compresses and causes ischemia of the lower medulla and C1 level of the spinal cord, resulting in autonomic paresis. This final insult is associated hypotension due to vasodilation from sympathectomy and vasopressin deficiency combined with left ventricular dysfunction as well as hypovolemia from diabetes insipidus. Much individual variability exists in these hemodynamic abnormalities, but in all cases, deterioration of cardiovascular status to cardiac arrest is likely if aggressive management is not proactively instituted. Evidence suggests that preventing or ameliorating the sympathetic storm may decrease cardiac and pulmonary injury associated with brain death.[52,53] When deterioration occurs, the authors' policy is to resuscitate aggressively, even including advanced cardiac life support and blood transfusion. It is our policy to maximally support every potential organ donor until and unless the family indicates the patient would not want to donate.

Physiologic abnormalities in brain death that require critical care are listed in **Box 6**. Management of brain dead patients and organ donors has been reviewed with established guidelines and innovative therapies offered.[38,54–57] Salim and colleagues[58] found that vasopressors were required in 97.1% of their series of brain dead patients and that coagulopathy, thrombocytopenia, and diabetes insipidus occurred in half. Hypovolemia is extremely common and requires aggressive treatment. Optimization of donor management goals yields a larger number of organs transplanted for each donor.[59,60] Aggressive management of potential organ donors may include steroids, thyroid hormone, peritoneal resuscitation, and even extracorporeal membrane oxygenation.[61–70]

We recommend early implementation of institutional catastrophic brain injury guidelines (CBIGs) before herniation. CBIGs provide an algorithm by which hemodynamic and hormonal support and management of other complications associated with brain death may be addressed. Donor management protocols are often provided by regional organ procurement organizations and can even be used before brain death. Most protocols are based on empiric guidelines, consensus statements or conferences, and case series from the literature.[59,71] A simplified algorithm for managing

---

Box 6
Common problems/complications in subjects who are brain dead that may need to be managed

1. Hemodynamic complications
   a. Bradycardia
   b. Hypotension
   c. Low cardiac output/stress cardiomyopathy

2. Arrhythmias

3. Diabetes insipidus
   a. Hypovolemia
   b. Hypernatremia

4. Pulmonary dysfunction and complications
   a. Pulmonary edema
   b. Traumatic lung injury
   c. Aspiration
   d. Infection

5. Endocrine deficiency

6. Hypothermia (rarely hyperthermia)

7. Hyperglycemia

8. Coagulopathy

9. Cyto- and endothelial dysfunction

10. Hypernatremia (adverse effect on liver allograft)

---

brain dead or dying patients is the "Rule of 100s." Maintain a systolic blood pressure greater than 100 mm Hg using vasoactive drugs, intravenous fluids, and blood products. Maintain Pao_2 greater than 100 mm Hg. Maintain urine output of approximately 100 mL/h by aggressively monitoring for and treating hypervolemia, hypovolemia, and diabetes insipidus. Equally important is monitoring for and aggressively treating coagulopathy and anemia.

The Society of Critical Care Medicine recommends a goal urine output of 1 mL/kg per minute and a MAP 60 mm Hg, ideally without high-dose vasopressors.[57] Invasive hemodynamic monitoring is used for goal-directed care of patients who are brain dead at our institution. Enteral nutrition should be considered, as it may diminish inflammatory effects of brain death on organ dysfunction.[72]

VARIABILITY IN BRAIN DEATH DETERMINATION AMONG NATIONS

In the United States, the UDDA makes the regulatory definition of death clear; however, in other countries such regulatory consistency is not always present. Although most European nations rely primarily on clinical examination and view brain death similar to the United States, in several European countries, ancillary testing is mandatory.[73] Cultural and religious differences between nations coincide with differences in the concept of the meaning of death. For this reason, an international consensus for declaration of brain death is unlikely.

BRAIN DEATH AND THE LAW

In 1978, as definitions regarding determinations of death were being increasingly scrutinized in criminal and civil litigation, the Uniform Law Commissioners created the

Uniform Brain Death Act. This Act was modified to become the UDDA in 1980. The UDDA sought to clarify terminology and added "irreversible cessation of circulatory and respiratory functions" as an alternative to the standards. The act is designed to address minimum reasonable standards and is intentionally vague. By recognizing cardiopulmonary and brain death as separate entities, it lends discretion on interpretation to the medical profession.

Each US state has formal criteria for determination of death, but the legal language provides woefully little specificity with regard to clinical brain death testing. State and federal law can provide guidance in unique situations, such as a pregnant mother who has suffered catastrophic brain injury or brain death but maintains a viable intrauterine pregnancy. Current US law requires and ethical and clinical practice guidelines advocate support of the intrauterine pregnancy until maturation of the fetus to the point at which delivery can be safely induced.[74–76]

BRAIN DEATH AND RELIGION

Early scholars of brain death asserted that its concept and practice were compatible with the beliefs of the world's principal religions.[77] Most Christians accept brain death without serious exception.[78] Before an International Transplant Society meeting in 2000, Pope John Paul II affirmed brain death to be compatible with Catholic beliefs.[79] A rabbinic debate persists in Judaism. Reform and Conservative rabbis accept brain death almost without exception but this is not the case within more traditional arms of Judaism. In contrast to a rather long history of opposition to the concept of brain death, religious authorities in several Islamic countries, including conservative Saudi Arabia, permit brain death and organ transplantation.[80] Hindu culture in India endorses brain death.[81] Following a lengthy social battle, Shinto-Confucian religious authorities in Japan also acknowledge the occurrence of brain death.[82] All states in the United States have enacted statutes or written administrative regulations permitting physicians to declare death by brain death determination[83] with only New Jersey and New York in the 1990s enacting escape clauses for those who may have religious or personal convictions against the concept.[83,84]

ETHICAL CHALLENGES

Ethical controversy exists among medical practitioners of the same specialty regarding the real meaning and definition of brain death. Even neurologists lack a consistent teleologic definition of brain death and argue about the optimal diagnostic tests for brain death. Almost half of neurologists accept brain death fundamentally as a state of permanent unconsciousness, but many do not consider brain death as equivalent to circulatory death.[85–87] Wijdicks writes "confirmatory tests do not confirm anything [because brain death] is synonymous with a certain clinical state [from which] there are no recoveries on record." These sentiments imply that our conceptual framework of brain death is, at least to a certain degree, based in theory rather than clear scientific basis, as we might think. For example, one would presume that cessation of brain flow would lead to significant cerebral tissue necrosis following arterial inflow occlusion but varying degrees of tissue necrosis have been reported in pathologic examination after brain death. Most recently, Wijdicks and Pfeifer[88] reported varying degrees of necrosis on microscopic examination and concluded that neuropathologic examination may not be diagnostic of brain death.

A wide range of specialists performing brain death testing with different policies and different techniques illustrates the broad ethical and contextual variability in brain death determination.[89] Similar variability regarding the determination of brain death can be found worldwide.[2] We must not accept our current understanding of brain death as the end-all. We must continuously challenge our scientific understanding of brain death through further research and ethical discussion.

SUMMARY

Brain death determination is a fundamental part of surgical critical care. It has an interesting history and continuing ethical implications. Statutory guidance is minimal. Practice guidelines exist but are not widely implemented. Significant policy and practice variation exists, putting the ill-informed or inexperienced intensivist at risk. The gravity of brain death determination is arguably the greatest of any clinical assessment we perform. We should feel confident in following our own guidelines but we should never be afraid to ask ourselves if we are making the correct decisions. We should remain open-minded and not be afraid to question our practice or compare our practices with those of others to ensure that our standards are most impeccable. Brain death testing should be performed rigorously, with attention to detail in clinical examination and with knowledgeable, deliberate application of ancillary tests where necessary. In all cases, we should aggressively deliver high-quality neuro-critical care. The outcome of our efforts is the very determination of life or death, for both our own patient and the potential organ donor recipient.

REFERENCES

1. Wijdicks EF. Determining brain death in adults. Neurology 1995;45(5):1003–11.
2. Wijdicks EF, Varelas PN, Gronseth GS, et al. Evidence-based guideline update: determining brain death in adults: report of the Quality Standards Subcommittee of the American Academy of Neurology. Neurology 2010;74:1911–8.
3. Nakagawa TA, Ashwal S, Mathur M, et al. Guidelines for the determination of brain death in infants and children: an update of the 1987 Task Force recommendations. Crit Care Med 2011;39:2139–55.
4. Wijdicks EFM. Brain death. 3rd edition. New York: Oxford University Press; 2017.
5. Teresi D. The undead. New York: Penguin Random House; 2012.
6. Practice parameters for determining brain death in adults (summary statement). The Quality Standards Subcommittee of the American Academy of Neurology. Neurology 1995;45(5):1012–4.
7. Chamoun RB, Robertson CS, Gopinath SP. Outcome in patients with blunt head trauma and a Glasgow Coma Scale score of 3 at presentation. J Neurosurg 2009; 111(4):683–7.
8. Wang HH, Varelas PN, Henderson GV, et al. Improving uniformity in brain death determination policies over time. Neurology 2017;88(6):562–8.
9. Greer DM, Wang HH, Robinson JD, et al. Variability of brain death policies in the United States. JAMA Neurol 2016;73(2):213–8.
10. Mollaret P, Goulon M. Le coma depassse. Rev Neurol (Paris) 1959;101:3–15.
11. Beecher H. A definition of irreversible coma: report of the Ad Hoc Committee of the Harvard Medical School to Examine the Definition of Brain Death. JAMA 1968; 205:337–40.
12. Mohandas A, Chou SN. Brain death: a clinical and pathological study. J Neurosurg 1971;35:211–8.
13. Diagnosis of brain death. Statement issued by the honorary secretary of the Conference of Medical Royal Colleges and their Faculties in the United Kingdom on 11 October 1976. Br Med J 1976;2:1187–8.

14. Lustbader D, O'Hara D, Wijdicks E, et al. Second brain death examination may negatively affect organ donation. Neurology 2011;76:119–24.
15. Koenig MA, Bryan M, Lewin JL, et al. Reversal of transtentorial herniation with hypertonic saline. Neurology 2008;70(13):1023–9.
16. Skoglund TS, Nellgard B. Long-time outcome after transient transtentorial herniation in patients with traumatic brain injury. Acta Anaesthesiol Scand 2005;49(3): 337–40.
17. Mauritz W, Leitgeb J, Wilbacher I, et al. Outcome of brain trauma patients who have Glasgow Coma Scale score of 3 and bilateral fixed and dilated pupils in the field. Eur J Emerg Med 2009;16(3):153–8.
18. Busl KM, Greer DM. Pitfalls in the diagnosis of brain death. Neurocrit Care 2009; 11(2):276–87.
19. Goudreau JL, Wijdicks EF, Emery SF. Complications during apnea testing in the determination of brain death: predisposing factors. Neurology 2000;55(7): 1045–8.
20. Levesque S, Lessard MR, Nicole PC, et al. Efficacy of a T-piece system and a continuous positive airway pressure system for apnea testing in the diagnosis of brain death. Crit Care Med 2006;34(8):2213–6.
21. Kramer AH, Couillard P, Bader R, et al. Prevention of hypoxemia during apnea testing: a comparison of oxygen insufflation and continuous positive airway pressure. Neurocrit Care 2017;27(1):60–7.
22. Saposnik G, Maurino J, Saizar R, et al. Spontaneous and reflex movements in 107 patients with brain death. Am J Med 2005;118(3):311–4.
23. Saposnik G, Basile VS, Young GB. Movements in brain death: a systematic review. Can J Neurol Sci 2009;36(2):154–60.
24. Wijdicks EF. The diagnosis of brain death. N Engl J Med 2001;344:1215–21.
25. Jain S, Degeorgia M. Brain death-associated reflexes and automatisms. Neurocrit Care 2005;3(2):122–6.
26. Patterson JR, Grabois M. Locked-in syndrome: a review of 139 cases. Stroke 1986;17:758–64.
27. Kotsoris H, Schleifer L, Menken M, et al. Total locked-in state resembling brain death in polyneuropathy. Ann Neurol 1984;16:150.
28. Danzl DF, Pozos RS. Accidental hypothermia. N Engl J Med 1994;331:1756–60.
29. Molina DK, McCutcheon JR, Rulon JJ. Head injuries, pentobarbital, and the determination of death. Am J Forensic Med Pathol 2009;30(1):75–7.
30. Hallbach JL, von Meyer L, Maurer HH. Recommendations from the Clinical Toxicology Committee of the Society for Toxicological and Forensic Chemistry (GTFCh) for toxicological analysis in the context of determining brain death. TIAFT Bulletin 2004;34:14–5. Available at: https://www.gtfch.org/cms/images/stories/RichtlinienBDeath.pdf. Accessed July 2, 2017.
31. Yang KL, Dantzker DR. Reversible brain death: a manifestation of amitriptyline overdose. Chest 1991;99:1037–8.
32. Roberts DJ, MacCulloch KA, Versnik EJ, et al. Should ancillary brain blood flow analyses play a larger role in the neurological determination of death? Can J Anaesth 2010;57(10):927–35.
33. Palaniswamy V, Sadhasivam S, Selvakumaran C, et al. Single-photon emission computed tomography imaging for brain death donor counseling. Indian J Crit Care Med 2016;20(8):477–9.
34. Palmer S, Bader MK. Brain tissue oxygenation in brain death. Neurocrit Care 2005;2(1):17–22.

35. DeCampo MP. Imaging of brain death in neonates and young infants. J Paediatr Child Health 1993;29:255–8.

36. Flowers WM, Patel BR. Persistence of cerebral blood flow after brain death. South Med J 2000;93(4):364–70.

37. Kurtek RW, Lai KK, Taue WN, et al. Tc-99m hexamethylpropylene amine oxime scintigraphy in the diagnosis of brain death and its implications for the harvesting of organs used for transplantation. Clin Nucl Med 2000;25(1):7.

38. Shemie SD, Ross H, Pagliarello J, et al. Organ donor management in Canada: recommendations of the forum on medical management to optimize donor organ potential. CMAJ 2006;174:S13–30.

39. Australian and New Zealand Intensive Care Society. The ANZICS statement on death and organ donation. Edition 3.2. Melbourne: ANZICS; 2013.

40. Heran M, Heran N, Shemie S. A review of ancillary tests in evaluating brain death. Can J Neurol Sci 2008;35:409–19.

41. Munari M, Zucchetta P, Carollo C, et al. Confirmatory tests in the diagnosis of brain death: comparison between SPECT and contrast angiography. Crit Care Med 2005;33(9):2068–73.

42. Donohoe KH, Agrawal G, Frey KA, et al. SNM practice guideline for brain death scintigraphy 2.0. J Nucl Med Technol 2012;40(3):198–203.

43. Conrad GR, Sinha P. Scintigraphy as a confirmatory test of brain death. Semin Nucl Med 2003;33(4):312–23.

44. Young GB, Lee D. A critique of ancillary tests for brain death. Neurocrit Care 2004;1(4):499–508.

45. Sharma D, Souter MJ, Moore AE, et al. Clinical experience with transcranial Doppler ultrasonography as a confirmatory test for brain death: a retrospective analysis. Neurocrit Care 2011;14:370–6.

46. Dupas B, Gayet-Delacroix M, Villers D, et al. Diagnosis of brain death using two-phase spiral CT. AJNR Am J Neuroradiol 1998;19(4):641–7.

47. Wijdicks EF. Brain death worldwide: accepted fact but no global consensus in diagnostic criteria. Neurology 2002;58(1):20–5.

48. Leclerc X, Taschner CA, Vidal A, et al. The role of spiral CT for the assessment of the intracranial circulation in suspected brain-death. J Neuroradiol 2006;33(2):90–5.

49. Frampas E, Videcoq E, deKerviler F, et al. CT angiography for brain death diagnosis. AJNR Am J Neuroradiol 2009;30(8):1566–70.

50. Berengeur CM, Davis FE, Howington JU. Brain death confirmation: comparison of computed tomographic angiography with nuclear medicine perfusion scan. J Trauma 2010;68(3):553–9.

51. ACR 2017 guideline updated 2016. Available at: www.acr.org/Quality-Safety/Standards-Guidelines/Practice-Guidelines-by-Modality.

52. Yeh T, Wechsler AS, Graham L, et al. Central sympathetic blockade ameliorates brain death-induced cardiotoxicity and associated changes in myocardial gene expression. J Thorac Cardiovasc Surg 2002;124(6):1087–98.

53. Audibert G, Charpentier C, Segin-Devaux C, et al. Improvement of donor myocardiac function after treatment of autonomic storm during brain death. Transplantation 2006;82(8):1031–6.

54. Smith M. Physiologic changes during brain stem death—lessons for management of the organ donor. J Heart Lung Transplant 2004;23(9s):S217–22.

55. Frontera JA, Kalb T. How I manage the adult potential organ donor: donation after neurological death. Neurocrit Care 2010;12(1):103–10, 111-116.

56. McKeown DW, Bonser RS, Kellum JA. Management of the heartbeating brain-dead organ donor. Br J Anaesth 2012;108(S1):i96–107.

57. Kotloff RM, Blosser S, Fulda GJ, et al. Management of the potential organ donor in the ICU: Society of Critical Care Medicine/American College of Chest Physicians/Association of Organ Procurement organizations consensus statement. Crit Care Med 2015;43(6):1291–325.

58. Salim A, Martin M, Brown C, et al. Complications of brain death: frequency and impact on organ retrieval. Am Surg 2006;72(5):377–81.

59. Franklin GA, Santos AP, Smith JW, et al. Optimization of donor management goals yields increased organ use. Am Surg 2010;76(6):587–94.

60. Malinoski DJ, Daly MC, Patel MS, et al. Achieving donor management goals before deceased donor procurement is associated with more organs transplanted per donor. J Trauma 2011;71(4):990–6.

61. Guglin M. How to increase the utilization of donor hearts? Heart Fail Rev 2015; 20(1):95–105.

62. Krishnamoorthy V, Borbely X, Rowhani-Rahbar A, et al. Cardiac dysfunction following brain death in children: prevalence, normalization, and transplantation. Pediatr Crit Care Med 2015;16(4):e107–12.

63. Mohamedali B, Bhat G, Tatooles A, et al. Neurogenic stress cardiomyopathy in heart donors. J Card Fail 2014;20(3):207–11.

64. Mohamedali B, Bhat G, Zelinger A. Frequency and pattern of left ventricular dysfunction in potential heart donors: implications regarding use of dysfunctional hearts for successful transplantation. J Am Coll Cardiol 2012;60(3):235–6.

65. Casartelli M, Bombardini T, Simion D, et al. Wait, treat and see: echocardiographic monitoring of brain-dead potential donors with stunned heart. Cardiovasc Ultrasound 2012;10:25.

66. Venkateswaran RV, Townend JN, Wilson IC, et al. Echocardiography in the potential heart donor. Transplantation 2010;89(7):894–901.

67. Berman M, Ali A, Ashley E, et al. Is stress cardiomyopathy the underlying cause of ventricular dysfunction associated with brain death? J Heart Lung Transplant 2010;29:957–65.

68. Dujardin KS, McCully RB, Wijdicks EF, et al. Myocardial dysfunction associated with brain death: clinical, echocardiographic, and pathologic features. J Heart Lung Transplant 2001;20(3):350–7.

69. Smith JW, Matheson P, Morgan G, et al. Addition of direct peritoneal lavage to human cadaver organ donor resuscitation improves organ procurement. J Am Coll Surg 2017;220(4):539–47.

70. Fan X, Chen Z, Nasralla D, et al. The organ preservation and enhancement of donation success ratio effect of extracorporeal membrane oxygenation in circulatory unstable brain death donor. Clin Transplant 2016;30(10):1306–13.

71. Salim A, Velmahos GC, Brown C, et al. Aggressive organ donor management significantly increases the number of organs available for transplantation. J Trauma 2005;58(5):991–4.

72. Singer P, Shapiro H, Cohen J. Brain death and organ damage: the modulating effects of nutrition. Transplantation 2005;80(10):1363–8.

73. Guignard NG, Gardner AI, Baker S, et al. Brain death determination in Australia and New Zealand: a survey of intensive care units. Crit Care Resusc 2011;13: 271–3.

74. Hussein I, Govenden V, Grant J, et al. Prolongation of pregnancy in a woman who sustained brain death at 26 weeks of gestation. BJOG 2006;113:120–2.

75. Powner DJ, Bernstein IM. Extended somatic support for pregnant women after brain death. Crit Care Med 2003;31(4):1241–9.

76. Esmaeilzadeh M, Dictus C, Kayvanpour E, et al. One life ends, another begins: management of a brain-dead pregnant mother—a systematic review. BMC Med 2010;8:74.

77. Veith FJ, Fein JM, Tendler MD, et al. Brain death—a status report of medical and ethical considerations. JAMA 1977;238:1651–5.

78. Campbell CS. Fundamentals of life and death: Christian fundamentalism and medical science. In: Youngner SJ, et al, editors. The definition of death: contemporary controversies. Baltimore (MD): Johns Hopkins University Press; 1999. p. 194–209.

79. Furton EJ. Brain death, the soul, and organic life. Natl Cathol Bioeth Q 2002;2(3): 455–70.

80. Yaqub BA, Al-Deeb SM. Brain death: current status in Saudi Arabia. Saudi Med J 1996;17:5–10.

81. Bernat JL, Beresford R. 1st Edition. Ethical and legal issues in neurology, vol. 118. New York: Elsevier; 2013.

82. Lock M. Contesting the natural in Japan: moral dilemmas and technologies of dying. Cult Med Psychiatry 1995;19(1):1–38.

83. Beresford HR. Brain death. Neurol Clin 1999;17(2):295.

84. Olick RS. Brain death, religious freedom, and public policy: New Jersey's landmark legislative initiative. Kennedy Inst Ethics J 1991;1(2):275–92.

85. Joffe AR, Anton NR, Duff JP, et al. A survey of American neurologists about brain death: understanding the conceptual basis and diagnostic tests for brain death. Ann Intensive Care 2012;2:4.

86. Souter M, van Norman G. Ethical controversies at end of life after traumatic brain injury: defining death and organ donation. Crit Care Med 2010;38(9Suppl): S502–9.

87. Controversies in the determination of Death. A white paper of the President's Council on Bioethics. Washing DC, 2008. Available at: https://bioethicsarchive. georgetown.edu/pcbe/reports/death/. Accessed July 2, 2017.

88. Wijdicks EF, Pfeifer EA. Neuropathology of brain death in the modern transplant era. Neurology 2008;70(15):1234–7.

89. Greer DM, Varelas PN, Haque S, et al. Variability of brain death determination guidelines in leading US neurologic institutions. Neurology 2008;70(4):284–9.

Goals of Care and End of Life in the ICU

Ana Berlin, MD, MPH, FACS

KEYWORDS

- Goals of care • Shared decision making • ICU • Functional and cognitive outcomes
- End-of-life care • Palliative care • Communication

KEY POINTS

- The trauma and long-term sequelae of critical illness affect not only patients but also their families and caregivers.
- Unrealistic expectations and erroneous assumptions about the outcomes acceptable to patients are important drivers of misguided and goal-discordant medical treatment.
- Compassionately delivering accurate and honest prognostic information inclusive of functional, cognitive, and psychosocial outcomes is crucial for helping patients and families understand what to expect from an episode of surgical crticial illness.
- Skilled communication and shared decision-making strategies ensure that treatments provided in the ICU are aligned with realistic and attainable patient goals.
- Attentive management of physical and nonphysical symptoms, including the psychosocial and spiritual needs of families and caregivers, eases suffering in the ICU and beyond.

INTRODUCTION

There is little doubt that the past half-century has seen tremendous advances in surgical critical care. The advent of lung-protective ventilation in the management of acute respiratory distress syndrome (ARDS), the evolution of balanced resuscitation strategies for the reduction of abdominal compartment syndrome, and the aggressive deployment of prevention and treatment strategies against the systemic inflammatory response syndrome and sepsis, along with many other technological innovations, have markedly reduced the morbidity and mortality associated with critical illness and multiorgan system failure. Nevertheless, at times even the

Disclosure Statement: Support for Dr A. Berlin's preparation of this article was provided by the New Jersey Medical School Hispanic Center of Excellence, Health Resources and Services Administration through Grant D34HP26020. She has no additional relevant financial disclosures.
Department of Surgery, Rutgers New Jersey Medical School, Medical Science Building G-506, 185 South Orange Avenue, Newark, NJ 07103, USA
E-mail address: Ana.Berlin@njms.rutgers.edu

Surg Clin N Am 97 (2017) 1275–1290
http://dx.doi.org/10.1016/j.suc.2017.07.005
0039-6109/17/© 2017 Elsevier Inc. All rights reserved.

surgical.theclinics.com

most aggressive measures fail to rescue patients from death or from life states that they would find unacceptable. It is an important role of the surgical intensivist to recognize when these situations might occur, to elicit patient values and identify appropriate goals of treatment of critically ill patients with poor or uncertain prognoses, to relieve the physical and nonphysical symptoms and family/caregiver distress that often accompany the end of life and the sequelae of critical illness, and to skillfully shepherd patients and families through appropriate transitions of care in the final weeks, days, and hours. This review addresses core principles and incorporates recent literature adding to the evidence base for improving the care of critically ill surgical patients at or near the end of life. The principles and evidence presented are not only relevant in the care of primarily surgical patients by surgical intensivists but also of critically ill patients with primarily medical diagnoses who develop surgical problems and require the attention of surgeons equipped to meet the challenges of prognostication, communication, and decision making in this population.

A few caveats deserve mention at the outset. First, end-of-life care is often falsely equated with palliative care. This is understandable in the context of the history and evolution of palliative medicine, which originated as an offshoot of the hospice movement focused on relief of suffering for the terminally ill. It is paramount, however, to recognize the distinctions between the two. Present-day palliative care is specialized medical care dedicated to improving the quality of life of patients with serious or life-limiting illness and their families.[1] Although relieving burdensome physical and nonphysical symptoms at the end of life is a component of palliative care, the expansion of the field of palliative medicine has resulted in a shift in focus from improving the quality of death and dying to helping patients live as best as they can for as long as they can—regardless of their stage of illness. Second, all too often, the phrase "goals of care" is narrowly invoked to imply a conversation regarding resuscitation preferences or withdrawal of life-sustaining treatment (WLST). However, establishing clear and realistic treatment goals and promoting care strategies concordant with those goals are important aims of both palliative and critical care, regardless of the specific treatment decision in question or a patient's prognosis for survival. With that in mind, this review is focused on the optimal care of critically ill surgical patients with serious underlying illness or at the end of life, and should by no means be construed as a comprehensive primer for palliative care or goal setting, broadly speaking, in the surgical ICU.

PROGNOSTICATION: HELPING CRITICALLY ILL PATIENTS AND THEIR CAREGIVERS UNDERSTAND WHAT TO EXPECT

Unrealistic expectations and erroneous assumptions about the outcomes acceptable to patients have been identified as important drivers of misguided and goal-discordant medical treatment in serious illness and at the end of life. The landmark Study to Understand Prognoses and Preferences for Outcomes and Risks of Treatments (SUPPORT) found that almost half of ICU patients experienced unwanted medical treatment, more than half were undertreated for pain, and many failed to have their therapeutic preferences identified or heeded by their treatment teams.[2] Thus, recognizing and avoiding overtreatment and under-treatment at the end of life is an important aspect of surgical critical care. Appropriate goal setting and decision making in surgical critical care require consideration of the respective likelihoods of a range of outcomes and a clear sense of which of those outcomes are acceptable to a patient and which are not. The relevant outcomes include not only hospital and short-term survivals but also long-term survival (extending beyond the customary 30 days to

6 months or 1 year or more), functional and cognitive status, health-related quality of life, and psychosocial outcomes for both patients and caregivers.

Multiple scoring systems are available to predict short-term mortality and sometimes ICU length of stay for critically ill patients. Based on degree of derangement in physiologic, clinical, and laboratory parameters, these scoring systems include the Acute Physiology and Chronic Health Evaluation scoring system, Sequential (Sepsis-related) Organ Failure Assessment instrument, the Simplified Acute Physiologic Score, and the Mortality Prediction Model. However, these scoring systems are not designed to forecast outcomes for single individuals but rather large populations of critically ill patients, limiting their utility for decision making on a case-by-case basis. In addition, mortality estimates based on 30-day or in-hospital outcomes often paint an incomplete picture of the health care trajectory for seriously ill surgical patients. For example, in a large retrospective cohort study of Medicare recipients, two-thirds of older patients who received prolonged mechanical ventilation after high-risk surgery were dead within the year; 30-day survivors had a 47% 1-year mortality rate and a 90% risk of discharge to dependent care.[3]

Because predictors of mortality are imperfect for individual patients and because patients and their caregivers care deeply about outcomes other than short-term mortality alone,[4] it is problematic to strategically offer or limit aggressive life-saving or life-sustaining critical care based on probabilistic life-or-death outcomes. Rather than focusing exclusively on survival, every effort should be made to accurately and honestly prognosticate about the nature of the future clinical course and the expected resulting health states, so that patients and their surrogates can make well-informed decisions about treatment options and their sequelae. Forecasting functional outcomes in particular is crucial for patients and caregivers and also has important impacts on clinician behavior. For instance, specifically documenting a patient's functional prognosis has been shown in a scenario-based randomized controlled trial to have significant bearing on the likelihood of a clinician subsequently broaching the subject of WLST.[5] In addition, acknowledging and anticipating expected functional outcomes affords clinical teams the opportunity to prospectively minimize and mitigate adverse sequelae of critical illness through targeted survivorship strategies.

ICU survival is no guarantee of a good outcome. Not only do mortality risks remain elevated for months after ICU discharge but also functional and cognitive deficits linger, and ongoing pain and other physical symptoms are unfortunately common among ICU survivors. These features characterize the syndrome of persistent infection and immunosuppression, neuropathy, myopathy, endocrinopathy, and cognitive dysfunction now recognized as chronic critical illness.[6] In a landmark 2004 study of patients with prolonged respiratory failure, Nelson and colleagues[7] reported prevalence rates of 50% to 95% for a range of chronic critical illness symptoms affecting survivors, including nausea, dyspnea, insomnia, and anxiety. In a large prospective cohort study of adults over 65 who spent greater than 24 hours in an ICU, including surgical ICUs, more than one-third of patients were dead at 6 months; health-related quality of life declined during the follow-up period for most older patients (86 years and older), whereas it tended to improve for younger patients (age 65–69).[8] In a follow-up to SUPPORT, investigators found that approximately half of survivors of severe acute respiratory failure needed help with at least 1 activity of daily living, and more than one-quarter rated their quality of life as poor or fair 5 years after ICU discharge.[9] Choi and colleagues[10] found that the vast majority of ICU survivors (89%–97%) self-reported at least 1 symptom, most commonly sleep disturbance, fatigue, weakness, and pain, across all time-points in a 4-month follow-up study. Additional investigators have documented significant persistent long-term functional disability as measured by impaired performance on 6-minute walk test, along with decreased physical quality of life and increased costs and use of health care services, in ARDS survivors 2 years to 5 years after discharge from the ICU.[11,12] Because duration of bed rest in the ICU is directly related to weakness over the course of 2-year follow-up, it is possible that interventions to reduce the duration of bed rest during critical illness may prove beneficial for reducing the prevalence and severity of chronic impairment among ICU survivors[12] (**Fig. 1**).

Diminished quality of life and functional impairment are closely tied to cognitive and psychosocial outcomes. In a retrospective cohort study of trauma patients admitted to the surgical ICU, of whom 50% had severe traumatic brain injuries, fewer than half of survivors who completed follow-up were able to return to work or school within 2 years to 5 years.[13] In a prospective cohort study, global cognitive deficits and impaired executive function comparable to moderate traumatic brain injury or mild Alzheimer disease were found in up to one-third of ICU survivors of shock or respiratory failure 1 year after discharge, despite a baseline cognitive impairment prevalence of only 6%.[14] The prospective longitudinal cohort study Bringing to light the Risk factors And Incidence of Neuropsychological dysfunction in ICU survivors (BRAIN-ICU) demonstrated that one-quarter of ICU survivors face deficits in both basic and instrumental activities of daily living up to 1 year postdischarge.[15] Approximately one-third of ICU survivors suffer from depression 1 year after discharge, and the prevalence of posttraumatic stress disorder (PTSD) is as high as 20% 6 months to 12 months after ICU discharge.[15–17] The pooled prevalence of cognitive impairment, mood disorders, and PTSDs has been measured at 20% among 5-year survivors of ARDS[18] (see **Fig. 1**).

Finally, outcomes among patient caregivers, including friends and family, must also be considered. The experience of having a loved one in the ICU is highly traumatic.

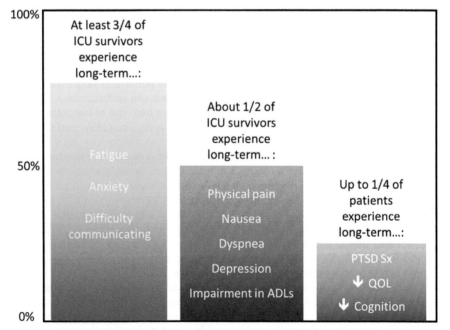

Fig. 1. Estimated prevalence of chronic symptoms in survivors of critical illness. ADLs, activities of daily living; Sx, symptom; QOL, quality of life. (*Data from* Refs.[6,8,9,13–16])

This trauma is compounded by grief and bereavement for the loved ones of decedents and ongoing distress for loved ones of survivors suffering from chronic critical illness and other post-ICU impairments. High rates of depressive symptoms, with a prevalence of up to 23% to 50% at 1 year, have been observed among caregivers of mechanically ventilated ICU survivors—exceeding the burden of depression seen among caregivers of patients with dementia. In addition, 3 months after discharge, symptoms suggesting a moderate to major risk of PTSD were found in one-third of family members of ICU patients overall and in more than 80% of family members who had shared in end-of-life decisions for an ICU decedent.[19,20] Caregiver-reported findings suggest that some of these burdens can be mitigated by increased contact and communication with physicians, improved counseling about what to expect, greater emotional support, and better symptom management for their loved ones in the ICU.[21]

COMMUNICATION AND DECISION MAKING: WORKING WITH CRITICALLY ILL PATIENTS AND THEIR CAREGIVERS TO CHOOSE THE BEST TREATMENTS FOR THEM

In the face of uncertainty about ICU outcomes, communication and decision-making skills become paramount for ensuring that patients receive treatments that are medically appropriate and concordant with their values, goals, and priorities. Structured communication interventions have been shown to improve end-of-life care for critically ill patients,[22,23] and shared decision making (SDM) has been established now for decades as a standard of patient-centered care in the ICU and is applicable for all treatment decisions that hinge on personal values and preferences.[24,25] Nevertheless, confusion persists as to the nature and optimal implementation of SDM. Too often, SDM is interpreted merely as shared burden of responsibility on the part of physician and patient for choosing from among a set of treatment options. This, however, can leave some patients and their surrogate decision makers feeling abandoned by their physician, who has abdicated an important professional responsibility in the name of patient autonomy that may not be desired. A more ethically and scientifically grounded interpretation of SDM is one in which the physician and the patient/surrogate share different roles and spheres of deliberation in the decision-making process, which is mediated by the physician or another trusted and invested member of the clinical care team. In general, patients and surrogates are best poised to contribute knowledge and information about what is important to them, whereas clinicians should contribute their knowledge of treatment options and their likely outcomes in the context of a patient's overall illness and articulate an interpretation of how each treatment option supports or undermines the values and priorities expressed by the patient and/or surrogate.[26]

The tenets of communication and SDM in the ICU involve timing, setting, core content, and key steps. First, especially when patients are unable to participate in discussions about their care, every effort should be made to reach out to family members, caregivers, and surrogates (herein referred to as "family") as early as possible in the ICU stay. Studies of family satisfaction and outcomes have noted improvements when family meetings are scheduled within 72 hours of admission to the ICU, and 5 days is now considered a minimum standard.[22,27–29] Among other benefits, meeting early helps avoid the pitfall of not having met until an acute life-threatening situation develops, forcing the encounter to take place suboptimally in the midst of a pressured crisis. Additional triggers for family meetings are discussed subsequently in this section and include changes in medical status, uncertainty or disagreements between or among family members and clinicians regarding the therapeutic goals and whether/how these can be achieved, and family requests (see **Table 2**).

Setting—including the location, individuals involved, and their expectations—plays an important role in the success of a communication intervention. Privacy, quiet, freedom from distractions, and ample seating options should be ensured. The patient should be included as much as possible but often is not able to participate due to the nature of critical illness. Decisional capacity should be objectively assessed and documented, and, when found lacking, the appropriate surrogate(s) or proxy(ies)—assuming they exist—need to be called on. Staff should be interspersed among the family, and those in attendance should reflect the makeup of the interdisciplinary team, including the physicians (intensivists, surgeons, and palliative care clinicians), nurse, social worker, chaplain, translator, and others involved in the patient's care as appropriate. Individuals should identify themselves clearly and understand each other's roles and the purpose of the meeting. Clinicians should prebrief with each other prior to the meeting to ensure that they all have a clear command of the relevant medical facts, to establish consensus as to the unified messages that will be conveyed to the family, to openly address and resolve their own biases or conflicts with respect to the appropriateness of various potential therapeutic options, and to agree on an appointed facilitator for the meeting.[30] Similarly, family meeting guides are available as printed hand-outs to help family members prepare for meetings with ICU clinicians and to facilitate comprehension, maximize efficiency, and ensure that feelings and concerns are appropriately addressed.[31]

Opening a family meeting or discussion of goals of care can feel awkward and intimidating to clinicians, but it is important to remember that the family members gathered may feel the same way. Beginning the meeting with an expression of gratitude for the participants' time and an open-ended question is an excellent way to set a relaxed and inviting tone and to gather clues about the family's emotional state and assess their informational and decision-making preferences—because not all patients want to share equally in SDM or any of its domains[32] (**Table 1** lists key meeting objectives and sample phrases to use and to avoid). Throughout the meeting, clinicians should resist the temptation to dominate the meeting or to seek intellectual refuge from strong emotions by providing lengthy clinical explanations, using medical jargon, and focusing on procedures. Instead, clinicians should not only encourage family members to contribute their perspectives and participate in determining the flow of the conversation but also allow time and space for silence and the nonverbal expression of emotion, which should be actively explored and validated throughout the conversation by members of the clinical team. Empathic statements—including expressions of naming, understanding, respecting, supporting, and exploring emotion (NURSE statements)—have been associated with greater family satisfaction in communication interventions.[33,34]

The next task in the conversation is to discuss prognosis. First, clinicians must elicit a patient's/family's understanding of the nature and expected course of the acute problem and any contributing underlying conditions. Again, open-ended questions are especially helpful (see **Table 1**). Then, the clinical team must compassionately and effectively communicate the prognostic assessment to the patient/family, explicitly addressing the life-threatening and life-altering nature of critical illness, and contextualizing this in terms of the overall health trajectory and functional status. The 6-step Set-up, Patient's Perception, Invitation, Knowledge, Emotions and Empathy, Strategy and Summary (SPIKES) protocol[35] has long been advocated as a strategy for breaking bad news, but recent investigators have emphasized the lack of evidence, in particular patient and caregiver-reported outcomes, in rigorously evaluating the effectiveness of this methodology. Nevertheless, it remains an important tool whose value may be enhanced through adaptation to individual patient preferences, clinician style, and cultural contexts.[36] Providing ranges of expected outcomes (eg, best case and worst case), acknowledging uncertainty, and emphasizing the rapidly evolving nature of critical illness can help prepare caregivers for the emotional trauma of a loved one's stay in the ICU. In addition, clinicians must deliver honest, consistent messages and avoid the common pitfall of mitigating the emotional impact of unwelcome news by providing false reassurances or encouraging unrealistic hopes. By anticipating and tracking nuanced characteristics of the strong emotions that are often triggered by the delivery of poor prognostic information, clinicians can be prepared to respond effectively using empathic strategies tailored to individuals' unique needs.[37]

After establishing a shared understanding of prognosis, clinicians should next seek to formulate a comprehensive mutual understanding of a patient's values and preferences. Exploratory questions should be used to elicit the patient's goals, values, and priorities as well as fears and worries. Furthermore, clinicians should explore what tradeoffs the patient would or would not be willing to make for the chance of a given outcome. The patient dignity question, "What do I need to know about [you/your loved one] as a person to take the best care of [you/him/her] that I can?" has shown promise for promoting patient-centeredness in the care of seriously ill patients across multiple settings, including acute hospitalization.[38,39] Exploration of goals should include an understanding of treatments that the patient wishes to avoid (eg, tracheostomy) or states that would be unacceptable to him or her (eg, severe communication impairment). Sample questions for exploring values, hopes, and fears are listed in **Table 1**.

The final steps in the goals of care conversation include outlining the therapeutic options, making a recommendation for treatment that is aligned with a patient's goals (including consideration of a time-limited trial, when appropriate [discussed later]), affirming that the clinical team is committed to caring for the patient and family regardless of the treatment course, and adjourning the meeting. Before proceeding, however, it is wise to assess the patient/caregiver for readiness to continue. It may be necessary to tailor the agenda of each meeting to the clinical context and situational needs. For example, delivering poor prognostic information or breaking bad news may dominate the initial meeting after a traumatic injury. In these instances, formulating a shared understanding of the patient's prognosis, establishing therapeutic rapport, providing emotional support, and probing for patient preferences may be the most important goals of the encounter; although families may initially be too overwhelmed to address specific treatment goals and participate in decision making about therapeutic options, a clear and specific follow-up interval should be agreed on at which point to continue the conversation.

Therapeutic options to be considered in the context of critical illness may include invasive procedures, such as bronchoscopy, tracheostomy, gastrostomy, or surgical interventions; continuing treatment, withholding treatment, or WLST (mechanical ventilation, renal replacement therapy, artificial nutrition and hydration, use of cardiac assistive technology); introduction, escalation, or withdrawal of therapeutic measures, such as vasopressors or antibiotics; and resuscitation status. The role of concurrent palliative or comfort-directed care should be stressed, and patients/caregivers should be reassured that aggressive symptom management will be pursued to the fullest extent allowed by the overarching therapeutic strategy. Treatments that cannot effectively meet the therapeutic goals should not be offered. Because preferences vary for patient/caregiver engagement in the decisional domain of SDM, clinicians should obtain an invitation to make a treatment recommendation if they believe they have

Table 1
Family meeting/goals of care conversation: key objectives and phrases to use and to avoid in the critical care setting

Objective	Sample Phrases to Use	Pitfalls to Avoid
Create the right setting and open the family meeting	"Thank you for taking the time to come in to talk about your mom. How are you doing with all of this?" "I want to make sure we all understand what we need to so that we can we give her the best care possible. Before we get started, are there any specific topics you want us to address?"	Setting a dominant tone; delivering an exhaustively detailed clinical summary
Probe for understanding	"Tell me what you know about your mother's condition right now."	Sharing information without assessing prior understanding: "I am not sure if any of the other doctors mentioned this, but your mother [has cancer/had a heart attack/etc.]…"
Deliver prognostic information	"Your mother is very sick. While we are doing everything possible to help her pull through, there is a very serious chance she might not make it… [PAUSE/ALLOW SILENCE]… …And if she does, she will likely be so weak and debilitated that she will not be able to go home for a very long time, if ever."	Offering false hope or mixed messages: "While things look very grave right now, you never know. Things could always turn around for the better."
Elicit goals/values and fears/worries	"Tell me about your mom. What kind of person is she? What kinds of things are important to her? What do I need to know about her as a person in order to provide her with the best possible care?" "What do you think she would have to say about this if she could speak for herself right now?" "Was there anything your mom was particularly looking forward to before this all happened?" "What worries you most?" "Can you think of any abilities or activities so crucial to your mom that she would find life without them intolerable?"	Focusing on treatments and procedures: "Do you want us to do the feeding tube or not?" Using language not grounded in reality: "What would your mom have wanted?"

Expect emotion; demonstrate empathy and respect	"Sometimes what is important to you might be different from what would be important to your mom. **Is it hard** for you to stay focused on her perspective?" "**I really respect** your ability to put aside your own priorities and be such an amazing advocate for her." "I see your eyes are welling up. This is very hard. Can you **tell me more** about what you are feeling right now?"	Assuming one understands: "**I know** how you must feel." Devaluing emotion: "**I understand** you are angry about what happened, **but** we need to focus on what to do next."
Make appropriate treatment recommendations grounded in patient goals and values; consider a time-limited trial Affirm commitment to patient and caregiver well-being	"Your mom took the trouble to let us know how she felt about treatments at the end of life. We should honor and respect what she told us." "Based on your mom's priorities, I recommend we start dialysis. Let's see how things go and plan to meet again in the next 48 h. If by the end of the week things don't turn around, we should discuss a plan B focused on maintaining what you've told me would be most important for her." "We will do everything possible that will help your mom. Her comfort and dignity will be our top priorities." "Let's talk about how we might be able to fulfill your mom's wish to die at home." "Looking back on this 6 months from now, I want you to know in your heart that we all did the best we could—you included." "Can you think of any religious services or spiritual support that would be helpful to you right now?"	Failing to provide a viable alternative; leaving decision up to the surrogate: "Do you still want us to keep **doing everything?**" Feeding into fears of abandonment and lack of caring: "I think we should **stop aggressive therapy**." "My recommendation is to **withdraw care.**"
Summarize, strategize, and adjourn	"I know this is a lot of information. It is normal to feel overwhelmed. Would you like some time to process this, before meeting again to discuss some next steps?" "Can you think of anything you wanted to talk about that we haven't addressed?" "I am sure you will think of additional questions. Please write them down so we can discuss them next time we meet." "Thank you so much for sharing what you did with me today. It has helped me understand and appreciate a lot more about your mom and how important she is to you." "Let's get together again on Friday for another update. Would that work for you?"	Prematurely closing the door to further questions or concerns: "If you have no more questions, I think that is about all we have to cover."

Data from Refs.[36,56–58]

the clinical certainty and sufficient data about a patient's preferences to do so. In making a recommendation, clinicians should emphasize how the recommended treatment aligns with what the patient's values and goals in the context of both the acute problem and premorbid health trajectory.

The time-limited trial is a practical and effective strategy for facilitating goal-oriented critical care in the context of uncertain prognoses. With demonstrated applicability to the surgical patient population, time-limited trials help mutualize expectations among clinicians and families, permit the initiation of treatment without a protracted commitment in the event of clinical failure, and provide a safe platform from which to fully explore the possibilities offered by life-saving and life-prolonging technology.[40,41] In a time-limited trial, clinicians and family/caregivers outline objective measures of improvement or deterioration—based on a patient's predetermined goals—to be assessed after a defined period of initial therapy (eg, 48 hours or 1 week). At the agreed-on interval, outcomes are evaluated and, depending on a patient's progress toward the desired goals, the intervention is either continued or discontinued, as previously decided. Regardless of whether a time-limited trial is pursued, closure of the meeting involves checking for shared understanding among all participants, actively encouraging family/caregivers to raise any lingering questions or concerns, and settling on a mutually convenient time for a subsequent encounter.

Finally, family meetings should be promptly and clearly documented in the medical chart or electronic health record. Such notes should be clearly identified so that other members of the treatment team can readily access important information about the goals of care and patient and family preferences. Structured note templates not only facilitate documentation but also may help prompt clinicians to address the important content areas. Such a template for an ICU family meeting should include the following core elements[31]:

- Location
- Patient participation
- Family/caregiver participants and their contact information
- Clinical team participants
- Preexisting advance directives or health care proxy documents identified
- The patient's/family's/surrogate's understanding of the prognosis
- Patient identity and values; patient/family hopes and worries/fears
- Specific therapeutic goals identified
- Plan/recommendations made
- Other content of meeting (such as emotional or spiritual support provided)
- Time involved in meeting

Note headers containing key search words or phrases, including "family meeting," "goals of care," or "palliative care," help distinguish documentation of important conversations from standard progress notes and may facilitate not only clinical care but also quality improvement and research endeavors.

When, how, and by whom should communication interventions and other more comprehensive palliative care services be deployed in the surgical ICU? Triggers for structured serious illness communication interventions and palliative care assessment are continually being developed and defined, largely based on prognostic criteria that ideally include not only mortality risk but also the potential for future distress and functional or cognitive impairment (**Table 2**).[42–45] Various service delivery models have also been described, including consultative, integrative, and mixed models. Mosenthal and colleagues[27] and Lambda and colleagues[28] described an integrative model for changing the culture around end-of-life care in the surgical ICU for both trauma and liver transplant

Table 2
Suggested triggers for ICU family meetings to discuss goals of care

Prognosis-Based Criteria	Procedure-Based Criteria
• Expected ICU length of stay >5 d • Admission to ICU after >10 d in hospital • Readmission to surgical ICU • Mortality risk >25% • Significant predicted decline in functional or cognitive status • Age >80 y • Presence of 2 or more life-limiting comorbidities (ESRD, COPD, CHF, stage IV malignancy, status post cardiac arrest, status post intracerebral hemorrhage requiring mechanical ventilation) • Physician answers "No" to question (current critical illness notwithstanding): *"Would you be surprised if this person were to die in the next year?"*	• Family request • Consideration of tracheostomy • Consideration of feeding tube placement • Consideration of renal replacement therapy • Consideration of LVAD or IABP therapy • Consideration of any surgical intervention in a critically ill patient

Abbreviations: CHF, congestive heart failure; COPD, chronic obstructive pulmonary disease; d, days; ESRD, end-stage renal disease; IABP, intra-aortic balloon pump; ICU, intensive care unit; LVAD, left ventricular assist device; y, years.
    Data from Refs.[21,22,42–44,59,60]

patients; in both populations, a program, including family support and assessment of prognosis and preferences at admission, along with an interdisciplinary family meeting within 72 hours, was successful in achieving earlier consensus on goals of care as well as decreasing length of stay for patients who died without affecting overall mortality.[27,28]

In addition, debate has stirred over the role of palliative care specialists versus generalist clinicians in performing communication interventions and palliative care assessments for critically ill patients. All physicians and health care professionals should be expected to have a command of basic palliative care skills, including routine prognostication, communication, and symptom management. Some especially complex or vulnerable patients, however, may require clinicians with specialized expertise in these areas.[46] Although the supply of palliative care specialists is increasing to meet rising demand, the triggers for specialist palliative care involvement must currently be titrated to the availability of clinicians to provide those services, and the remainder of the system's need must at this time be met by generalists (or continue unaddressed). Simply deploying palliative care specialists for one-off interventions likely is ineffective in supporting patients with serious illness and their caregivers. A recent randomized controlled trial showed that palliative care specialist–led family meetings for patients requiring greater than 7 days of mechanical ventilation failed to reduce anxiety and depression symptoms among caregivers and may have increased symptoms of PTSD. These meetings were highly scripted for the delivery of prognostic information as the primary communication goal and generally did not involve an ICU physician or other members of the ICU clinical team.[47] Thus, who performs the communication interventions may be secondary to how these interventions are carried out. These findings highlight the shortcomings of a blanket strategy reliant on specialized consultative services divested from the longitudinal relationships and therapeutic alliances that should be fostered between ICU clinicians and family caregivers and emphasizes the importance of equipping primary providers with the interpersonal and communication skills required to meet the basic needs of most patients.

Surgeons with palliative care expertise may be uniquely poised to facilitate SDM for critically ill surgical patients perioperatively.[48]

SYMPTOM MANAGEMENT: EASING PHYSICAL AND NONPHYSICAL SUFFERING IN THE ICU AND BEYOND

The goals of symptom management in the ICU include not only relieving suffering in the present and providing a quality end-of-life experience for decedents and their families but also minimizing future burdens for survivors. Pain should be aggressively managed and controlled for all patients. Although opioids remain the mainstay, non-opioid adjuncts—including local anesthetics, nonsteroidal anti-inflammatory drugs, acetaminophen, ketamine, and other neuropathic drugs—also may be considered as appropriate. Dyspnea is also treated with opioids, in addition to addressing underlying correctable factors and providing humidified oxygen. Delirium should be carefully assessed, and contributing factors, including sleep and circadian rhythm disturbance, should be mitigated. Hypoactive delirium is best managed with reorienting stimuli and reassurance (for both patient and family/caregivers), whereas patients with hyperactive delirium and unmanageable agitation are treated with antipsychotics. Benzodiazepines, which can worsen disorientation and further disinhibit patients, and restraints, which can worsen agitation, should generally be avoided.[49]

Most patients who die in the ICU do so only after withholding life-sustaining treatment WLST.[50] Ideally, this decision is reached through the communication and SDM strategy outlined previously. Because the transition from curative to comfort-oriented treatment can be difficult for patients and loved ones, extra emotional and spiritual support should be available at this time. In addition, it should be recognized that organ donation can help soothe the grief of family and caregivers, especially when this act represents the fulfillment of a patient's dying wish. In this context, when appropriate, patients should be referred to the regional organ procurement organization prior to WLST for further evaluation related to donation while the ICU team continues to care for the patient in his or her best interest. Palliative extubation generally involves placement of an active order to allow natural death/do not resuscitate/do not intubate; discontinuation of neuromuscular blocking agents; administration of appropriate medications for relief of dyspnea, agitation, and other symptoms; extubation with or without prior incremental reduction of ventilator support; and ongoing family/caregiver support.[51]

Actively dying patients may experience noisy respirations caused by uncleared upper airway secretions pooling in the posterior pharynx; these are likely to be more distressing for family and caregivers than for an unconscious or minimally conscious patient and generally can be managed with glycopyrrolate and positioning. Similarly, family members concerned about their loved one's dry mucous membranes will be reassured to learn that dry mouth is not representative of thirst in the dying patient but may nevertheless derive comfort from providing oral care with moist sponges. Dying patients and their families often grapple with existential concerns surrounding meaning ("Why am I suffering?" "What has my life meant?"), value ("What value do I still have for my family/workplace/community?"), and relationships ("Whom have I loved?" "Whom must I forgive?"). The ICU team can facilitate the "work" of the dying through efforts to maintain comfort and cognition, being available for listening and emotional support, encouraging family presence, allowing for grieving, and providing as peaceful as possible a setting for the dying patient and his or her family. Invasive and noninvasive monitoring, pulse oximetry, suctioning, laboratory draws, and all non-beneficial treatments should be discontinued. The so-called doctrine of double effect legally and ethically empowers physicians to provide medications and therapies intended to relieve suffering (eg, opioids for pain and dyspnea and anxiolytics for agitation), even if these hasten death as a collateral consequence of their use.[52] Transition to home or inpatient hospice should be facilitated if possible and concordant with a patient's wishes, although moving patients in the last hours of life is generally discouraged. Medical/Provider Orders for Life-Sustaining Treatment (MOLST/POLST) forms, representing actionable orders reflective of the SDM and advance care planning that has taken place in the ICU, should be completed prior to such transfers to ensure that patient preferences are honored across all health care settings.

Helping critically ill patients and their caregivers prepare for and cope with a future outside the ICU is an important challenge at the frontier of critical care. The practice of reflective writing in ICU diaries is one intervention shown to have reduced symptoms of PTSD among European survivors or critical illness, and efforts to understand what benefits it offers to family are ongoing.[17] Depression screening for caregivers at ICU admission, during the ICU course, or in follow-up after discharge is the subject of ongoing investigation into ways of improving caregiver outcomes and should be considered.[19,53] Families of ICU decedents, particularly when children are involved, are ideally referred to bereavement support groups. Caregivers report increased satisfaction associated with receiving spiritual support services, condolence cards from the treating team, and clinician attendance at their loved one's funeral.[54] Periodic interdisciplinary memorial services, or ICU death rounds, may be effective in building resilience and combatting burnout among critical care providers.[38,55,56] Ultimately, these palliative efforts, as adjuncts to high-quality prognostication, communication, and decision making, help yield positive critical care outcomes for all those whose lives are touched by the ICU.

SUMMARY

Critical illness is traumatic for patients and their families and caregivers. Unrealistic expectations and mistaken assumptions about patients' goals of care often drive burdensome and unwanted treatment of those with serious illness or at the end of life. Compassionately delivering accurate and honest prognostic information inclusive of functional, cognitive, and psychosocial outcomes is crucial for helping patients and families understand what to expect from an ICU stay. Interdisciplinary strategies to develop a shared understanding of patient values and priorities as related to potential future health states and available therapeutic options help ensure that chosen treatments in the ICU are aligned with realistic and attainable patient goals. Focusing critical care efforts broadly on the well-being of the patient and family unit through optimal symptom management and attention to psychosocial and spiritual needs is important for easing physical and nonphysical suffering in the ICU and beyond. Attention to these 3 domains of care for critically ill patients and their caregivers helps ensure the best possible outcomes, independent of survival.

REFERENCES

1. The Center to Advance Palliative Care (CAPC). About palliative care. Available at: https://www.capc.org/about/palliative-care/. Accessed May 24, 2017.

2. The Writing Group for the SUPPORT Investigators. A Controlled trial to improve care for seriously ill hospitalized patients. The study to understand prognoses and preferences for outcomes and risks of treatments (SUPPORT). JAMA 1995;274(20):1591–8.

3. Nabozny MJ, Barnato AE, Rathouz PJ, et al. Trajectories and prognosis of older patients who have prolonged mechanical ventilation after high-risk surgery. Crit Care Med 2016;44(6):1091–7.

4. Schwarze ML, Brasel KJ, Mosenthal AC. Beyond 30-day mortality: aligning surgical quality with outcomes that patients value. JAMA Surg 2014;149(7):631–2.

5. Turnbull AE, Krall JR, Ruhl AP, et al. A scenario-based, randomized trial of patient values and functional prognosis on intensivist intent to discuss withdrawing life support. Crit Care Med 2014;42(6):1455–62.

6. Cooper Z, Bernacki RE, Divo M. Chronic critical illness: a review for surgeons. Curr Probl Surg 2011;48(1):12–57.

7. Nelson JE, Meier DE, Litke A, et al. The symptom burden of chronic critical illness. Crit Care Med 2004;32(7):1527–34.

8. Khouli H, Astua A, Dombrowski W, et al. Changes in health-related quality of life and factors predicting long-term outcomes in older adults admitted to intensive care units. Crit Care Med 2011;39(4):731–7.

9. Garland A, Dawson NV, Altmann I, et al, SUPPORT Investigators. Outcomes up to 5 years after severe, acute respiratory failure. Chest 2004;126(6):1897–904.

10. Choi J, Hoffman LA, Schulz R, et al. Self-reported physical symptoms in intensive care unit (ICU) survivors: pilot exploration over four months post-ICU discharge. J Pain Symptom Manage 2014;47(2):257–70.

11. Herridge MS, Tansey CM, Matté A, et al, Canadian Critical Care Trials Group. Functional disability 5 years after acute respiratory distress syndrome. N Engl J Med 2011;364(14):1293–304.

12. Fan E, Dowdy DW, Colantuoni E, et al. Physical complications in acute lung injury survivors: a two-year longitudinal prospective study. Crit Care Med 2014;42(4):849–59.

13. Livingston DH, Tripp T, Biggs C, et al. A fate worse than death? Long-term outcome of trauma patients admitted to the surgical intensive care unit. J Trauma 2009;67(2):341–8 [discussion: 348–9].

14. Pandharipande PP, Girard TD, Jackson JC, et al. Long-term cognitive impairment after critical illness. N Engl J Med 2013;369(14):1306–16.

15. Jackson JC, Pandharipande PP, Girard TD, et al, Bringing to light the Risk Factors And Incidence of Neuropsychological dysfunction in ICU survivors (BRAIN-ICU) study investigators. Depression, post-traumatic stress disorder, and functional disability in survivors of critical illness in the BRAIN-ICU study: a longitudinal cohort study. Lancet Respir Med 2014;2(5):369–79.

16. Wintermann GB, Brunkhorst FM, Petrowski K, et al. Stress disorders following prolonged critical illness in survivors of severe sepsis. Crit Care Med 2015;43(6):1213–22.

17. Parker AM, Sricharoenchai T, Raparla S, et al. Posttraumatic stress disorder in critical illness survivors: a metaanalysis. Crit Care Med 2015;43(5):1121–9.

18. Herridge MS, Moss M, Hough CL, et al. Recovery and outcomes after the acute respiratory distress syndrome (ARDS) in patients and their family caregivers. Intensive Care Med 2016;42(5):725–38.

19. Haines KJ, Denehy L, Skinner EH, et al. Psychosocial outcomes in informal caregivers of the critically ill: a systematic review. Crit Care Med 2015;43(5):1112–20.

20. Cameron JI, Chu LM, Matte A, et al, RECOVER Program Investigators (Phase 1: towards RECOVER), Canadian Critical Care Trials Group. One-year outcomes in caregivers of critically ill patients. N Engl J Med 2016;374(19):1831–41.

21. Teno JM, Clarridge BR, Casey V, et al. Family perspectives on end-of-life care at the last place of care. JAMA 2004;291(1):88–93.

22. Lilly CM, De Meo DL, Sonna LA, et al. An intensive communication intervention for the critically ill. Am J Med 2000;109(6):469–75.
23. Campbell ML, Guzman JA. Impact of a proactive approach to improve end-of-life care in a medical ICU. Chest 2003;123(1):266–71.
24. Charles C, Gafni A, Whelan T. Shared decision-making in the medical encounter: what does it mean? (or it takes at least two to tango). Soc Sci Med 1997;44(5): 681–92.
25. Davidson JE, Powers K, Hedayat KM, et al, American College of Critical Care Medicine Task Force 2004-2005, Society of Critical Care Medicine. Clinical practice guidelines for support of the family in the patient-centered intensive care unit: American College of Critical Care Medicine Task Force 2004-2005. Crit Care Med 2007;35(2):605–22.
26. Kon AA, Davidson JE, Morrison W, et al, American College of Critical Care Medicine, American Thoracic Society. Shared decision making in ICUs: an American College of Critical Care Medicine and American Thoracic Society Policy Statement. Crit Care Med 2016;44(1):188–201.
27. Mosenthal AC, Murphy PA, Barker LK, et al. Changing the culture around end-of-life care in the trauma intensive care unit. J Trauma 2008;64(6):1587–93.
28. Lamba S, Murphy P, McVicker S, et al. Changing end-of-life care practice for liver transplant service patients: structured palliative care intervention in the surgical intensive care unit. J Pain Symptom Manage 2012;44(4):508–19.
29. Nelson JE, Mulkerin CM, Adams LL, et al. Improving comfort and communication in the ICU: a practical new tool for palliative care performance measurement and feedback. Qual Saf Health Care 2006;15(4):264–71.
30. Hwang DY, Yagoda D, Perrey HM, et al. Consistency of communication among intensive care unit staff as perceived by family members of patients surviving to discharge. J Crit Care 2014;29(1):134–8.
31. Nelson JE, Walker AS, Luhrs CA, et al. Family meetings made simpler: a toolkit for the intensive care unit. J Crit Care 2009;24(4):626.e7-14.
32. Levinson W, Kao A, Kuby A, et al. Not all patients want to participate in decision making. A national study of public preferences. J Gen Intern Med 2005;20(6): 531–5.
33. Selph RB, Shiang J, Engelberg R, et al. Empathy and life support decisions in intensive care units. J Gen Intern Med 2008;23(9):1311–7.
34. Back AL, Arnold RM, Baile WF, et al. Approaching difficult communication tasks in oncology. CA Cancer J Clin 2005;55(3):164–77.
35. Buckman R. Breaking bad news: a guide for health care professionals. Baltimore (MD): Johns Hopkins University Press; 1992.
36. Dean A, Willis S. The use of protocol in breaking bad news: evidence and ethos. Int J Palliat Nurs 2016;22(6):265–71.
37. Back AL, Arnold RM. "Isn't there anything more you can do?": when empathic statements work, and when they don't. J Palliat Med 2013;16(11):1429–32.
38. Cook D, Rocker G. Dying with dignity in the intensive care unit. N Engl J Med 2014;370(26):2506–14.
39. Johnston B, Pringle J, Gaffney M, et al. The dignified approach to care: a pilot study using the patient dignity question as an intervention to enhance dignity and person-centred care for people with palliative care needs in the acute hospital setting. BMC Palliat Care 2015;14:9.
40. Neuman MD, Allen S, Schwarze ML, et al. Using time-limited trials to improve surgical care for frail older adults. Ann Surg 2015;261(4):639–41.

41. Quill TE, Holloway R. Time-limited trials near the end of life. JAMA 2011;306(13): 1483–4.
42. Weissman DE, Meier DE. Identifying patients in need of a palliative care assessment in the hospital setting: a consensus report from the Center to Advance Palliative Care. J Palliat Med 2011;14(1):17–23.
43. Hua MS, Li G, Blinderman CD, et al. Estimates of the need for palliative care consultation across united states intensive care units using a trigger-based model. Am J Respir Crit Care Med 2014;189(4):428–36.
44. Bernacki RE, Block SD, American College of Physicians High Value Care Task Force. Communication about serious illness care goals: a review and synthesis of best practices. JAMA Intern Med 2014;174(12):1994–2003.
45. Finkelstein M, Goldstein NE, Horton JR, et al. Developing triggers for the surgical intensive care unit for palliative care integration. J Crit Care 2016;35:7–11.
46. Quill TE, Abernethy AP. Generalist plus specialist palliative care–creating a more sustainable model. N Engl J Med 2013;368(13):1173–5.
47. Carson SS, Cox CE, Wallenstein S, et al. Effect of palliative care-led meetings for families of patients with chronic critical illness: a randomized clinical trial. JAMA 2016;316(1):51–62.
48. Berlin A, Kunac A, Mosenthal AC. Perioperative goal-setting consultations by surgical colleagues: a new model for supporting patients, families, and surgeons in shared decision making. Ann Palliat Med 2017;6(2):178–82.
49. Blinderman CD, Billings JA. Comfort care for patients dying in the hospital. N Engl J Med 2015;373(26):2549–61.
50. Mark NM, Rayner SG, Lee NJ, et al. Global variability in withholding and withdrawal of life-sustaining treatment in the intensive care unit: a systematic review. Intensive Care Med 2015;41(9):1572–85.
51. Campbell ML, Yarandi HN, Mendez M. A two-group trial of a terminal ventilator withdrawal algorithm: pilot testing. J Palliat Med 2015;18(9):781–5.
52. Dunn GP, Martensen R, Weissman D, editors. Surgical palliative care: a resident's guide. Chicago: American College of Surgeons and Cunniff-Dixon Foundation; 2009. p. 231–7.
53. van Beusekom I, Bakhshi-Raiez F, de Keizer NF, et al. Reported burden on informal caregivers of ICU survivors: a literature review. Crit Care 2016;20:16.
54. Prigerson HG, Jacobs SC. Perspectives on care at the close of life. Caring for bereaved patients: "all the doctors just suddenly go". JAMA 2001;286(11): 1369–76.
55. Hough CL, Hudson LD, Salud A, et al. Death rounds: end-of-life discussions among medical residents in the intensive care unit. J Crit Care 2005;20(1):20–5.
56. Lee KJ, Forbes ML, Lukasiewicz GJ, et al. Promoting Staff resilience in the pediatric intensive care unit. Am J Crit Care 2015;24(5):422–30.
57. Stone MJ. Goals of care at the end of life. Proc (Bayl Univ Med Cent) 2001;14(2): 134–7.
58. Stapleton RD, Engelberg RA, Wenrich MD, et al. Clinician statements and family satisfaction with family conferences in the intensive care unit. Crit Care Med 2006; 34(6):1679–85.
59. Schwarze ML, Campbell TC, Cunningham TV, et al. You can't get what you want: innovation for end-of-life communication in the intensive care unit. Am J Respir Crit Care Med 2016;193(1):14–6.
60. Norton SA, Hogan LA, Holloway RG, et al. Proactive palliative care in the medical intensive care unit: effects on length of stay for selected high-risk patients. Crit Care Med 2007;35(6):1530–5.

Indications and Methods of Anticoagulation Reversal

Jeremy L. Holzmacher, MD, Babak Sarani, MD*

KEYWORDS

- Anticoagulation reversal • Direct oral anticoagulants • Warfarin
- Prothrombin complex concentrate • Protamine • Idarucizumab • Andexanet alfa
- Aripazine

KEY POINTS

- Understanding the mechanisms of action and pharmacology of anticoagulant drugs is required to maximize the ability to reverse anticoagulation when needed.
- Reversing anticoagulation for invasive procedures should weigh the patient-related risks for thrombosis against the potential for bleeding.
- The approval of idarucizumab for dabigatran reversal and the impending development of specific and non-specific anti-factor Xa reversal agents now comprise a key strategy in the treatment of anticoagulant-associated hemorrhage and perioperative treatment.

INTRODUCTION

The use of anticoagulants within the United States is on the rise with specific direct oral anticoagulant (DOAC) medications gaining Food and Drug Administration (FDA) approval for the prevention of thromboembolic complications, including stroke prevention associated with atrial fibrillation and in the treatment of venous thromboembolism.[1] Normal hemostasis is a tightly controlled and highly regulated process that uses enzyme activation and amplification along with endothelial and platelet interactions to activate thrombin and propagate fibrin formation and cross-linking (**Fig. 1**).[2] Anticoagulant medications disrupt this process directly by inhibiting clotting factor activity, indirectly by depleting vitamin K–dependent clotting factors, or by amplifying native anticoagulant pathways through antithrombin III (ATIII).[2] Historically, the most common anticoagulant prescribed was warfarin, and standard reversal strategy was based on factor repletion using plasma and vitamin K.[2–4] The advent of both oral

Disclosure Statement: The authors have nothing to disclose.
Center for Trauma and Critical Care, Department of Surgery, George Washington University Medical Center, 2150 Pennsylvania Avenue Northwest, Suite 6B, Washington, DC 20037, USA
* Corresponding author. 2150 Pennsylvania Avenue Northwest, Suite 6B, Washington, DC 20037.
E-mail address: bsarani@mfa.gwu.edu

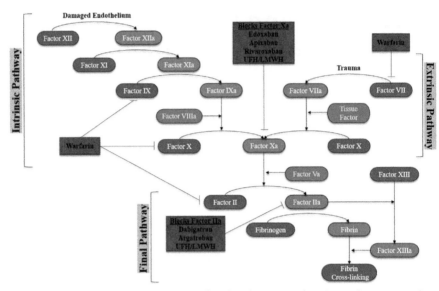

Fig. 1. Coagulation cascade and targets of oral and parenteral anticoagulant agents. (*Data from* Ferreira JL, Wipf JE. Pharmacologic therapies in anticoagulation. Med Clin North Am 2016;100(4):695–718.)

and parenteral direct anti–factor Xa and thrombin (factor IIa) inhibitors, however, has required the development of alternative reversal methods.

In 2010, the FDA approved dabigatran, a direct thrombin inhibitor, for the prevention of stroke in patients with nonvalvular atrial fibrillation. Shortly thereafter, 3 additional DOACs—rivaroxaban, apixaban, and edoxaban—were approved for similar indications.[2] The benefits of DOAC drugs were the immediacy of full anticoagulation without the need for routine blood monitoring and better overall bleeding profiles; however, DOAC-specific antidotes have been slow to development, have limited availability, and are expensive.[5] As such, reversal strategies for these newer medications are either newly formed or still forming.

Considering the evolving nature of anticoagulation and need for cogent and evidenced based reversal strategies, this article reviews the mechanisms of action of the commonly used anticoagulants as well as the indications for and current methodologies of anticoagulation reversal. Although many patients on full anticoagulation may also be taking antiplatelet medications, the methods for mitigating their effects on hemostasis are beyond the scope of this article. Similarly, postprocedural resumption of anticoagulation and periprocedural bridging are not discussed.

REVERSAL STRATEGIES FOR ALL ANTICOAGULANTS

Underlying any decision to reverse a patient's anticoagulation status is the risk-benefit analysis weighing possible thrombosis against potential bleeding (**Fig. 2**). With this understanding, anticoagulation reversal can be divided into 3 categories depending on the urgency needed to restore hemostasis: (1) emergent or urgent requiring reversal in less than an hour, (2) semiurgent requiring reversal within hours, or (3) nonurgent reversal that can typically happen over a matter of days. Regardless of the urgency, reversing any anticoagulant starts by withholding the offending agent. In emergent and semiurgent circumstances, considerations should be given toward administering

Assess Patient Bleeding Risk:
• Major bleed or ICH <3 mo
• Quantitative or Qualitative Platelet Abnormality
• INR above therapeutic range
• Prior bleeding with bridging or during similar procedure

Assess Patient Thrombosis Risk:
• **Low:** CHA$_2$DS$_2$-VASc 1–4, no prior TE
• **Moderate:** CHA$_2$DS$_2$-VASc 5–6 *or* prior TE >3 mo
• **High:** CHA$_2$DS$_2$-VASc ≥7 *or* prior TE ≤3 mo

Risk of Bleeding   **Risk of Thrombosis**

Fig. 2. Balancing risk of bleeding against risk of thrombosis. ICH, intracranial hemorrhage; TE, thromboembolism. (*Data from* Doherty JU, Gluckman TJ, Hucker WJ, et al. 2017 ACC expert consensus decision pathway for periprocedural management of anticoagulation in patients with nonvalvular atrial fibrillation. J Am Coll Cardiol 2017;69(7):871–98; and Rechenmacher SJ, Fang JC. Bridging anticoagulation. J Am Coll Cardiol 2015;66(12):1392–403.)

agent-specific antidotes if available or concentrated factor depending on the expediency of effect. It is also important to take into context the need for anticoagulation reversal. For instance, bleeding wounds or traumatic injuries may be amenable to local measures, including topical hemostatic agents, manual pressure, or tourniquets. Appropriate laboratory testing should be done to establish degree of coagulopathy on presentation and monitor the efficacy of reversal methods if possible. Unfortunately, there is currently no commercially available, reliable means to measure the degree of coagulopathy from DOAC use. Nonetheless, this point is especially relevant because some interventions have a shorter duration of effect (eg, plasma) compared with the anticoagulant used resulting in potential rebound of the anticoagulant effect over time. Lastly, it is important to remember that in emergent or urgent cases, therapy can and often should be initiated prior to laboratory results becoming available.

PARENTERAL ANTICOAGULANTS

Parenteral anticoagulants can be divided into 2 categories depending on the mechanism of action: (1) indirect anticoagulants, which act as cofactors with ATIII to inactivate factor Xa and/or thrombin, and (2) direct anticoagulants, which specifically target and inactivate thrombin.[2] The former are comprised of unfractionated heparin (UFH) and the low-molecular-weight heparins (LMWHs), including enoxaparin and fondaparinux, whereas the latter represent argatroban and bivalirudin.

UNFRACTIONATED HEPARIN
Mechanism of Action and Pharmacology

UFH acts as an indirect anticoagulant by amplifying the activity of ATIII to inactivate factors Xa and thrombin and thereby hinder thrombus formation (**Table 1**). Routes of delivery vary between subcutaneous injection and intravenous (IV) infusion with variable dosing depending on the indication of use and the route of administration.[2] Typical prophylactic dosages are given as 5000 U to 7500 U subcutaneous injections in 8-hour or 12-hour intervals whereas therapeutic dosing is weight based and titrated to an activated partial thromboplastin time (aPTT) 1.5 times to 2.0 times of control.[2,6] Some

Table 1
Parenteral anticoagulants —mechanism of action, pharmacology, and reversal

Agent	Mechanism	Pharmacology	Reversal Method

UFH	Cofactor with ATIII, inactivates factors Xa and thrombin	• Elimination: Hepatic Dose dependent
		• Half-life: 60–90 min
		• Monitor: aPPT (1.5–2.0 times control)
			Nonurgent:
			• Hold infusion for 4–6 h results in near-complete reversal
			Emergent/urgent:
			• Protamine sulfate
			  ○ 1 mg/80–100 U UFH if within 15 min of UFH infusion
			  ○ 0.5 mg/80–100 U within 60 min or
			  ○ 0.25 mg/80–100 U within 2 h
			  ○ Maximum 50 mg dose

Enoxaparin	Cofactor to ATIII, inactivates factor Xa and thrombin	• Elimination: renal
		• Half-life: ~4–8 h
		• Monitor: Anti- Xa levels ($\geq$0.5 IU/mL constitutes therapeutic)
			Nonurgent:
			• Time dependent, ~24 h
			Emergent/urgent:
			• PCC at 20 U/kg
			• Partial reversal with protamine, but degree unclear
			  ○ If dosed $\leq$8 h: 1 mg/1 mg enoxaparin
			  ○ If dosed >8 h: 0.5 mg/1 mg enoxaparin

Fondaparinux	Cofactor to ATIII, inactivates factor Xa, less activity toward factor IIa	• Elimination: renal • Half-life ~17–21 h • Monitor: anti- Xa levels ($\geq$0.5 IU/mL constitutes therapeutic)	Nonurgent • Time dependent: ~24 h Emergent/urgent: • PCC at 20 U/kg • Protamine has not been shown to be effective
Argatroban	Direct thrombin inhibitor	• Elimination: hepatic • Half-life: ~30–60 min • Monitor: aPTT ○ INR can be falsely elevated	Nonurgent: • Time dependent: full reversal in ~4–6 h Emergent/urgent: • No effective means of reversal has been established

Data from Baglin T, Barrowcliffe TW, Cohen A, et al, the British Committee for Standards in Haematology. Guidelines on the use and monitoring of heparin. Br J Haematol 2006;133(1):19–34; and Di Nisio M, Middeldorp S, Büller HR. Direct thrombin inhibitors. N Engl J Med 2005;353(10):1028–40.

institutions, however, monitor anti–factor Xa levels with therapeutic anticoagulation defined as greater than or equal to 0.5 IU/kg.[2,6] UFH is metabolized by the liver and undergoes dose-dependent elimination with a half-life of approximately 60 minutes to 90 minutes.[3] Bioavailability differs depending on the route of delivery, with subcutaneous administration having a bioavailability of 50% or less whereas IV use confers 100% bioavailability.[6] Therefore, although no monitoring is typically required for subcutaneous dosing, IV use requires regular monitoring of the aPTT or anti–factor Xa levels.[6]

Reversal

UFH can be reversed in several ways depending on the clinical scenario. For nonurgent or planned reversals, simple discontinuation of an UFH infusion suffices because the half-life of IV heparin is approximately 60 minutes to 90 minutes.[7] UFH is eliminated in a dose-dependent manner; therefore, holding infusions for 4 hours to 6 hours results in near-complete reversal of the anticoagulant. For more urgent reversal, protamine sulfate can be given at a dose of 1 mg per 80 U to 100 U of UFH to a maximal dose of 50 mg when administered within 15 minutes of IV heparin and halved for every additional 60 minutes up to 2 hours (see **Table 3**).[6] Protamine sulfate chemically combines with heparin to form inactive salts; therefore, when dosed appropriately, protamine reverses UFH to infinity and beyond. It is important to remember, however, that because the half-life of IV UFH is approximately 1 hour to 1.5 hours, the dose of heparin administered within the last few hours should be used to calculate the dose of protamine required (eg, if a patient had been receiving 1250 IU/h of IV UFH over 2 hours, then 25 mg of protamine should be given). aPTT should be followed every 4 hours to 6 hours to assess the efficacy of reversal and assess for potential rebound.

LOW-MOLECULAR-WEIGHT HEPARINS: ENOXAPARIN AND FONDAPARINUX

Like UFH, LMWHs (ie, enoxaparin) act as cofactors to ATIII to inactivate factors Xa and thrombin (see **Table 1**). Unlike UFH, however, LMWHs exhibit 90% bioavailability when given subcutaneously with a 4-hour to 8-hour half-life and are primarily eliminated by the kidneys.[8] Although there is no FDA-approved antidote for the anticoagulant effects of LMWH, protamine sulfate has exhibited some ability to partially reversal the anti-factor IIa effects of LMWH.[7,9]

Fondaparinux is a synthetic LMWH, which uses the same mechanisms of action as enoxaparin but with less activity toward factor IIa (see **Table 1**).[8] Unlike enoxaparin, however, fondaparinux has a significantly longer half-life of 17 hours to 21 hours but undergoes similar renal elimination. To date, there are no FDA-approved antidotes to fondaparinux.

PARENTERAL DIRECT THROMBIN INHIBITORS: ARGATROBAN
Mechanism of Action and Pharmacology

Argatroban and bivalirudin are highly selective, reversible direct thrombin inhibitors used primarily for the treatment of heparin-induced thrombocytopenia with or without thrombosis syndrome or during percutaneous coronary (see **Table 1**).[10,11] Plasma concentrations reach peak effect within 1 hour to 3 hours, and it has a half-life of approximately 30 minutes to 1 hour, allowing for quick dissipation of its anticoagulant effect after withholding infusion.[10,12] The clearance of argatroban, however, is mediated by hepatic metabolism; therefore, dosages need to be reduced in those with hepatic impairment and caution needs to be exercised in those with liver dysfunction.[10] Monitoring can done with serial testing of the aPTT because the degree of derangement in the aPTT correlates with clinically evident coagulopathy.[12] Bivalirudin has a half-life of 25 minutes and eliminated primarily through proteolytic cleavage and renal metabolism; therefore, caution should be exercised in patients with renal insufficiency.[13]

Reversal

Aripazine, a synthetic molecule that inhibits nearly all parenteral and oral anticoagulants, is in development and theoretically can serve as an antidote to in the direct thrombin inhibitors incidences of bleeding (see **Table 3**).[12,14] Its mechanism of action is direct binding to anticoagulants, thereby neutralizing them. When presented with hemorrhage, argatroban and bivalirudin infusion should be discontinued immediately. There are currently no FDA-approved specific reversal agents for the parenteral direct thrombin inhibitors; however, given the short half-life of both agents, a specific antidote may not be necessary except in severe circumstances.[12,14]

WARFARIN
Mechanism of Action and Pharmacology

The vitamin K antagonist warfarin has been the workhorse of the oral anticoagulants since the 1960s and remains one of the most widely used anticoagulant medications.[15] Pharmacologically, warfarin competitively inhibits vitamin K epoxide reductase (VKORC1) and blocks the conversion of oxidized vitamin K to its reduced form, thereby limiting its availability for subsequent γ-carboxylation of the procoagulant factors II, VII, IX, and X as well as the anticoagulant proteins C and S (**Table 2**).[15] The anticoagulant effect of warfarin can be monitored through the international normalized ratio (INR) with anticoagulation typically defined as an INR greater than 2.0.[15] Warfarin is primarily metabolized by the liver through the cytochrome P450 (CYP) system, primarily by CYP2C9, and its effect on the INR can vary with polymorphisms in VKORC1. Therefore, both the half-life and bioactivity of warfarin are dependent on the age of the patient, polymorphisms within CYP2C9 and VKORC1 alleles, and medication interactions that either activate or suppress the CYP pathway. Thus, after warfarin has been discontinued, INR levels can take 3 days to 7 days to normalize.[3]

Nonurgent Reversal

In nonurgent circumstances, such as elective surgery or supratherapeutic INR without accompanying hemorrhage, stopping warfarin until the INR normalizes or returns to therapeutic range is sufficient. Administering oral vitamin K can also aid in nonurgent reversal (**Table 3**). Routine daily INR testing, however, is not cost effective and no studies have validated routine preoperative INR monitoring on intraoperative or postoperative bleeding, deferral in surgery, or reductions in blood product utilization to reverse residual anticoagulation.[3] Some indirect evidence suggests that INR testing the day prior to surgery may minimize intraoperative blood product usage or aid in the deferral of surgery if INR values are elevated, but this should be considered on a case-by-case basis.[16,17] As stated previously, the half-life of warfarin can vary between patients; however, first-order elimination should result in a 50% residual anticoagulation effect after 1 half-life, 25% after 2 half-lives, and so on.[6] In a prospective cohort study assessing patients who had warfarin interruption 5 days prior to surgery without the use of vitamin K, fewer than 10% of patients had an INR greater than 1.5.[18] Conversely, retrospective case series have identified that short intervals of warfarin interruption lead to insufficient normalization of the INR.[19] Similarly, a randomized trial where patients had warfarin held 5 days versus 1 day prior to surgery had significantly higher INR in the short interval group (1.24; 95% CI, 1.19–1.24, vs 1.61; 95% CI, 1.50–1.71).[20] Therefore, in instances where nonurgent and full reversal is desired, warfarin should be discontinued 5 days prior to procedures.

Some patients do not require anticoagulation reversal prior to invasive surgery, whereas conversely others may require bridging therapy through parenteral adjuncts. The large determinant of continuation or bridging is guided by the perioperative bleeding risk and risk for thromboembolism (see **Fig. 2**). Patients undergoing procedures with low perioperative risk of bleeding, such as minor dental procedures (eg,

Table 2
Oral anticoagulants —mechanism of action, pharmacology, and reversal

Agent	Mechanism	Pharmacology	Reversal Method

Apixaban	Direct anti–factor Xa inhibitor	• Elimination:
		  25% renal
		  75% hepatic
		• Half-life: 8–15 h[b]
		• Onset: 1–3 h
			Nonurgent:
			• Time: 24 h for low-risk procedure, longer for higher-risk procedure or decrease CrCl
			Emergent/urgent:
			• Can consider 25–50 U/kg 4F-PCC or aPCC

Dabigatran	Direct thrombin inhibitor	• Elimination:
		  80% renal elimination
		  20% bile
		• Half-life: 12–14 h[b]
		• Onset: 0.5–2 h
			Nonurgent:
			• Time: 24-h for low-risk procedure, longer for higher-risk procedure or decrease CrCl
			Emergent/urgent:
			• Idarucizumab: 5 mg IV bolus/5 min
			• Can consider 25–50 U/kg 4F-PCC
			• Can consider hemodialysis

Edoxaban	Direct anti–factor Xa inhibitor	• Elimination:
		  50% renal
		  50% hepatic
		• Half-life: 9–11 h[b]
		• Onset: 1–2 h
			Nonurgent:
			• Time: 24 h for low-risk procedure, longer for higher-risk procedure or decrease CrCl
			Emergent/urgent:
			• Can consider 25–50 U/kg 4F-PCC or aPCC

Rivaroxaban	Direct anti–factor Xa inhibitor	• Elimination:
		  75% renal
		  25% hepatic
		• Half-life: 7–13 h[b]
		• Onset: 2–4 h
			Nonurgent:
			• Time: 24 h for low-risk procedure, longer for higher-risk procedure or decrease CrCl
			Emergent/urgent:
			• Can consider 25–50 U/kg 4F-PCC or aPCC

Warfarin	Inhibits reduction of vitamin K, limiting γ-carboxylation of factors X, IX, VII, and II as well as proteins C and S	• Elimination: hepatic metabolism by CYP enzymes
		• Half-life: 36–48 h
		• Onset: 3–5 d
		• Monitoring: INR
			Nonurgent:
			• Time: hold for 5 d, INR normalization variable depending on age, dose, and drug/enzyme interactions
			• If not bleeding and INR >10
			  ○ Oral vitamin K (1–5 mg)
			Emergent/urgent:
			• Minor bleeding with any INR:
			  ○ IV vitamin K (1 mg–3 mg)
			• Major bleeding with any INR or impending surgery
			  ○ 4F-PCC[a] + IV vitamin K (5–10 mg)
			  ○ FFP at 20 mL/kg can be given if PCC unavailable or in need of volume for resuscitation

Abbreviation: CrCl, creatinine clearance.
 [a] 4F-PCC dosing based on weight and INR value; see **Table 3.**
 [b] DOAC half-life can vary depending on the CrCl.
Data from Tummala R, Kavtaradze A, Gupta A, et al. Specific antidotes against direct oral anticoagulants: a comprehensive review of clinical trials data. Int J Cardiol 2016;214:292–8; and Garcia DA, Crowther MA. Reversal of warfarin. Circulation 2012;125(23):2944–7.

Table 3
Reversal agents—mechanism of action, pharmacology, and dosage

Agent	Mechanism	Pharmacology	Dosages/Descriptions
Andexanet alfa	rF Xa decoy protein	• Target: LMWH, anti-Xa inhibitors • Onset: immediate • Duration: ~6 h	• 400–800 mg IV bolus (30 mg/min) followed by 4-mg/min argatroban 8-mg/min infusion • Lower dose for apixaban, higher for rivaroxaban • FDA approval pending
Aripazine	Synthetic, water-soluble inhibitory molecule	• Target: UFH, LMWHs, argatroban, DOACs • Onset: 5–10 min • Duration: ~24 h	• 100–300 mg IV bolus • FDA approval pending
Idarucizumab	Neutralizing antibody specific for dabigatran	• Target: dabigatran • Onset: immediate • Duration: ~24 h	• 5-mg IV bolus over 5 min • Low potential for rebound
FFP	Replace coagulation inactive factors X, IX, VII, and II	• Target: warfarin • Onset: variable depending on the dose and the magnitude of anticoagulation • Duration: 4–6 h • Monitor: INR	• Typically given empirically in 2–4 U increments • Can also be given in a 10–20 mL/kg infusion to provide reversal. Expect 20%–30% increase in plasma clotting factor concentrations. • Potential for rebound anticoagulation depending on the half-life of anticoagulant used • Do not give for DOAC reversal.
PCCs	Replaces factors X, IX, VII, and II at a concentration 25× FFP	• Target: warfarin • Onset: immediate • Duration: 12–24 h	INR level: • <4: 25 IU/kg • 4–6: 35 IU/kg • >6: 50 IU/kg
Protamine sulfate	Combines chemically with heparin to form inactive salts	• Target: UFH, partially LMWH • Onset: ~5 min • Duration: Up to 2 h • Monitor: aPTT	IV UFH • 1 mg/100 U UFH (max dose 50 mg) • If infusion held ≥60 min, give 0.5 mg/100 U. • If infusion held ≥2 h, give 0.25 mg/100 U. • Rapid infusion causes hypotension, flash pulmonary edema, and allergic reactions: limit to 5 mg/min.

Vitamin K	Leads to in vivo production of functional factors X, IX, VII, and II	• Target: warfarin
		• Onset:
		  ○ PO 12–24 h
		  ○ IV 4–6 h
		• Duration: dependent on degree of coagulopathy
			PO dosing: typically given in nonemergent circumstances
			IV dosing
			• 10 mg: ICH, severe hemorrhage
			• 2–5 mg: urgent reversal for nonmajor/major bleeding
			• 0.25–1 mg: typically given for nonemergent partial reversal of a high INR

Abbreviation: ICH, intracranial hemorrhage.
Data from Refs.[3,29,55]

tooth extractions or root canals with local prohemostatic measures), cataract surgery, or minor dermatologic procedures (eg, excision of basal or squamous cell skin cancers), can likely continue therapy with little risk.[3] Meanwhile, warfarin patients at high risk for thrombosis, such as atrial fibrillation patients with CHA_2DS_2-VASc scores greater than 7 or thromboembolism within the last 3 months, should continue with periprocedural anticoagulation using bridging therapy.[1] Patients at moderate risk for thrombosis should be stratified by the periprocedural bleeding risk, and patients at increased risk should not undergo bridging therapy.[1–3,21]

Emergent or Urgent Reversal

In cases of ongoing major bleeding or in preparation of an emergent procedure with a moderate risk to high risk of bleeding, time-dependent elimination is not a viable option for reversal. In such instances, the effects of warfarin need to be counteracted quickly and effectively. Historically, this has been accomplished with the use of fresh frozen plasma (FFP) to replenish factors X, IX, VII, and II (see **Table 3**).[22] Plasma also provides intravascular volume, which may be beneficial in bleeding patients. FFP is however, not without its drawbacks, including the potential for transfusion-associated lung injury, transfusion-associated circulatory overload (TACO), and potential anticoagulation rebound.[15,22,23] Moreover, the time to effect can be severely hindered because FFP takes time to infuse and the volume of plasma needed to reestablish normal coagulation capability increases directly with the degree of anticoagulation present.[15,24] There is little consensus on the appropriate dosing of FFP to reverse warfarin-induced coagulopathy, which has led to empirical treatment strategies based on serial laboratory testing and clinical gestalt rather than robust evidence-based guidelines.[5,15,24,25] In practice, this results in 2 U to 4 U of FFP given to decrease INR values or a dosage of 10 mL/kg to 20 mL/kg to increase plasma levels of clotting factor by 20% to 30% (see **Table 3**).[26]

Prothrombin complex concentrates (PCCs) have several distinct advantages compared with FFP, including rapid administration, balanced delivery of clotting factors at higher concentrations than plasma, and greater durability (see **Table 3**).[24] In 1 retrospective comparison, PCC was found to reverse INR nearly twice as fast as FFP (11.8 vs 5.7 hours, $P<.001$), and FFP was associated with a 2-fold increase in the relative risk of serious adverse events compared with PCC (relative risk; 2.0; 95% CI, 1.1–3.5). There are 2 major variants of PCC depending on the factors present within: 3-factor (3F)-PCC consists of factors II, IX, and X but only has trace factor VII, whereas 4-factor (4F)-PCC contains factors II, VII, IX, and X.[4] To date, the FDA has only approved the 4F-PCC Kcentra (CSL Behring, King of Prussia, Pennsylvania) for the emergent reversal of warfarin; however, the 3F-PCC Profilnine SD (Grifols, Emeryville, California) has been used off-label for warfarin reversal.[4]

Several studies have compared 4F-PCC to 3F-PCC combined with recombinant factor (rF) VIIa. In 1 retrospective cohort study 3F-PCC combined with rFVIIa had greater reductions in INR compared with 4F-PCC, although both achieved reductions of INR below 1.5; however, patients receiving 3F-PCC with rFVIIa had a near 10-fold higher incidence of deep venous thrombosis compared with 4F-PCC patients.[4] Other studies have also demonstrated high rates of thrombotic complications despite durable INR reversal after 3F-PCC with rFVIIa.[4,27,28] Conversely, 4F-PCC has been approved by the FDA for warfarin reversal since 2013 and has demonstrated efficient and effective reductions in INR with low thromboembolic events.[4,24,26–29] In a prospective, multicenter, observational trial detailing 256 patients who received PCC, no incidences of thromboembolic adverse events were found after 4F-PCC administration.[30]

In cases of bleeding, vitamin K administration helps replete stores of clotting factors II, IV, IX, and X, thereby increasing the speed of reversal and reducing the INR over 4 hours to 6 hours for IV infusion and up to 24 hours for oral administration (see **Table 3**).[8,15] When emergent reversal is required, IV vitamin K should be given with PCC or FFP to prevent rebound because FFP's half-life is 4 hours to 6 hours whereas the half-life of PCC is dependent on the clotting factors present, ranging from 4 hours for factor VII to 60 hours for factor II.[8,20]

DIRECT ORAL ANTICOAGULANTS: RIVAROXABAN, APIXABAN, EDOXABAN, AND DABIGATRAN

Within the past decade, 4 DOACs have received FDA approval for the prevention of stroke in nonvalvular atrial fibrillation and in the treatment of venous thromboembolisms. These include 3F Xa inhibitors (rivaroxaban, apixaban, and edoxaban) and the direct thrombin inhibitor dabigatran (see **Table 2**).[31] In contrast to warfarin, which targets clotting factors within the intrinsic and extrinsic pathways, DOACs target clotting factors specific to the common pathway (see **Fig. 1**). As such, monitoring of the anticoagulant effect of these drugs can be problematic because conventional coagulation testing (eg, prothrombin time/INR or partial thromboplastin time/aPTT) either remains unaffected or produces variable results depending on the medication in use and the patient's renal function.[31] Therefore, alternative DOAC-specific monitoring tests have been developed to quantify the degree of anticoagulation. For instance, the direct thrombin inhibitors can be monitored using the diluted thrombin time (dTT) or the ecarin clotting time (ECT), both of which are highly sensitive for dabigatran use.[31,32] The dTT and ECT, however, do not reflect the degree of anticoagulation of the anti–factor Xa inhibitors rivaroxaban, apixaban, and edoxaban. Instead, anti–factor Xa chromogenic assays can correlate with plasma concentrations of anti–factor Xa DOACs, although the assay must be calibrated to each specific anti-Xa inhibitor and is not widely available.[31,32]

Two randomized clinical trials evaluating the use of apixaban and dabigatran (the Apixabn for Reduction in Stroke and Other Thromboembolic Events in atrial fibrillation and the Randomized Evaluation of Long Term Anticoagulant Therapy with Dabigatran Etexilate trials, respectively) demonstrated reduced risk of major bleeding events and reductions in the relative risk of intracranial hemorrhage compared with warfarin; however, DOACs have higher rates of major gastrointestinal bleeding within these same studies.[33,34] Following suit, numerous other studies demonstrated that the relative risk of major bleeding and fatal bleeding was reduced in DOACs compared with warfarin.[31,35–41] Therefore, although the bleeding profile associated with the DOACs is better compared with warfarin, clinicians should be cognizant of potential gastrointestinal bleed.

Nonspecific Reversal Strategies

Similar to warfarin, withholding DOACs in anticipation of an elective procedure should take into account the periprocedural bleeding risk and patient-related risk factors for thrombosis (see **Fig. 2**). For procedures with a low risk of bleeding, both dabigatran and the anti-Xa inhibitors can be held for approximately 24 hours with little risk of hemorrhage.[1] Caution is advised, however, because the half-lives of the DOACs vary depending on the creatinine clearance of the patient. As the creatinine clearance decreases, the half-life of all DOACs increase, however, notably with dabigatran because it is primarily eliminated by the kidneys (see **Table 3**). Therefore, caution is advised in patients with renal insufficiency or chronic kidney disease and longer wait times or checking anti-Xa chromogenic assay levels may be necessary to assure acceptable reversal is achieved.

Four-factor PCCs have proved highly effective for reversal of warfarin-induced anticoagulation by repletion of factors II, VII, IX, and X, but 3F-PCC reversal for DOACs has produced inconsistent results.[31,41,42] Activated PCCs (aPCCs) contain the same factors present in 4F-PCC but in both active and inactive forms, producing a more robust procoagulant effect. aPCCs, however, also have elevated risks of thromboembolic complications.[43] Moreover, there are few data to support PCC use in DOAC reversal, although several small randomized trials demonstrated a dose-dependent relationship of PCC reversal in healthy volunteers when administered 50 U/kg and partial reversal with 25 U/kg for rivaroxaban and edoxaban.[42,44] Plasma should not be used to reverse the anticoagulant effects of DOACs because it contains an insufficient concentration of clotting factors to be effective, and the increased volume load may precipitate TACO.[42] Instead, FFP use in DOAC-associated bleeding may be used as a plasma volume expander with preference given to PCCs for factor replacement. Similarly, vitamin K has no role in the management of DOAC-associated bleeding because the mechanism of action for all FDA-approved DOACs does not influence the plasma concentrations of vitamin K–dependent clotting factors. The use of rFVIIa may provide some reversal for the anticoagulant effects of DOACs, but available data are based on in vitro and ex vivo studies and the high thromboembolic risk associated with use likely makes the risk of rFVIIa outweigh the benefits.[44,45] Lastly, dabigatran exhibits low protein binding in vivo, making hemodialysis a potential avenue for drug removal when concerned for overdose or in the setting of ongoing bleeding.[46,47] Unfortunately, dialysis access in presence of full anticoagulation and ongoing bleeding may not be achievable, and there is evidence that tissue rebound may result in anticoagulation rebound after cessation of therapy, likely leaving a narrow group of patients who may benefit from dialysis-mediated dabigatran clearance.[47,48]

Specific Reversal Agent

Idarucizumab
Idarucizumab is a humanized monoclonal antibody that binds both free and thrombin-bound dabigatran with an affinity 350 times higher than the binding affinity of dabigatran for thrombin, in effect neutralizing anticoagulation through kidney excretion of idarucizumab-dabigatran complexes.[31,49] In a randomized, placebo-controlled, double-blind, proof-of-concept phase 1 trial, healthy volunteers were randomized to receive 1 of 4 dosing regimens of idarucizumab after receiving 220 mg of dabigatran for 4 days. The primary endpoint was an incidence of drug-related adverse events with the secondary endpoints reversal of dTT (direct thrombin time), ECT, aPTT, and thrombin time.[50] In all volunteers, no significant adverse reactions were observed, and idarucizumab immediately reversed all secondary endpoints. A follow-up phase III clinical trial evaluated patients on dabigatran who were either bleeding or undergoing an urgent procedure and assessed anticoagulation reversal as a primary endpoint 4 hours after administration of idarucizumab with a second but equally important outcome, the restoration of hemostasis.[51] Of patients with elevated dTT and ECT, 100% (95% CI, 100–100) had dTT and ECT return to baseline, and 68% of bleeding patients and 84% of patients undergoing an urgent procedure had restoration of hemostasis with 12 hours or intraoperatively, respectively. Idarucizumab was given FDA approval for reversal of anticoagulation mediated by dabigatran in October of 2015.

Andexanet alfa
Andexanet alfa is an rFXa decoy protein that binds and neutralizes the direct oral factor Xa and thrombin inhibitors as well as LMWHs, including fondaparinux.[42,52] Initial phase 2 clinical trials demonstrated rapid, dose-dependent reversal of

DOAC-mediated anticoagulation in healthy volunteers when andexanet alfa was given as a bolus followed by a 2-hour infusion, with no thrombotic or other adverse events observed.[53,54] Based on these findings, 2 parallel randomized, double-blind, placebo-controlled trials were undertaken evaluating the efficacy of andexanet alfa to reverse apixaban–mediated (Andexanet Alfa, a Novel Antidote to the Anticoagulant Effects of FXA Inhibitors [ANNEXA]-A) and rivaroxaban (ANNEXA-R)–mediated anticoagulation in healthy volunteers ages 50 to 75 years old.[52] Dosages were given based on findings in previous phase 2 studies with apixaban patients receiving a 400 mg bolus followed by a continuous 4-mg/min infusion for 120 minutes whereas rivaroxaban patients received an 800 mg bolus followed by a continuous 8-mg/min infusion for 120 minutes. Within both trials the primary endpoint (the percent change in anti–factor Xa activity from baseline to nadir) was achieved rapidly and effectively compared with placebo (92% and 94%, respectively, compared with 18% and 21%, respectively; $P<.001$). Moreover, reversal was achieved within 2 minutes to 5 minutes of bolus and sustained during infusion. Currently, phase 3 clinical trials are ongoing (http://www.clinicaltrials. gov, NCT02329327) to evaluate the efficacy and safety of andexanet alfa in patients taking anti–factor Xa inhibitors with acute major bleeding. To date, FDA approval is pending.

Aripazine

Aripazine (ciraparantag, PER977) is a synthetic, water-soluble molecule that binds both direct and indirect parenteral and oral anticoagulants, including UFH, LMWHs, and all the DOACs.[42,44] In animal studies, aripazine reduced bleeding and reversed the effects of both direct factor Xa and factor IIa inhibitors.[14,42,44] A phase 1 dose-ranging study demonstrated 100-mg to 300-mg doses of aripazine decreased whole-blood clotting time to near-normal value in healthy volunteers who were given a single dose of edoxaban, 60 mg. Although still early in development, aripazine has been granted fast track designation by the FDA, a status that facilitates the development and expedition of drugs intended to treat serious or life-threatening conditions and that demonstrate potential to address unmet clinical needs.[41] Additional clinical trials are ongoing with FDA approval pending.

SUMMARY

As the population continues to age and the number of indications requiring anticoagulation grows, anticoagulant use will rise. In recent years, clinicians have benefited from a growing armamentarium of available reversal agents, and the advent of targeted therapies like idarucizumab will undoubtedly herald a new regard toward the management of anticoagulant-associated bleeding and periprocedural reversal. Ongoing trials evaluating andexanet alfa and aripazine will hopefully only continue to broaden the available regimen of safe and effective agent-specific therapy. The decision to reverse a patient's anticoagulation status, however, must weigh the benefits of reversal against the risks of thrombosis, which requires practical understanding not only of anticoagulants in use but also of their respective antidotes.

REFERENCES

1. Doherty JU, Gluckman TJ, Hucker WJ, et al. 2017 ACC expert consensus decision pathway for periprocedural management of anticoagulation in patients with nonvalvular atrial fibrillation. J Am Coll Cardiol 2017;69(7):871–98.
2. Ferreira JL, Wipf JE. Pharmacologic therapies in anticoagulation. Med Clin North Am 2016;100(4):695–718.

3. Douketis JD, Spyropoulos AC, Spencer FA, et al. Perioperative management of antithrombotic therapy. Chest 2012;141(2):e326S–350.

4. Martin DT, Barton CA, Dodgion C, et al. Emergent reversal of vitamin K antagonists: addressing all the factors. Am J Surg 2016;211(5):919–25.

5. Rechenmacher SJ, Fang JC. Bridging anticoagulation. J Am Coll Cardiol 2015; 66(12):1392–403.

6. Baglin T, Barrowcliffe TW, Cohen A, et al, the British Committee for Standards in Haematology. Guidelines on the use and monitoring of heparin. Br J Haematol 2006;133(1):19–34.

7. Pai M, Crowther MA. Neutralization of heparin activity. Handb Exp Pharmacol 2012;207:265–77.

8. Gordon JL, Fabian TC, Lee MD, et al. Anticoagulant and antiplatelet medications encountered in emergency surgery patients: a review of reversal strategies. J Trauma Acute Care Surg 2013;75(3):475–86.

9. Garcia DA, Baglin TP, Weitz JI, et al, American College of Chest Physicians. Parenteral anticoagulants: antithrombotic therapy and prevention of thrombosis, 9th ed: American College of Chest Physicians Evidence-Based Clinical Practice Guidelines. Chest 2012;141(2 Suppl):e24S–43.

10. Dhillon S. Argatroban: a review of its use in the management of heparin-induced thrombocytopenia. Am J Cardiovasc Drugs 2009;9(4):261–82.

11. Di Nisio M, Middeldorp S, Büller HR. Direct thrombin inhibitors. N Engl J Med 2005;353(10):1028–40.

12. Greinacher A, Thiele T, Selleng K. Reversal of anticoagulants: an overview of current developments. Thromb Haemost 2015;113(5):931–42.

13. Wiedermann CJ, Stockner I. Warfarin-induced bleeding complications - clinical presentation and therapeutic options. Thromb Res 2008;122(Suppl 2):S13–8.

14. Woods K, Douketis JD, Kathirgamanathan K, et al. Low-dose oral vitamin K to normalize the international normalized ratio prior to surgery in patients who require temporary interruption of warfarin. J Thromb Thrombolysis 2007;24(2): 93–7.

15. Jones HU, Muhlestein JB, Jones KW, et al. Preoperative use of enoxaparin compared with unfractionated heparin increases the incidence of re-exploration for postoperative bleeding after open-heart surgery in patients who present with an acute coronary syndrome: clinical investigation and reports. Circulation 2002;106(12 Suppl 1):I19–22.

16. Kovacs MJ, Kearon C, Rodger M, et al. Single-arm study of bridging therapy with low-molecular-weight heparin for patients at risk of arterial embolism who require temporary interruption of warfarin. Circulation 2004;110(12):1658–63.

17. Larson BJG, Zumberg MS, Kitchens CS. A feasibility study of continuing dose-reduced warfarin for invasive procedures in patients with high thromboembolic risk. Chest 2005;127(3):922–7.

18. Steib A, Barre J, Mertes M, et al. Can oral vitamin K before elective surgery substitute for preoperative heparin bridging in patients on vitamin K antagonists? J Thromb Haemost 2010;8(3):499–503.

19. Douketis JD, Spyropoulos AC, Kaatz S, et al. Perioperative bridging anticoagulation in patients with atrial fibrillation. N Engl J Med 2015;373(9):823–33.

20. Johansen M, Wikkelsø A, Lunde J, et al. Prothrombin complex concentrate for reversal of vitamin K antagonist treatment in bleeding and non-bleeding patients. Cochrane Database Syst Rev 2015;(7):CD010555.

21. Hickey M, Gatien M, Taljaard M, et al. Outcomes of urgent warfarin reversal with frozen plasma versus prothrombin complex concentrate in the emergency department. Circulation 2013;128(4):360–4.

22. Sarode R, Milling TJ, Refaai MA, et al. Efficacy and safety of a 4-factor prothrombin complex concentrate in patients on vitamin K antagonists presenting with major bleeding: a randomized, plasma-controlled, phase IIIb study. Circulation 2013;128(11):1234–43.

23. Rashidi A, Tahhan HR. Fresh frozen plasma dosing for warfarin reversal: a practical formula. Mayo Clin Proc 2013;88(3):244–50.

24. Kalus JS. Pharmacologic interventions for reversing the effects of oral anticoagulants. Am J Health Syst Pharm 2013;70(10 Suppl 1):S12–21.

25. Barton CA, Johnson NB, Case J, et al. Risk of thromboembolic events after protocolized warfarin reversal with 3-factor PCC and factor VIIa. Am J Emerg Med 2015;33(11):1562–6.

26. DeLoughery E, Avery B, DeLoughery TG. Retrospective study of rFVIIa, 4-factor PCC, and a rFVIIa and 3-factor PCC combination in improving bleeding outcomes in the warfarin and non-warfarin patient. Am J Hematol 2016;91(7):705–8.

27. Pabinger I, Brenner B, Kalina U, et al. Prothrombin complex concentrate (Beriplex P/N) for emergency anticoagulation reversal: a prospective multinational clinical trial. J Thromb Haemost 2008;6(4):622–31.

28. Desmettre T, Dubart A-E, Capellier G, et al. Emergency reversal of anticoagulation: the real use of prothrombin complex concentrates: a prospective multicenter two year French study from 2006 to 2008. Thromb Res 2012;130(3):e178–83.

29. Tummala R, Kavtaradze A, Gupta A, et al. Specific antidotes against direct oral anticoagulants: a comprehensive review of clinical trials data. Int J Cardiol 2016;214:292–8.

30. Adcock DM, Gosselin R. Direct oral anticoagulants (DOACs) in the laboratory: 2015 review. Thromb Res 2015;136(1):7–12.

31. Granger CB, Alexander JH, McMurray JJV, et al. Apixaban versus warfarin in patients with atrial fibrillation. N Engl J Med 2011;365(11):981–92.

32. Connolly SJ, Ezekowitz MD, Yusuf S, et al. Dabigatran versus warfarin in patients with atrial fibrillation. N Engl J Med 2009;361(12):1139–51.

33. Bouillon K, Bertrand M, Maura G, et al. Risk of bleeding and arterial thromboembolism in patients with non-valvular atrial fibrillation either maintained on a vitamin K antagonist or switched to a non-vitamin K-antagonist oral anticoagulant: a retrospective, matched-cohort study. Lancet Haematol 2015;2(4):e150–9.

34. Schulman S, Kearon C, Kakkar AK, et al. Dabigatran versus warfarin in the treatment of acute venous thromboembolism. N Engl J Med 2009;361(24):2342–52.

35. Schulman S, Kakkar AK, Goldhaber SZ, et al. Treatment of acute venous thromboembolism with dabigatran or warfarin and pooled analysis. Circulation 2014; 129(7):764–72.

36. Investigators TE. Oral rivaroxaban for symptomatic venous thromboembolism. N Engl J Med 2010;363(26):2499–510.

37. Investigators TE-P. Oral rivaroxaban for the treatment of symptomatic pulmonary embolism. N Engl J Med 2012;366(14):1287–97.

38. Majeed A, Hwang H-G, Connolly SJ, et al. Management and outcomes of major bleeding during treatment with dabigatran or warfarin. Circulation 2013;128(21): 2325–32.

39. Palareti G. Direct oral anticoagulants and bleeding risk (in comparison to vitamin K antagonists and heparins), and the treatment of bleeding. Semin Hematol 2014;51(2):102–11.

40. Ruff CT, Giugliano RP, Antman EM. Management of bleeding with non–vitamin K antagonist oral anticoagulants in the era of specific reversal agents. Circulation 2016;134(3):248–61.
41. Siegal DM, Garcia DA, Crowther MA. How I treat target-specific oral anticoagulant-associated bleeding. Blood 2014;123(8):1152–8.
42. Yorkgitis BK. Non–vitamin K antagonist oral anticoagulant reversal: hope is on the horizon. Am J Surg 2016;212(1):160–4.
43. Lee FMH, Chan AKC, Lau KK, et al. Reversal of new, factor-specific oral anticoagulants by rFVIIa, prothrombin complex concentrate and activated prothrombin complex concentrate: a review of animal and human studies. Thromb Res 2014; 133(5):705–13.
44. Alikhan R, Rayment R, Keeling D, et al. The acute management of haemorrhage, surgery and overdose in patients receiving dabigatran. Emerg Med J 2014;31(2): 163–8.
45. Singh T, Maw TT, Henry BL, et al. Extracorporeal therapy for dabigatran removal in the treatment of acute bleeding: a single center experience. Clin J Am Soc Nephrol 2013;8(9):1533–9.
46. Chang DN, Dager WE, Chin AI. Removal of dabigatran by hemodialysis. Am J Kidney Dis 2013;61(3):487–9.
47. Pollack CVJ, Reilly PA, Eikelboom J, et al. Idarucizumab for dabigatran reversal. N Engl J Med 2015;373(6):511–20.
48. Stangier J, Rathgen K, Stähle H, et al. Influence of renal impairment on the pharmacokinetics and pharmacodynamics of oral dabigatran etexilate: an open-label, parallel-group, single-centre study. Clin Pharmacokinet 2010;49(4):259–68.
49. Glund S, Stangier J, Schmohl M, et al. Safety, tolerability, and efficacy of idarucizumab for the reversal of the anticoagulant effect of dabigatran in healthy male volunteers: a randomised, placebo-controlled, double-blind phase 1 trial. Lancet 2015;386(9994):680–90.
50. Siegal DM, Curnutte JT, Connolly SJ, et al. Andexanet Alfa for the reversal of factor Xa inhibitor activity. N Engl J Med 2015;373(25):2413–24.
51. Crowther M, Levy GG, Lu G, et al. A phase 2 randomized, double-blind, placebo-controlled trial demonstrating reversal of edoxaban-induced anticoagulation in healthy subjects by Andexanet Alfa (PRT064445), a Universal Antidote for Factor Xa (fXa) Inhibitors. Blood 2014;124(21):4269.
52. Vandana M, Michael K, Genmin L, et al. A phase 2 randomized, double-blind, placebo-controlled trial demonstrating reversal of rivaroxaban-induced anticoagulation in healthy subjects by Andexanet Alfa (PRT064445), an antidote for Fxa inhibitors. Blood 2013;122(21):3636.
53. Crowther M, Lu G, Conley P, et al. Reversal of factor Xa inhibitors-induced anticoagulation in healthy subjects by Andexanet Alfa. Crit Care Med 2014;42: A1469.
54. Ansell JE, Bakhru SH, Laulicht BE, et al. Use of PER977 to reverse the anticoagulant effect of edoxaban. N Engl J Med 2014;371(22):2141–2.
55. Garcia DA, Crowther MA. Reversal of warfarin. Circulation 2012;125(23):2944–7.

Resuscitation for Hypovolemic Shock

Kyle J. Kalkwarf, MD[a],*, Bryan A. Cotton, MD[a]

KEYWORDS

- Hemorrhagic shock • Trauma • Coagulopathy • Damage control resuscitation
- Massive transfusion • Visoelastic hemostatic assays

KEY POINTS

- Massive hemorrhage in trauma causes inadequate tissue perfusion and coagulopathy.
- Early transfusion with balanced ratios of blood products results in improved coagulation profiles, less product and transfusions improved outcomes in trauma patients requiring massive transfusion.
- Damage control resuscitation for patients in hemorrhagic shock results in decreased morbidity and improved survival.
- Monitoring coagulation and basing resuscitation on visoelastic hemostatic assays results in decreased transfusions and improved survival.

INTRODUCTION: HISTORY OF HEMORRHAGIC SHOCK RESUSCITATION

The term "shock" originates from "choc," which was coined by French surgeon Henri François Le Dran in the eighteenth century to describe the destructive impact of gunshot.[1] It subsequently evolved to signify the suddenly worsening condition that can ensue after major trauma. In modern medical literature, shock denotes a lack of end-organ perfusion, which can result from multiple etiologies, but hemorrhage is the cause of acute hypovolemic shock resulting from nonburn trauma.

The first recorded human blood transfusion occurred in 1819,[2] but its use did not become common until almost 100 years later when the discovery of blood types[3] and development of techniques to crossmatch blood[4] allowed for widespread use. Crystalloid became the standard resuscitation fluid used for hemorrhagic shock in the nineteenth and early twentieth centuries[5–7] because of its availability and safety. However, with the high volume of severely injured combatants encountered during

Disclosure Statement: Dr B.A. Cotton has served as a consultant for Haemonetics Corporation, Braintree, MA, makers of TEG thromboelastogram. Dr K.J. Kalkwarf has no disclosures or conflicts.
[a] Department of Surgery, University of Texas, McGovern Medical School at UTHealth, 6431 Fannin Street, MSB 4.286, Houston, TX 77030, USA
* Corresponding author.
E-mail address: Kyle.Kalkwarf@gmail.com

World War I (WWI), Allied physicians soon that realized crystalloid transfusions resulted in "unsatisfactory" results because of dilution.[8] They preferred using limited whole-blood transfusions to maintain a low blood pressure and rewarming the patient.[9] This became the standard of care for resuscitation for the last 8 months of the Great War.[10] WWII physicians described similar practices of giving enough whole blood to achieve a systolic blood pressure of 85 mm Hg, along with appropriate skin color and warmth, while working to quickly stop bleeding.[11,12] They also used transfusions of recently developed reconstituted dried plasma to maintain blood pressure while preparing whole blood.[13]

By the time of the Vietnam War, there was a renewed interest in crystalloid administration based on subsequently refuted basic science[14,15] and animal models[16–19] of hemorrhage shock that showed improved survival from infusing Ringer lactate (LR) before whole-blood transfusion. As a result, trauma patients began receiving increasing quantities of crystalloid. Simultaneously, new blood fractionation techniques were being developed that allowed for whole blood to be separated into units of red blood cells (RBCs), plasma, and platelets. The ability to treat multiple patients with one unit of whole blood and the risk of hepatitis[20,21] associated with plasma at that time prompted medical leaders and groups[22,23] to advocate for specific component blood therapy for all transfusions despite no rigorous studies demonstrating the effects of such therapy in massively bleeding patients.[24,25] Although some studies performed at that time suggested "noninferiority in elective surgical cases," not a single study showed hemostatic potential in bleeding patients. Blood bankers demonstrated that they could administer component therapy safely, not necessarily that they should.

Trends away from whole-blood transfusions and toward large-volume crystalloid and RBC resuscitation continued throughout the last three decades of the twentieth century as a result of studies that said LR and more than six units of RBCs could be used without causing coagulopathy,[26] and others saying it was not important to augment blood transfusions with plasma[27,28] or platelets[29] unless there was clinical or laboratory coagulopathy. Another study declaring that it was safe to administer 2 L of crystalloid while waiting for blood[30] was widely propagated when it was adopted by the Advanced Trauma Life Support course.[31] Often forgotten is that these studies were conducted in patients receiving whole blood rather than RBCs and LR, as had become the standard practice in some busy trauma centers as early as the mid-1970s.[32] Concerns about human immunodeficiency virus transmission[33,34] and goals of therapy targeting "supranormal" resuscitation[35–40] led to continued propagation of transfusing large volumes of only crystalloid and RBCs during the 1980s and 1990s despite new tests making blood transfusions safe and large multicenter trails that showed no survival advantage to supranormal resuscitation.[41,42]

When examined critically, large-volume transfusion strategies resulted in increased morbidity including decreased intestinal perfusion along with increased abdominal compartment syndrome, cardiopulmonary dysfunction, multiple organ dysfunction, and death.[43–45] At the same time, coagulopathy was being identified in severely injured patients, independent of resuscitation,[46–48] and was found to be associated with increased mortality.[47,49,50] As a result, military surgeons returned to resuscitation techniques attempting to replicate the whole blood used in previous wars by including high ratios of plasma and platelets to RBCs. Results from data collected during conflicts in Afghanistan and Iraq showed that patients who received high ratios of plasma to RBCs had improved survival compared with those who received lower ratios.[51] As a result, the military developed damage control resuscitation (DCR) to reduce blood loss and coagulopathy. DCR is focused on limiting crystalloids, delivering whole blood or high ratios of plasma and platelets, and maintaining permissive hypotension (**Fig. 1**). Massive transfusion (MT) protocols (MTP) were developed to achieve these goals of DCR and, in some instances, have been shown to improve survival independent of ratios. Finally, experts have recommended avoiding hypothermia and rapidly controlling hemorrhage with surgery and appropriate hemostatic adjuncts.[52]

DAMAGE CONTROL RESUSCITATION
Limit Crystalloid

Of all the three tenets of DCR, some trauma surgeons argue that the reduction in crystalloids over the last decade has had the greatest impact of improving survival. Despite decades of liberal use treating trauma patients, it is now known that infusing large volumes of crystalloid as a replacement for lost blood worsens the "vicious cycle of coagulopathy" resulting from hypoxia, acidosis, and hypothermia that was originally described 35 years ago.[32,53] Intravenous fluids are known to dilute clotting factors,[54] cool patients,[55] and create acidosis.[56] They also cause edema[57,58] and end-organ dysfunction[59] by disrupting cellular mechanisms and causing inflammation. This results in several complications including cardiac,[44] respiratory,[53] gastrointestinal,[60] and immune dysfunction; decreased wound healing[45]; increased anastomotic leak[44,61]; abdominal compartment syndrome[43,62]; open abdomens[53,63]; hyperfibrinolysis[64]; and mortality.[44,53,65] Limiting crystalloid also results in fewer overall blood transfusions for those with life-threatening injuries.[66–68]

Permissive Hypotension

The origins of the second tenet reach back to WWI and WWII, where physicians described increased blood loss and rebleeding when normal blood pressure is achieved before hemorrhage control.[9,11] The protective effect of hypotension was confirmed in animal models that showed decreased blood loss and improved mortality with limited resuscitation.[24,69–72] A study in swine demonstrated that rebleeding occurs at an average systolic blood pressure of 94 mm Hg and a mean arterial pressure of 64 mm Hg.[73] Randomized controlled trials confirmed the improvement in mortality from delaying resuscitation to a normal blood pressure until after operative control of

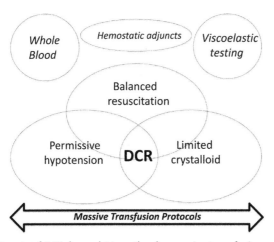

Fig. 1. The three tenets of DCR, brought together by massive transfusion protocols, and supported by several adjuncts.

bleeding[74] in penetrating[75] and blunt trauma patients.[76] A study in the 1990s from Houston randomized to receive prehospital fluid resuscitation (crystalloids) versus none in penetrating torso patients presenting with hypotension (blood pressure ≤90 mm Hg).[74] Fluid resuscitation in the "no fluids" arm was withheld until the patient entered the operating room. The patients who received delayed resuscitation had improved survival compared with those who received immediate fluid resuscitation.

Balanced (1:1:1) Resuscitation

The third and final tenet of DCR is the one that has been the most studied and most noted. The initial call to arms for DCR strongly advocated for a ratio of blood products that approximated whole blood (1:1:1).[52] Following publication of the initial military experience describing improved survival for those receiving higher ratios of plasma to RBCs,[53] the findings were replicated in the military experience[77] and multiple retrospective trials in civilians.[49,78–81] of those receiving a ratio or platelets: plasma/RBC (1:1:1). These studies included patients injured by blunt[82] and penetrating[83] mechanisms. The improvement in outcomes from plasma transfusions is attributed to decreasing inflammation, edema, and vascular permeability by repairing tight junctions and the glycocalyx of the vascular endothelium,[84,85] in addition to improving platelet function and clot formation.[86] Plasma also decreases blood hypercoagulability by modulating thrombin generation.[87] A limiting factor in fresh frozen plasma (FFP) administration has traditionally been the 45 minutes required to thaw it before transfusion. Prethawed[88] or liquid plasma[89] can be used to decrease this time[90,91] and 69% of level I and II American College of Surgeons Trauma Quality Improvement Program trauma centers now have plasma immediately available for MTP activations.[92] This has been shown to allow for earlier transfusions, balanced resuscitation, decreased overall blood product transfusions, and improved mortality.[90,93] Similar to higher ratios of transfused plasma, multiple studies have demonstrated improved survival for patients receiving balanced ratios of platelets.[94–99] Platelet inhibition and dysfunction is common after brain injury[100] and minor trauma.[101] It is associated with increased morbidity and mortality[102] because platelets improve wound healing, vascular integrity, and immune response.[98]

With the accumulation of trials demonstrating improved outcomes with balanced resuscitation, these practices quickly spread to civilian trauma practices throughout the United States, with MTP using a 1:1:1 ratio of plasma/platelets/RBCs blossoming from just a few institutions a decade ago[103] to more than 85% of major trauma centers today.[104] Retrospective reviews from trauma centers that implemented DCR showed an almost 50% reduction in crystalloid use at one center,[105] whereas another showed significantly less use of crystalloid and all blood components.[53] DRC is also associated with decreased morbidity from abdominal compartment syndrome,[63,105] infection,[105] and organ failure[106] and reduced mortality[53,105] from hemorrhage.[107]

In 2009, a study examining the time to transfusion of different blood components demonstrated a limitation of retrospective studies. Because of the time required to thaw FFP, the time to first transfusion of FFP (93 minutes) was significantly greater than the time to first RBC transfusion (18 minutes), despite attempting to achieve balanced ratios. As a result, patients who died early received RBCs but were not able to receive the appropriate ratio of FFP and platelets to achieve a balanced transfusion. In contrast, those who survived were eventually able to achieve the goal ratios, thus creating a survival bias.[108] The PROPPR trial was designed as a prospective, randomized, multicenter trial to overcome the selection bias of retrospective trials by evaluating the two most common resuscitation ratios[99] as determined by the

PROMMTT study, which observed transfusion practices in 10 level 1 trauma centers.[99] Although the PROPPR study showed no improvement in 24-hour survival for 1:1:1 versus 1:1:2 (plasma/platelet/RBC), it did show less death from exsanguination at 24 hours for higher ratios of plasma and platelets (9.2% in 1:1:1 group vs 14.6% in 1:1:2 group) and found no difference in complications for the group receiving higher ratios of plasma and platelets, alleviating concerns about their transfusion. The balanced plasma to RBC group also had decreased mortality at 3 hours, which is the median time to hemorrhagic death.[107,109–111]

ADJUNCTS TO DAMAGE CONTROL RESUSCITATION
Whole Blood

Whole blood is the optimal resuscitation fluid for patients who are massively bleeding. After first being successfully used to treat hemorrhagic shock in WWI, military doctors have successfully transfused more than a million units of whole blood during conflicts over the past century and it was preferentially used in civilian trauma until the 1970s when it fell out of favor because of concerns about safety and waste.[4,10,112,113] Recent military conflicts in Iraq and Afghanistan led to a resurgence of whole blood where more than 10,000 units were transfused[34] to the most severely injured patients.[114] Retrospective reviews of those who were transfused with warm fresh whole blood showed that it increased 24-hour and 30-day survival when compared with balanced component therapy.[115,116] These findings are supported by an in vitro study that showed whole blood is more hemostatic[117] and a pilot prospective randomized trial that showed it resulted in less transfusions of RBC, plasma, and platelets when patients with nonsurvivable head injuries were excluded.[118] The reason for the superiority is that a 500-mL unit of fresh whole blood has a hematocrit of 38% to 50%, a total of 150,000 to 400,000 platelets per microliter with full activity,[119] and 100% activity of clotting factors.[112] By comparison, transfusing one unit of plasma, platelets, and RBCs results in 660 mL of fluid with a hematocrit of 29%, a total of 88,000 platelets per microliter, 65% coagulation factor activity with reduced flow characteristics, and increased additives including anticoagulants (**Table 1**).[34,112]

Massive Transfusion Protocols

Based on experiences in WWII, Beecher[11] wrote, "about 2.5% (sic) of those wounded would fall into the group that is in bad enough condition to require special resuscitative care." That proportion of civilian trauma admissions currently requires more than 10 units of blood within 24 hours of admission,[120] but two to three times that percentage of injured modern military combatants require an MT.[53,95] The mortality for patients

Table 1			
Comparison of whole blood unit versus component therapy (reconstituted whole blood)			
	Whole Blood (1 U)	**1:1:1 Component Therapy (1 U Plasma, 1 U Platelets, 1 U RBC, 1 U Cryoprecipitate)**	**1:1:2 Component Therapy (1 U Plasma, 1 U Platelets, 2 U RBC, 1 U Cryoprecipitate)**
Volume, mL	500	680	900
Hematocrit,%	38–50	29	38
Platelet count	>150,000	80,000	60,000
Coagulation factors, %	100	65	52
Fibrinogen, mg	1000	1000	1000

receiving MT is 20% to 65%,[53,120–121] but instituting MTPs has decreased mortality rates by more than 50%.[53,106,122,123] There are, however, side effects and risks associated with blood transfusions. Therefore, DCR should be reserved for patients who are in hemorrhagic shock or will require an MT.[124] The problem is determining which patients will eventually require an MT and which will not.

During WWII, Beecher[11] used increasing pulse, decreasing blood pressure, and cool skin as indications for a blood transfusion.[11] Based on this and experiences from previous wars,[8] the US military showed that a patient's baseline mental status (assuming no head injury)[125] and a normal radial pulse[126] could be used to reliability predict the need for transfusion and a life-saving intervention.[127] When ultrasound is available, the ABC Score is able to predict the need for an MT based on a scoring system that gives points for penetrating mechanism, positive focused assessment sonography for trauma, systolic blood pressure less than or equal to 90 mm Hg, and an arrival heart rate greater than 120 beats per minute.[128] This scoring system was verified in a rural hospital[129] and in a multicenter trial.[130] It is currently being used in civilian medical transport helicopters to determine if blood products should be given in the prehospital setting.[131] Although it has a tendency to overactivate the MTP, it misses less than 5% of MT or substantial bleeding scenarios.[130]

Viscoelastic Hemostatic Assays

Thrombelastography (TEG) was developed almost 70 years ago[132] to evaluate clot initiation, formation, strength, stability, and breakdown[57,133] in addition to evaluating the patient for hypocoagulable and hypercoagulable states.[134,135] It was not used to guide therapy for trauma patients until half a century later when it was shown to be easier to use, more cost efficient, and a better prognosticator of blood transfusion than conventional coagulation tests (CCT)[132,136] because it is able to evaluate the entire coagulation cascade[133] rather than just plasma.[134] There are two commercially available viscoelastic hemostatic assays (VHA): TEG and rotational thromboelastometry. Both use whole blood and rotation, but TEG rotates a cup with a fixed metal piston suspended in the blood sample, whereas rotational thromboelastometry rotates a metal pin in a blood sample contained in a stationary cup.[137] Rapid TEG (r-TEG) introduces tissue factor as an additional activator[138] and is thus able to provide initial results to guide resuscitation within 5 minutes, an almost 10-fold improvement over CCT and traditional TEG.[139] A series of retrospective trials demonstrate the superiority of VHA to CCT.[135,140,141] More recently, the Denver group noted improved survival for MTP patients that were randomized to resuscitation with VHA versus CCT.[142] In addition, r-TEG-guided resuscitation resulted in decreased transfusions of plasma, platelet, and cryoprecipitate compared with CCT. Both the Denver and Houston groups have published recommended treatment thresholds for r-TEG (**Table 2**).

Hemostatic Adjuncts

In addition to describing clot formation, VHA also provides information on fibrinolysis, or clot breakdown, that is not afforded by CCT. Posttraumatic fibrinolysis is a spectrum with excessive clot breakdown resulting in uncontrolled bleeding to one extreme and shutdown resulting in thrombus formation and subsequent organ dysfunction to the other.[143] Both extremes are associated with increased mortality and are diagnosed based on TEG LY30. Hyperfibrinolysis is a highly lethal state, commonly present on the verge of exsanguination,[143] for which mortality increases significantly with each percentage increase in LY30.[64] It is treated with tranexamic acid, a synthetic antifibrinolytic derivative that blocks plasminogen from binding with fibrin and thus inhibits dissolution of the fibrin clot.[144] Tranexamic acid is administered in the first

Table 2
Summary of recommended thresholds for treatment by r-TEG from two level-1 centers with extensive experience with r-TEG guided resuscitation

r-TEG Parameter	Interpretation	Treatment
ACT ≥128 s	Prolonged with factor deficiency, severe hemodilution	Plasma
K-time ≥2.5 min	Increased with hypofibrinogenemia ± platelet dysfunction	Plasma ± cryoprecipitate
α-angle ≤65°	Decreased with hypofibrinogenemia or platelet dysfunction	Cryoprecipitate (or fibrinogen concentrate)
MA ≤55 mm	Decreased with platelet dysfunction ± hypofibrinogenemia	Platelets ± cryoprecipitate
LY-30 ≥3%	Increased with accelerated fibrinolysis	Tranexamic acid or aminocaproic acid

Abbreviations: ACT, activated clotting time; LY-30, lysis 30 min after MA greater than 20 mm; MA, maximal amplitude.

3 hours after injury to patients with LY30 values greater than 3%, the percentage at which mortality increases significantly,[64,143] without increasing mortality.[145] Other hemostatic adjuncts for bleeding patients include prothrombin complex concentrate[146] and recombinant activated factor VII.[147]

Avoiding Hypothermia

In addition to providing the proper resuscitation fluid, it is also important to limit other causes of coagulopathy and blood loss by correcting hypothermia, not causing unnecessarily high blood pressure, and stopping surgical bleeding. Severely injured trauma patients are frequently hypothermic because of exposure and infusion of cold fluids. This worsens coagulopathy and increases mortality[32,148–150] because of decreased fibrinogen synthesis[151] and reduced platelet function.[152] As a result, it is necessary to implement warming techniques, including warmed intravenous fluids and heating blankets, to patients with hypothermia.[58]

SUMMARY

The current practice of hypovolemic shock resuscitation for trauma is similar to the protocols developed while treating thousands of severely injured soldiers during WWI and WWII. Deviation from these practices in the second half of the twentieth century has been rejected based on experiences and trials conducted over the last decade. Continued expansion of DCR into civilian practice will result some in some changes, but it is hoped not to the point that inferior care is provided and clinicians are not forced to relearn the same lessons in the future.

REFERENCES

1. Parrillo, Dellinger. Critical care medicine: principles of diagnosis and management in the adult. 4th edition. Philadelphia: Elsevier Health Sciences, 2013. p. 299.
2. Blundell J. Some account of a case of obstinate vomiting, in which an attempt was made to prolong life by the injection of blood into the veins. Med Chir Trans 1819;10(Pt 2):296–311.

3. Schmidt PJ. Transfusion in America in the eighteenth and nineteenth centuries. N Engl J Med 1968;279(24):1319–20.

4. Spinella PC. Warm fresh whole blood transfusion for severe hemorrhage: US military and potential civilian applications. Crit Care Med 2008;36(7):S340–5.

5. Jennings CE. The intra-venous injection of fluid for severe hæmorrhage. Lancet 1882;120(3081):436–7.

6. Jennings CE. The intra-venous injection of fluid for severe hæmorrhage. Lancet 1883;121(3102):228–9.

7. Pye-Smith RJ. Sheffield public hospital and dispensary: five cases of intravenous injection of saline fluid for hæmorrhage and collapse. Lancet 1892; 139(3582):913–5.

8. Fraser J, Cowell EM. Clinical study of blood pressure in wound conditions. JAMA 1918;70(8):520–35.

9. Cannon WB. Traumatic shock. New York: D. Appleton; 1923.

10. Hess JR, Thomas MJ. Blood use in war and disaster: lessons from the past century. Transfusion 2003;43(11):1622–33.

11. Beecher HK. Preparation of battle casualties for surgery. Ann Surg 1945;121(6): 769–92.

12. Beecher HK. Early care of the seriously wounded man. J Am Med Assoc 1951; 145(4):193–200.

13. Beecher HK. Resuscitation, and anesthesia for wounded men, the management of traumatic shock. Springfield (IL): Charles C. Thomas; 1949.

14. Shires T, Williams J, Brown F. Acute change in extracellular fluids associated with major surgical procedures. Ann Surg 1961;154:803–10.

15. Shires T, Jackson DE. Postoperative salt tolerance. Arch Surg 1962;84:703–6.

16. Fogelman MJ, Wilson BJ. A different concept of volume replacement in traumatic hypovolemia observations on injured man and animal. Am J Surg 1960; 99(5):694–701.

17. Wolfman EF, Neill SA, Heaps DK, et al. Donor blood and isotonic salt solution. Effect on survival after hemorrhagic shock and operation. Arch Surg 1963;86: 869–73.

18. Shires T, Coln D, Carrico J, et al. Fluid therapy in hemorrhagic shock. Arch Surg 1964;88:688–93.

19. McClelland RN, Shires GT, Baxter CR, et al. Balanced salt solution in the treatment of hemorrhagic shock. JAMA 1967;199:830–4.

20. Davidsohn I. Speculation on future use of blood or blood component therapy. JAMA 1967;202(10):970–2.

21. Chaplin H Jr. Packed red blood cells. N Engl J Med 1969;281(7):364–7.

22. AMA Committee on Transfusion and Transplantation. Something old, something new. JAMA 1970;212(1):147.

23. Westphal RG. Rational alternatives to the use of whole blood. Ann Intern Med 1972;76(6):987–90.

24. Holcomb JB. Fluid resuscitation in modern combat casualty care: lessons learned from Somalia [review]. J Trauma 2003;54(5 Suppl):S46–51.

25. Holcomb JB. Reconstitution: reverse engineering. J Trauma 2011;70(5 Suppl): S65–7.

26. Shackford SR, Virgilio RW, Peters RM. Whole blood versus packed-cell transfusions: a physiologic comparison. Ann Surg 1981;193(3):337–40.

27. Counts RB, Haisch C, Simon TL, et al. Hemostasis in massively transfused trauma patients. Ann Surg 1979;190(1):91–9.

28. Lucas CE, Ledgerwood AM. Clinical significance of altered coagulation tests after massive transfusion for trauma. Am Surg 1981;47(3):125–30.

29. Reed RL 2nd, Ciavarella D, Heimbach DM, et al. Prophylactic platelet administration during massive transfusion. A prospective, randomized, double-blind clinical study. Ann Surg 1986;203:40–8.

30. Carrico CJ, Canizaro PC, Shires GT. Fluid resuscitation following injury: rationale for the use of balanced salt solutions. Crit Care Med 1976;4(2):46–54.

31. American College of Surgeons. Advanced trauma life support (ATLS) student course manual. 9th edition. Chicago: American College of Surgeons; 2012. p. 62–81.

32. Kashuk JL, Moore EE, Millikan JS, et al. Major abdominal vascular trauma-a unified approach. J Trauma Acute Care Surg 1982;22(8):672–9. RJ Lowe in Discussion.

33. Lee L, Moore EE, Hansen KC, et al. It's not your grandfather's field plasma. Surgery 2013;153(6):857–60.

34. Spinella PC, Pidcoke HF, Strandenes G, et al. Whole blood for hemostatic resuscitation of major bleeding. Transfusion 2016;56(S2):S190–202.

35. Bland R, Shoemaker WC, Shabot MM. Physiologic monitoring goals for the critically ill patient. Surg Gynecol Obstet 1978;147(6):833–41.

36. Shoemaker WC, Appel PL, Kram HB. Tissue oxygen debt as a determinant of lethal and nonlethal postoperative organ failure. Crit Care Med 1988;16(11):1117–20.

37. Fleming A, Bishop M, Shoemaker W, et al. Prospective trial of supranormal values as goals of resuscitation in severe trauma. Arch Surg 1992;127:1175–9 [discussion: 1179–81].

38. Bishop MH, Wo CCJ, Appel PL, et al. Relationship between supranormal circulatory values, time delays, and outcome in severely traumatized patients. Crit Care Med 1993;21:56–60.

39. Boyd O, Grounds RM, Bennett ED. A randomized clinical trial of the effect of deliberate perioperative increase of oxygen delivery on mortality in high-risk surgical patients. JAMA 1993;270(22):2699–707.

40. Bishop MH, Shoemaker WC, Appel PL, et al. Prospective, randomized trial of survivor values of cardiac index, oxygen delivery, and oxygen consumption as resuscitation endpoints in severe trauma. J Trauma 1995;38(5):780–7.

41. Gattinoni L, Brazzi L, Pelosi P, et al. A trial of goal-oriented hemodynamic therapy in critically ill patients. N Engl J Med 1995;333(16):1025–32.

42. Velmahos GC, Demetriades D, Shoemaker WC, et al. Endpoints of resuscitation of critically injured patients: normal or supranormal?: a prospective randomized trial. Ann Surg 2000;232(3):409–18.

43. Balogh Z, McKinley BA, Cocanour CS, et al. Supranormal trauma resuscitation causes more cases of abdominal compartment syndrome. Arch Surg 2003;138:637–42.

44. Brandstrup B, Tønnesen H, Beier-Holgersen R, et al. Effects of intravenous fluid restriction on postoperative complications: comparison of two perioperative fluid regimens: a randomized assessor-blinded multicenter trial. Ann Surg 2003;238(5):641.

45. Cotton BA, Guy JS, Morris JA Jr, et al. The cellular, metabolic, and systemic consequences of aggressive fluid resuscitation strategies. Shock 2006;26:115–21.

46. MacLeod JB, Lynn M, McKenney MG, et al. Early coagulopathy predicts mortality in trauma. J Trauma 2003;55(1):39–44.

47. Brohi K, Singh J, Heron M, et al. Acute traumatic coagulopathy. J Trauma 2003; 54:1127–30.
48. Niles SE, McLaughlin DF, Perkins JG, et al. Increased mortality associated with the early coagulopathy of trauma in combat casualties. J Trauma 2008;64(6): 1459–63 [discussion: 1463–5].
49. Gunter OL Jr, Au BK, Isbell JM, et al. Optimizing outcomes in damage control resuscitation: identifying blood product ratios associated with improved survival. J Trauma 2008;65(3):527–34.
50. Pidcoke HF, Aden JK, Mora AG, et al. Ten-year analysis of transfusion in Operation Iraqi Freedom and Operation Enduring Freedom: increased plasma and platelet use correlates with improved survival. J Trauma Acute Care Surg 2012;73(6):S445–52.
51. Borgman MA, Spinella PC, Perkins JG, et al. The ratio of blood products transfused affects mortality in patients receiving massive transfusions at a combat support hospital. J Trauma 2007;63(4):805–13.
52. Holcomb JB, Jenkins D, Rhee P, et al. Damage control resuscitation: directly addressing the early coagulopathy of trauma. J Trauma Acute Care Surg 2007; 62(2):307–10.
53. Cotton BA, Reddy N, Hatch QM, et al. Damage control resuscitation is associated with a reduction in resuscitation volumes and improvement in survival in 390 damage control laparotomy patients. Ann Surg 2011;254(4):598–605.
54. Maegele M, Lefering R, Yucel N, et al, AG Polytrauma of the German Trauma Society (DGU). Early coagulopathy in multiple injury: an analysis from the German Trauma Registry on 8724 patients. Injury 2007;38:298.
55. Tieu BH, Holcomb JB, Schreiber MA. Coagulopathy: its pathophysiology and treatment in the injured patient. World J Surg 2007;31:1055–64.
56. Myburgh JA, Mythen MG. Resuscitation fluids. N Engl J Med 2013;369:1243–51.
57. Feinman M, Cotton BA, Haut ER. Optimal fluid resuscitation in trauma: type, timing, and total. Curr Opin Crit Care 2014;20(4):366–72.
58. Duchesne JC, Kimonis K, Marr AB, et al. Damage control resuscitation in combination with damage control laparotomy: a survival advantage. J Trauma 2010; 69:46–52.
59. Shah SK, Uray KS, Stewart RH, et al. Resuscitation-induced intestinal edema and related dysfunction: state of the science. J Surg Res 2011;166(1):120–30.
60. Lobo DN, Bostock KA, Neal KR, et al. Effect of salt and water balance on recovery of gastrointestinal function after elective colonic resection: a randomized control trial. Lancet 2002;359:1812–8.
61. Schnüriger B, Inaba K, Wu T, et al. Crystalloids after primary colon resection and anastomosis at initial trauma laparotomy: excessive volumes are associated with anastomotic leakage. J Trauma Acute Care Surg 2011;70(3):603–10.
62. Balogh Z, McKinley BA, Cocanour CS, et al. Secondary abdominal compartment syndrome is an elusive early complication of traumatic shock resuscitation. Am J Surg 2002;184(6):538–43 [discussion: 543–4].
63. Hatch QM, Osterhout LM, Ashraf A, et al. Current use of damage control laparotomy, closure rates, and predictors of early fascial closure at the first takeback. J Trauma 2011;70(6):1429–36.
64. Cotton BA, Harvin JA, Kostousouv V, et al. Hyperfibrinolysis at admission is an uncommon but highly lethal event associated with shock and prehospital fluid administration. J Trauma Acute Care Surg 2012 Aug;73(2):365–70 [discussion: 370].

65. Ley EJ, Clond MA, Srour MK, et al. Emergency department crystalloid resuscitation of 1.5 L or more is associated with increased mortality in elderly and non-elderly trauma patients. J Trauma 2011;70:398–400.

66. Spinella PC, Perkins JG, Grathwohl KW, et al. Fresh whole blood transfusions in coalition military, foreign national, and enemy combatant patients during Operation Iraqi Freedom at a US combat support hospital. World J Surg 2008;32(1): 2–6.

67. Duchesne JC, Heaney J, Guidry C, et al. Diluting the benefits of hemostatic resuscitation: a multi-institutional analysis. J Trauma Acute Care Surg 2013; 75(1):76–82.

68. Shrestha B, Holcomb JB, Camp EA, et al. Damage-control resuscitation increases successful nonoperative management rates and survival after severe blunt liver injury. J Trauma Acute Care Surg 2015;78(2):336–41.

69. Kowalenko T, Stern S, Dronen S, et al. Improved outcome with hypotensive resuscitation of uncontrolled hemorrhagic shock in a swine model. J Trauma Acute Care Surg 1992;33(3):349–53.

70. Mabry RL, Holcomb JB, Baker AM, et al. United States army rangers in Somalia: an analysis of combat casualties on an urban battlefield. J Trauma Acute Care Surg 2000;49(3):515–29.

71. Burris D, Rhee P, Kaufmann C, et al. Controlled resuscitation for uncontrolled hemorrhagic shock. J Trauma 1999;46:216–23.

72. Holmes JF, Sakles JC, Lewis G, et al. Effects of delaying fluid resuscitation on an injury to the systemic arterial vasculature. Acad Emerg Med 2002;9:267–74.

73. Sondeen JL, Coppes VG, Holcomb JB. Blood pressure at which rebleeding occurs after resuscitation in swine with aortic injury. J Trauma 2003;54(5 Suppl): S110–7.

74. Bickell WH, Wall MJ Jr, Pepe PE, et al. Immediate versus delayed fluid resuscitation for hypotensive patients with penetrating torso injuries. N Engl J Med 1994;331(17):1105–9.

75. Wall MJ Jr, Granchi TS, Liscum K, et al. Delayed versus immediate fluid resuscitation in patients with penetrating trauma: subgroup analysis. J Trauma 1995; 39:173.

76. Schreiber MA, Meier EN, Tisherman SA, et al. A controlled resuscitation strategy is feasible and safe in hypotensive trauma patients: results of a prospective randomized pilot trial. J Trauma Acute Care Surg 2015;78(4):687.

77. Spinella PC, Perkins JG, Grathwohl KW, et al. Effect of plasma and red blood cell transfusions on survival in patients with combat related traumatic injuries. J Trauma 2008;64(2 Suppl):S69–77 [discussion: S77–8].

78. Duchesne JC, Hunt JP, Wahl G, et al. Review of current blood transfusions strategies in a mature level I trauma center: were we wrong for the last 60 years. J Trauma 2008;65:272–6 [discussion: 276–8].

79. Maegele M, Lefering R, Paffrath T, et al, Working Group on Polytrauma of the German Society of Trauma Surgery (DGU). Red-blood-cell to plasma ratios transfused during massive transfusion are associated with mortality in severe multiple injury: a retrospective analysis from the Trauma Registry of the Deutsche Gesellschaft für Unfallchirurgie. Vox Sang 2008;95(2):112–9.

80. Teixeira PG, Inaba K, Shulman I, et al. Impact of plasma transfusion in massively transfused trauma patients. J Trauma 2009;66(3):693–7.

81. Brown LM, Aro SO, Cohen MJ, et al. A high fresh frozen plasma: packed red blood cell transfusion ratio decreases mortality in all massively transfused trauma

patients regardless of admission international normalized ratio. J Trauma 2011; 71(2 Suppl 3):S358–63.

82. Sperry JL, Ochoa JB, Gunn SR, et al. Inflammation the Host Response to Injury Investigators. An FFP: PRBC transfusion ratio >/=1:1.5 is associated with a lower risk of mortality after massive transfusion. J Trauma 2008;65:986.

83. Rowell SE, Barbosa RR, Diggs BS, et al. Effect of high product ratio massive transfusion on mortality in blunt and penetrating trauma patients. J Trauma 2011;71(2 Suppl 3):S353–7.

84. Pati S, Matijevic N, Doursout MF, et al. Protective effects of fresh frozen plasma on vascular endothelial permeability, coagulation, and resuscitation after hemorrhagic shock are time dependent and diminish between days 0 and 5 after thaw. J Trauma 2010;69(Suppl 1):S55–63.

85. Watson JJ, Pati S, Schreiber MA. Plasma transfusion: history, current realities, and novel improvements. Shock 2016;46(5):468–79.

86. Sillesen M, Johansson PI, Rasmussen LS, et al. Fresh frozen plasma resuscitation attenuates platelet dysfunction compared with normal saline in a large animal model of multisystem trauma. J Trauma Acute Care Surg 2014;76(4): 998–1007.

87. Cardenas JC, Cap AP, Swartz MD, et al. Plasma resuscitation promotes coagulation homeostasis following shock-induced hypercoagulability. Shock 2016; 45(2):166–73.

88. Zielinski MD, Johnson PM, Jenkins D, et al. Emergency use of prethawed Group A plasma in trauma patients. J Trauma Acute Care Surg 2013;74(1):69–75.

89. Matijevic N, Wang YW, Cotton BA, et al. Better hemostatic profiles of never-frozen liquid plasma compared with thawed fresh frozen plasma. J Trauma Acute Care Surg 2013;74(1):84–90 [discussion: 90–1].

90. Radwan ZA, Bai Y, Matijevic N, et al. An emergency department thawed plasma protocol for severely injured patients. JAMA Surg 2013;148(2):170–5.

91. Novak DJ, Bai Y, Cooke RK, et al. Making thawed universal donor plasma available rapidly for massively bleeding trauma patients: experience from the Pragmatic, Randomized Optimal Platelets and Plasma Ratios (PROPPR) trial. Transfusion 2015;55(6):1331–9.

92. Camazine MN, Hemmila MR, Leonard JC, et al. Massive transfusion policies at trauma centers participating in the American College of Surgeons Trauma Quality Improvement Program. J Trauma Acute Care Surg 2015;78(6):S48–53.

93. Holcomb JB, Pati S. Optimal trauma resuscitation with plasma as the primary resuscitative fluid: the surgeon's perspective. Hematology Am Soc Hematol Educ Program 2013;2013:656–9.

94. Holcomb JB, Wade CE, Michalek JE, et al. Increased plasma and platelet to red blood cell ratios improves outcome in 466 massively transfused civilian trauma patients. Ann Surg 2008;248(3):447–58.

95. Perkins JG, Cap AP, Spinella PC, et al. An evaluation of the impact of apheresis platelets used in the setting of massively transfused trauma patients. J Trauma 2009;66:S77–85.

96. Zink KA, Sambasivan CN, Holcomb JB, et al. A high ratio of plasma and platelets to packed red blood cells in the first 6 hours of massive transfusion improves outcomes in a large multicenter study. Am J Surg 2009 May;197(5): 565–70 [discussion: 570].

97. Inaba K, Lustenberger T, Rhee P, et al. The impact of platelet transfusion in massively transfused trauma patients. J Am Coll Surg 2010;211:573–9.

98. Holcomb JB, Zarzabal LA, Michalek JE, et al. Increased platelet:RBC ratios are associated with improved survival after massive transfusion. J Trauma 2011; 71(2 Suppl 3):S318–28.

99. Holcomb JB, del Junco DJ, Fox EE, et al, PROMMTT Study Group. The prospective, observational, multicenter, major trauma transfusion (PROMMTT) study: comparative effectiveness of a time-varying treatment with competing risks. JAMA Surg 2013;148(2):127–36.

100. Jacoby RC, Owings JT, Holmes J, et al. Platelet activation and function after trauma. J Trauma 2001;51:639–47.

101. Sirajuddin S, Valdez C, DePalma L, et al. Inhibition of platelet function is common following even minor injury. J Trauma Acute Care Surg 2016;81(2):328–32.

102. Wohlauer MV, Moore EE, Thomas S, et al. Early platelet dysfunction: an unrecognized role in the acute coagulopathy of trauma. J Am Coll Surg 2012; 214(5):739–46.

103. Malone DL, Hess JR, Fingerhut A. Massive transfusion practices around the globe and a suggestion for a common massive transfusion protocol. J Trauma 2006;60(6 Suppl):S91–6.

104. Hess JR, Holcomb JB. Resuscitating PROPPRly. Transfusion 2015;55(6): 1362–4.

105. Joseph B, Azim A, Zangbar B, et al. Improving mortality in trauma laparotomy through the evolution of damage control resuscitation: analysis of 1,030 consecutive trauma laparotomies. J Trauma Acute Care Surg 2017;82(2):328–33.

106. Cotton BA, Dossett LA, Au BK, et al. Room for (performance) improvement: provider-related factors associated with poor outcomes in massive transfusion. J Trauma 2009;67:1004–12.

107. Oyeniyi BT, Fox EE, Scerbo M, et al. Trends in 1029 trauma deaths at a level 1 trauma center: Impact of a bleeding control bundle of care. Injury 2017;48(1): 5–12.

108. Snyder CW, Weinberg JA, McGwin G Jr, et al. The relationship of blood product ratio to mortality: survival benefit or survival bias. J Trauma 2009;66(2):358–62.

109. Holcomb JB, Tilley BC, Baraniuk S, et al, PROPPR Study Group. Transfusion of plasma, platelets, and red blood cells in a 1:1:1 vs a 1:1:2 ratio and mortality in patients with severe trauma: the PROPPR randomized clinical trial. JAMA 2015; 313(5):471–82.

110. Demetriades D, Kimbrell B, Salim A, et al. Trauma deaths in a mature urban trauma system: is "trimodal" distribution a valid concept? J Am Coll Surg 2005;201(3):343–8.

111. Fox EE, Holcomb JB, Wade CE, et al, PROPPR Study Group. Earlier endpoints are required for hemorrhagic shock trials among severely injured patients. Shock 2017;47(5):567–73.

112. Kauvar DS, Holcomb JB, Norris GC, et al. Fresh whole blood transfusion: a controversial military practice. J Trauma 2006;61(1):181–4.

113. Murdock AD, BersÈus O, Hervig T, et al. Whole blood: the future of traumatic hemorrhagic shock resuscitation. Shock 2014;41:62–9.

114. Holcomb JB. Damage control resuscitation [review]. J Trauma 2007;62(6 Suppl):S36–7.

115. Spinella PC, Perkins JG, Grathwohl KW, et al. Warm fresh whole blood is independently associated with improved survival for patients with combat-related traumatic injuries. J Trauma 2009;66(4 Suppl):S69–76.

116. Holcomb JB, Spinella PC. Optimal use of blood in trauma patients. Biologicals 2010;38(1):72–7.

117. Golan M, Modan M, Lavee J, et al. Transfusion of fresh whole blood stored (4 degrees C) for short period fails to improve platelet aggregation on extracellular matrix and clinical hemostasis after cardiopulmonary bypass. J Thorac Cardiovasc Surg 1990;99(2):354–60.

118. Cotton BA, Podbielski J, Camp E, et al, Early Whole Blood Investigators. A randomized controlled pilot trial of modified whole blood versus component therapy in severely injured patients requiring large volume transfusions. Ann Surg 2013;258(4):527–32 [discussion: 532–3].

119. Repine TB, Perkins JG, Kauvar DS, et al. The use of fresh whole blood in massive transfusion. J Trauma 2006;60(6 suppl):S59–69.

120. Como JJ, Dutton RP, Scalea TM, et al. Blood transfusion rates in the care of acute trauma. Transfusion 2004;44(6):809–13.

121. Perkins JG, Schreiber MA, Wade CE, et al. Early versus late recombinant factor VIIa in combat trauma patients requiring massive transfusion. J Trauma 2007; 62(5):1095–9.

122. Biffl WL, Smith WR, Moore EE, et al. Evolution of a multidisciplinary clinical pathway for the management of unstable patients with pelvic fractures. Ann Surg 2001;233(6):843–50.

123. Riskin DJ, Tsai TC, Riskin L, et al. Massive transfusion protocols: the role of aggressive resuscitation versus product ratio in mortality reduction. J Am Coll Surg 2009;209:198–205.

124. Holcomb JB. Traditional transfusion practices are changing. Crit Care 2010; 14(3):162.

125. Meredith W, Rutledge R, Hansen AR, et al. Field triage of trauma patients based upon the ability to follow commands: a study in 29,573 injured patients. J Trauma Acute Care Surg 1995;38(1):129–35.

126. McManus J, Yershov AL, Ludwig D, et al. Radial pulse character relationships to systolic blood pressure and trauma outcomes. Prehosp Emerg Care 2005;9(4): 423–8.

127. Holcomb JB. Manual vital signs reliably predict need for lifesaving interventions in trauma patients. J Trauma 2005;59:821–9.

128. Nunez TC, Voskresensky IV, Dossett LA, et al. Early prediction of massive transfusion in trauma: simple as ABC (assessment of blood consumption). J Trauma 2009;66:346.

129. Krumrei NJ, Park MS, Cotton BA, et al. Comparison of massive blood transfusion predictive models in the rural setting. J Trauma Acute Care Surg 2012;72(1): 211–5.

130. Cotton BA, Dosseett LA, Haut EH, et al. Multicenter validation of a simplified score to predict massive transfusion in trauma. J Trauma 2010;69:S33–9.

131. Holcomb JB, Donathan DP, Cotton BA, et al. Prehospital transfusion of plasma and red blood cells in trauma patients. Prehosp Emerg Care 2015;19(1):1–9.

132. Plotkin AJ, Wade CE, Jenkins DH, et al. A reduction in clot formation rate and strength assessed by thrombelastography is indicative of transfusion requirements in patients with penetrating injuries. J Trauma 2008;64(2 Suppl):S64–8.

133. Spinella PC, Holcomb JB. Resuscitation and transfusion principles for traumatic hemorrhagic shock. Blood Rev 2009;23(6):231–40.

134. Cotton BA, Minei KM, Radwan ZA, et al. Admission rapid thrombelastography predicts development of pulmonary embolism in trauma patients. J Trauma Acute Care Surg 2012;72(6):1470–5.

135. Holcomb JB, Minei KM, Scerbo ML, et al. Admission rapid thrombelastography can replace conventional coagulation tests in the emergency department: experience with 1974 consecutive trauma patients. Ann Surg 2012;256(3):476–86.

136. Kaufmann CR, Dwyer KM, Crews J, et al. Usefulness of thrombelastography in assessment of trauma patient coagulation. J Trauma 1997;42:716–22.

137. Cotton BA, Faz G, Hatch QM, et al. Rapid thrombelastography delivers real-time results that predict transfusion within 1 hour of admission. J Trauma 2011;71(2): 407–14 [discussion: 414–7].

138. Kashuk JL, Moore EE, Sawyer M, et al. Postinjury coagulopathy management: goal directed resuscitation via POC thrombelastography. Ann Surg 2010; 251(4):604–14.

139. Johansson PI, Stensballe J, Oliveri R, et al. How I treat patients with massive hemorrhage. Blood 2014;124(20):3052–8.

140. Kashuk JL, Moore EE, Wohlauer M, et al. Initial experiences with point-of-care rapid thrombelastography for management of life-threatening postinjury coagulopathy. Transfusion 2012;52:23.

141. Tapia NM, Chang A, Norman M, et al. TEG-guided resuscitation is superior to standardized MTP resuscitation in massively transfused penetrating trauma patients. J Trauma Acute Care Surg 2013;74(2):378–86.

142. Gonzalez E, Moore EE, Moore HB, et al. Goal-directed hemostatic resuscitation of trauma-induced coagulopathy: a pragmatic randomized clinical trial comparing a viscoelastic assay to conventional coagulation assays. Ann Surg 2016;263(6):1051–9.

143. Moore EE, Moore HB, Gonzalez E, et al. Rationale for the selective administration of tranexamic acid to inhibit fibrinolysis in the severely injured patient. Transfusion 2016;56(Suppl 2):S110–4.

144. Napolitano LM, Cohen MJ, Cotton BA, et al. Tranexamic acid in trauma: how should we use it? J Trauma Acute Care Surg 2013;74(6):1575–86.

145. CRASH-2 Collaborators, Roberts I, Shakur H, Afolabi A, et al. The importance of early treatment with tranexamic acid in bleeding trauma patients: an exploratory analysis of the CRASH-2 randomised controlled trial. Lancet 2011;377: 1096–101.

146. Joseph B, Amini A, Friese RS, et al. Factor IX complex for the correction of traumatic coagulopathy. J Trauma Acute Care Surg 2012;72(4):828–34.

147. Spinella PC, Perkins JG, McLaughlin DF, et al. The effect of recombinant activated factor VII on mortality in combat-related casualties with severe trauma and massive transfusion. J Trauma 2008;64(2):286–93 [discussion: 293–4].

148. Jurkovich GJ, Greiser WB, Luterman A, et al. Hypothermia In trauma victims: an ominous predictor of survival. J Trauma 1987;27(9):1019–24.

149. Ferrara A, MacArthur JD, Wright HK, et al. Hypothermia and acidosis worsen coagulopathy in the patient requiring massive transfusion. Am J Surg 1990; 160:515–8.

150. Cosgriff NM, Ernest E, Sauaia A, et al. Predicting life-threatening coagulopathy in the massively transfused patient: hypothermia and acidosis revisited. J Trauma 1997;42(5):857–62.

151. Martini WZ, Holcomb JB. Acidosis and coagulopathy: the differential effects on fibrinogen synthesis and breakdown in pigs. Ann Surg 2007;246(5):831–5.

152. Hess JR, Holcomb JB. Transfusion practice in military trauma. Transfus Med 2008;18(3):143–50.

Ultrasound and Other Innovations for Fluid Management in the ICU

Mark Blum, MD, Paula Ferrada, MD*

KEYWORDS

- Image based resuscitation • Ultrasound • Echocardiogram

KEY POINTS

- Ultrasound is a user-dependent tool that can help guide therapy.
- The use of ultrasound to guide central line placement decreases complication rates.
- Cardiac ultrasound can help with the diagnosis of cases of hypotension.
- Lung ultrasound and pleura ultrasound are useful adjuncts for diagnosis causes of desaturation.
- Abdominal ultrasound can help in rapid visitation of fluid and intra-abdominal structures.

INTRODUCTION

Guiding therapy for a rapidly deteriorating patient continues to be an issue of interest in critical care. Having a tool that can aid in the decision making to treat shock expeditiously can be lifesaving in some instances. Please see Bracken A. Armstrong and colleagues' article, "Sepsis and Septic Shock Strategies," in this issue, for a discussion on the uses of ultrasound to rapidly diagnose causes of deterioration and guide therapy.

ULTRASOUND TO GUIDE THERAPY IN THE ICU

Ultrasound has been introduced in the past couple decades as a tool to guide therapy for critically ill patients.[1] The advantages of this technique are that it offers imaging immediately, it is portable, and it does not carry ionizing energy; therefore, the consequences of repeating the test are minimal.[2] It is, however, operator dependent. Because it is a diagnostic modality that depends on the transition of sound waves into the tissues, anything that interferes with the sound waves can result in poor

The authors have nothing to disclose.
Trauma, Critical Care and Emergency Surgery, Department of Surgery, VCU, PO Box 980454, Richmond, VA 23298-0454, USA
* Corresponding author. West Hospital, 15th Floor, East Wing, 1200 East Broad Street, Richmond, VA 23298.
E-mail address: pferrada@mcvh-vcu.edu

Surg Clin N Am 97 (2017) 1323–1337
http://dx.doi.org/10.1016/j.suc.2017.07.009
0039-6109/17/© 2017 Elsevier Inc. All rights reserved.

visualization. Air is not a good conductor of sound; large individuals can be more difficult to image as well as patients with subcutaneous edema and emphysema.[3]

The use of this tools extends from guiding procedures to volume status assessment. This article describes the basics of and technique for performing the test on each organ system.

FUNDAMENTALS

Ultrasound is a mechanical wave that requires a medium to travel. In the case of diagnostic ultrasound, these waves travel through human tissue.[2,4,5] Fluid is a good conductor of ultrasound and can provide a good interface to visualize organs around what otherwise is not visible. An example of this is visualizing the lung in the presence of a pleural effusion.

Ultrasound machines consist of electric pulse generators, transducers, systems for processing received echoes, and image display screens. The key elements of transducers (probes) are piezoelectric crystals, matching layers, backing material, cases, and electrical cables.

There are several transducer types. This article discusses phased array, linear array, and curved array.

The cardiac probe or phased array transducer has a low-frequency capacity and more penetration to tissues (2–4 MHz on average). It also has small footprints that produce images of sector format through small acoustic windows (eg, cardiac and cranial applications). Because these probes have more crystals than a curvilinear probe, the image is crisper. If an operator does not have a curvilinear probe, the phased array transducer can be used to obtain abdominal images as well.

Linear array transducers are traditionally used to visualize superficial structures because of their higher frequency and lower penetration (7–15 MHz in average). These probes are also useful to evaluate muscle and the pleura (**Fig. 1**).

Curvilinear transducers are optimal for abdominal imaging. They have lower frequencies and higher penetration (2–6 MHz). It is hard to place these probes in the thoracic cavity since their shape against the ribs. If an operator does not have a cardiac probe, however, these can also be used for cardiac visualization.

B mode refers to brightness. It uses the amplitude of the reflected ultrasound signals, which is converted into a gray-scale image. M mode measures the movement of structures along a single line (axis of the ultrasound beam). It is useful in evaluating heart wall or valve motion (echocardiography), hemodynamic status (inferior vena cava [IVC] diameter and motion), and lung sliding or movement of the diaphragm.

Doppler mode measures changes in frequency caused by sound reflections off a moving target (Doppler effect), usually blood, in common bedside practice. There are different versions of Doppler mode, including Doppler duplex, continuous-wave Doppler, and pulsed-wave Doppler[6–11] (**Fig. 2**).

VASCULAR ULTRASOUND

Ultrasound is used in many settings in critical care medicine in evaluating, diagnosing, and treating vascular disease. Ultrasound is essential in the ICU for procedures done with its guidance for safer and more efficient patient care.

Arterial

Aorta
Although CT scan is currently the confirmatory study to evaluate for aortic pathology, ultrasound can be used to visualize many different aortic disease processes and often is a useful adjunct in its work-up.

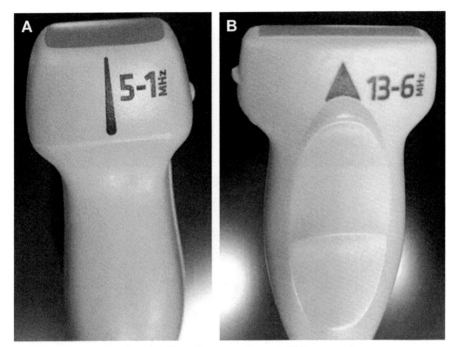

Fig. 1. Two types of probes. (*A*) Phased array probe and (*B*) linear probe.

Abdominal aortic aneurysm is a disease in which there is localized enlargement of the abdominal aorta, generally leading to weakening of wall strength and risking rupture. Ultrasound can be used to estimate the anteroposterior and transverse abdominal aortic aneurysm diameter from outer wall to outer wall. It can also visualize thrombus, plaque, intramural hematoma, or leakage with free fluid in the abdomen and/or retroperitoneum.

Aortic dissection is defined as separation of the aortic intima from the media. Transesophageal echocardiography (TEE) is the ultrasound modality of choice to visualize an intimal flap, which is defined as an echogenic band floating in an anechoic lumen. True and false lumens can be distinguished with duplex ultrasound, in which the false lumen shows decreased flow or absent flow in the case of thrombosis.

Peripheral arterial disease can be caused by atherosclerosis, thromboembolism, or vasospasm. It is more common in the lower extremities, with the superficial femoral artery the most common site of stenosis. B mode imaging can be used to visualize arterial wall thickening, lumen narrowing, or filling defects, whereas duplex ultrasound is used to determine the peak systolic velocity, flow direction, and changes in flow (triphasic to biphasic or monophasic).

Pseudoaneurysms are defined as a pulsatile encapsulated hematomas in communication with the lumen of a ruptured vessel via a patent neck, and their walls may consist of adventitia, hematoma, and fibrous tissue. Duplex imaging shows a yin-yang sign, or the bidirectional flow due to swirling of blood within the aneurysm. They are generally caused by catheterization of the vessel or trauma. Pseudoaneurysms can be treated with ultrasound-guided compression (60%–90% success rate) or with injection of thrombin into the neck of the pseudoaneurysm.[12–14]

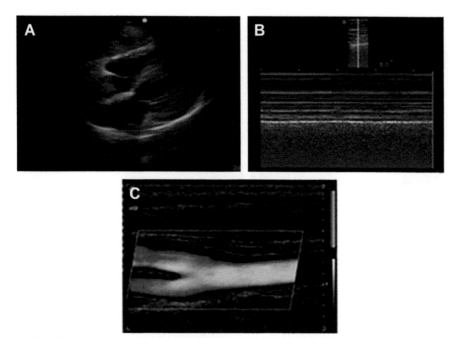

Fig. 2. Different modes of ultrasound. (*A*) B mode, also referred to as brightness mode, which is the regular 2-D mode, used to see when performing ultrasound. This particular window shows the subcostal view of the heart, 4 chambers, and the liver superiorly. The right ventricle is the structure located close to the liver edge. (*B*) M mode or motion. This particular image shows the normal lung with the seashore sign. (*C*) Color Doppler mode. Notice it is yellow because of the amount of turbulence captured by the image. Color Doppler is red when the structure imaged is moving toward the probe and blue when moving away. Other colors show when turbulence is captured either because of turbulent flow or because of the probe positioning related to the flow itself.

Ultrasound to guide arterial line placement

Arterial catheterization can be supplemented by use of ultrasound guidance. Ultrasound-guided arterial catheterization increases first-pass success rates by 71% over landmark techniques. Sites that can be visualized with ultrasound (high-frequency transducer) include the radial, femoral, axillary, and dorsalis pedis arteries.

For the purpose of ICU ultrasound, evaluation of the extremities can help when guiding procedures as well as identifying injury.

Venous

The deep venous system is assessed with ultrasound to evaluate for deep venous thrombosis (DVT). This is executed with a high-frequency linear probe (5–10 MHz) with the use of compression ultrasonography. Studies are performed in a transverse orientation, because errors can be produced in longitudinal axis.

Compressible veins are considered patent and without thrombus, whereas noncompressible veins are diagnostic of thrombus. If a thrombus is visible within the vein, compression is not required and may be rarely associated with dislodgement of the thrombus. Doppler and spectral analysis can be added to study but has not been shown to increase accuracy over compression ultrasound alone. DVT studies can be performed in both the upper and lower extremities.

For upper extremity studies, the patient should be positioned supine, in Trendelenburg position with the arm externally rotated and abducted 90° from the chest. The head should be rotated to the contralateral side and elevated above the extremity to avoid external compression of the distal subclavian vein between the first rib and clavicle. Target vessels are the internal jugular, subclavian, axillary, and brachial veins.

The examination is started by finding the paired brachial veins in the antecubital fossa. Compression should be performed every few centimeters caudal until the subclavian vein is reached. At this point, compression cannot be performed due to the clavicle preventing compression. Although the basilic vein is a superficial vein, a large clot burden at its junction with the brachial vein to form the axillary vein may be of clinical significance. Sequential compression of the internal jugular vein should be performed next in a similar fashion.

To evaluate the subclavian vein, changes in size of the superior vena cava and IVC with respiration and the sniff maneuver should be noted. A collapse of at least 60% should be expected. With complete thrombosis, there should be no response to these respiratory maneuvers as well as asymmetrically dilation when compared with the opposite side.

To study the lower extremity, patient position should be supine, reverse Trendelenburg position with flexion of the knee and external rotation of the hip. The popliteal vein can be imaged in prone position, with knee flexion of 45° or in lateral decubitus position. Compression ultrasound begins in the groin at the level of the inguinal ligament to identify the common femoral vein (CFV). The probe is the sequentially moved every few centimeters, checking for compressibility. The important compression points needed for an adequate study include

- CFV at inguinal ligament
- Junction of great saphenous vein and CFV
- Bifurcation of CFV into superficial femoral vein and deep femoral vein
- Popliteal vein
- Trifurcation of popliteal vein

The examination can also include compression ultrasound of the whole length of the superficial femoral vein and below-the-knee veins, including the soleal, gastrocnemius, and peroneal veins, although thrombus in these veins is often observed and not treated initially unless symptomatic or multiple.[15]

Central line placement under ultrasound

Ultrasound-guided central venous access greatly improves patient safety by reducing complications by reducing the number of attempts and duration. A linear array transducer (7–15 MHz) is generally used due to the high resolution and superficial location of the veins.

Vascular scanning prior to the procedure helps identify anatomy and any abnormalities, such as thrombosis or anatomic barriers (small size and location in relation to artery). Veins are typically elliptical or ovoid, thin walled, and readily collapsible, whereas arteries are circular, thick walled, less compressible, and pulsatile.

Internal jugular vein cannulation via ultrasound guidance is the standard of care currently in the ICU. Multiple studies show an increase successful placement and first attempt rates, along with decreased arterial puncture rate. This can be performed with transducer in longitudinal or transverse mode.

The procedure is done with direct visualization of needle entering the vein while at the same time getting flashback of venous blood in the syringe. A wire is then inserted into the needle and advanced with no resistance. Using a Seldinger technique, a dilator and then the catheter itself are placed into the vein and secured in place with sutures. Cardiac monitoring should be performed to watch for ectopy when advancing the wire or the catheter.

Femoral vein catheterization is assisted by ultrasound guidance with many of the same features as internal jugular cannulation. It improves first attempt rates and decreased arterial puncture rates. The procedure is performed in a similar fashion to jugular vein catheterization.

Subclavian vein cannulation can also be guided under ultrasound when done distally because the clavicle can produce shadowing allowing for poor visualization of the vessel.[16] (**Fig. 3**).

ABDOMINAL ULTRASOUND

Abdominal ultrasonography is performed with a phased array (1–5 Mhz) or curvilinear (1–3 Mhz) probe. It can be used in the diagnosis and treatment of many different organ pathologies.

In trauma management, the focused assessment with sonography for trauma (FAST) examination is commonly used a screening test to evaluate for fluid in the abdomen in the unstable patient. It consists of 4 views: subxyphoid, perihepatic, persplenic, and pelvis.

The subxyphoid view is used to evaluate for pericardial effusion and cardiac function. Perihepatic views can visualize fluid in the right pleural cavity, subphrenic, and

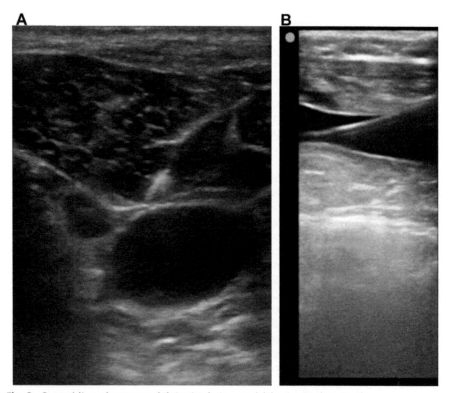

Fig. 3. Central line placement. (*A*) Sagittal view and (*B*) wire in the vessel.

Morison pouch, with the perisplenic view showing any fluid in the left upper quadrant or paracolic gutter. The pelvic view visualizes fluid by the pelvic organs, including bladder, uterus, and rectum (**Fig. 4**).

Ultrasound can be used as both a diagnostic and therapeutic tool in the management of ascites. Ascites can be tapped or drained under ultrasound guidance at the bedside.

Ultrasound is also the first line of imaging recommended in the work-up of biliary conditions. In evaluating the gallbladder, the probe is placed in the right upper quadrant, just below the costal margin in a transverse or longitudinal orientation. In these windows, biliary pathology, including gallstones, gallbladder sludge, thickened gallbladder wall, pericholecystic fluid, and dilated common bile ducts and stones, can be diagnosed.

The urinary system can also be evaluated using ultrasound. Renal ultrasound is performed in the midaxillary line, in approximately the ninth interspace for the right kidney and slightly more cephalad for the left kidney (seventh to eighth interspaces) in both longitudinal and transverse orientations.

Renal imaging includes visualization of the outer renal parenchyma and inner hypoechoic renal sinus. Generally, the ureter and collecting system in not easily visualized under ultrasound but with obstruction can be seen as hydronephrosis. Duplex imaging of the kidney is also performed and can evaluate renal artery flows and intraparenchymal flow and resistive index, which can be useful in the work-up of acute renal failure.

Bladder ultrasound can be used to evaluate for urinary retention and work-up of low urine output. Anatomic causes, such as tumor, clot, diverticulum, and stones, can be easily visualized. A fluid-filled bladder is best to delineate the bladder wall if needed.

Scrotal ultrasounds are performed with a high-frequency linear transducer (7–15 MHz). They are used in the evaluation of epididymis, testicular torsion, and scrotal trauma. Using B-mode and Doppler signals, evaluation of arterial and venous flow, testicular vascularity, and scrotal fluid hydrocele or hematocele can be performed.[2,3,13,14,17]

LUNG AND PLEURA

Ultrasound examination of the pleural cavity, when compared with CT or x-ray technology, is inexpensive and avoids ionizing radiation exposure.

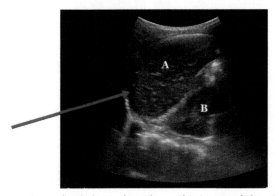

Fig. 4. The red arrow shows fluid above the spleen. This is one of the pitfalls of the FAST examination and the reason why it is important to visualize the entire spleen. A represents the spleen, B represents the kidney. Above the arrow, the diaphragm can be seen as a very bright liner structure.

The performance of bedside ultrasound precludes the need to transport acutely ill patients. The quality and sensitivity of ultrasound imaging for the diagnosis of pneumothorax are exceptional, in contrast to portable chest x-ray films that can have a sensitivity as low as 30% in some series.

Ultrasound has also proved effective in determining the presence and cause of effusions, based on the internal fluid echogenicity and associated changes in pleura and adjacent lung parenchyma.

A lines result from ultrasound reverberations that take place between the pleural interface and the transducer surface, producing repetitive horizontal hyperechoic lines, depicted distal to the pleura at equally spaced intervals. This is found in normal lung imaging.

B lines (also known as comet tails or lung rockets) are ultrasound artifacts caused by the reflection of ultrasound beams within thickened interlobular septa just under the pleura and are seen as hyperechoic vertical lines arising from the pleural line. A predominance of B lines can be indicative of pulmonary edema. B lines are 3 mm or less apart in cardiogenic or fluid overload whereas B lines that are 7 mm apart generally represent interstitial pulmonary edema (**Fig. 5**).

Lung sliding is defined as the motion of the visceral pleura against the parietal pleura as a result of inspiration and expiration. M mode (seashore sign) is viewed as continuous hyperechoic horizontal lines above the pleura representing the static chest wall, followed by a granulous pattern below the pleural line. This sandy pattern is created by the moving lung tissue during respiration.

Pneumothorax can be evaluated using ultrasound in clinically stable and unstable patients. Lung point is an ultrasound imaging finding in which the boundary of the noncollapsed part of the lung moves into the air-filled thorax replacing the signs of pneumothorax. The presence of lung point together with the lack of lung sliding 100% specific for identifying pneumothorax.

Lung pulse refers to subtle lung tissue motion (vibration) normally caused by the cardiac pulse. This appears as distinctive vertical bands in M mode and is most easily

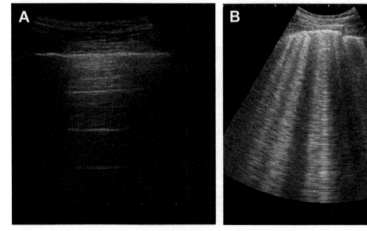

Fig. 5. An example of (*A*) A lines, as horizontal lines; these are an artifact produced by air in the thoracic cavity. (*B*) B lines; these are also called comet tails, start at the pleural surface, and shine down into the thoracic cavity. Abundance of B lines can be seen in patients with pulmonary edema.

viewed with a hyperinflated lung. The absence of lung pulse may imply the loss of lung tissue and is an additional clue for pneumothorax.

Pleural effusion is usually seen in the lateral and posterior basal windows as a hypo-echoic or anechoic space with the compressed lung base floating within. Septations within the effusion, swirling appearance, bilayer effect, and increased echogenicity are highly suggestive of exudate, empyema, or hemothorax. Under ultrasound guidance, this fluid can drained via thoracentesis or with placement of a chest tube. The chest tube can be placed via Seldinger technique with many different sizes of tube available, from 16F to 28F. The chest tube can also be placed via the tradition open technique after visualization of the fluid under ultrasound.[2,3]

Pneumothorax

Use of ultrasound for detection of pneumothorax is extensively validated. The presence of lung sliding in an area spanning 3 intercostal spaces has been shown to have a negative predictive value of 100% by Lichtenstein and colleagues.[18] Another prospective study by the same group in 73 ICU patients revealed that presence of A lines (horizontal artifacts) had a sensitivity and a negative predictive value of 100% and a specificity of 60% for the diagnosis of pneumothorax. When the presence of A line and absent lung sliding are combined, they had a sensitivity and a negative predictive value of 100% and a specificity of 96.5%.[2,3,6,19]

Technique

Using the linear high-frequency probe, start scanning obtaining images from the second intercostal space on the midclavicular line. Then lower the probe to the fourth intercostal space on anterior axillary line. Continue to the sixth intercostal space on the midaxillary line and, the eighth intercostal space on the posterior axillary line.

Air usually rises to the top when a patient is supine. Scanning patients from top down allows for a prompt diagnosis.

Fluid in the Pleural Space

Gravity brings the fluid down to the back with a patient in supine. This can allow for rapid visualization in the most dependent anatomic locations, such as fluid in the thoracic cavity (**Fig. 6**).

Technique

Use the low-frequency probe (curvilinear or phased array). Place it in the posterior axillary line on the vertical position with the cursor pointing superiorly. This view in both sides allows for visualization of the diaphragm and the lung. If there is a pleural effusion, the fluid and the lung bathing in this fluid can be seen.

Other Lung Pathology

The excessive presence of B lines can signify pulmonary edema. With the low-frequency probe it is possible to visualize a consolidation or a complete lobe collapse.

Once an operator is comfortable using this tool, more diagnostic applications become available.[2,3,6,19]

CARDIAC

All cardiac imaging should be performed with a phased array, low-frequency probe (typically 2–5 MHz). The ideal windows for this test are parasternal long axis, parasternal short axis, apical 4-chamber, subxyphoid long axis, and subxyphoid IVC.

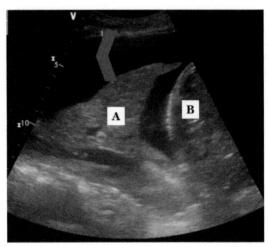

Fig. 6. Pleural effusion delineated by the red arrow. (*A*) The collapsed lung and (*B*) the liver below the diagram.

To perform the parasternal long axis view, the transducer marker should point toward the right shoulder with the probe placed next to the sternum, between the third and fifth intercostal spaces. The resultant view allows 2-D and M-mode evaluation of structures, including the left ventricle, outflow tract, and aortic root. Color Doppler is usually also applied to the aortic and mitral valves. Zoomed views of the aortic and mitral valves may also allow more detailed structural and functional evaluation. By angling the transducer, it may also be possible to acquire right ventricular inflow and pulmonary artery long axis views. From the parasternal long axis view, the proximal ascending aorta is potentially visualized by moving the transducer up 1 interspace.

The parasternal short axis view is done by rotating the probe is rotated until it is at 90° from the initial long axis position. This window is used to observe the left ventricle, in particular contractility and filling. Right ventricular enlargement can be seen in this window, such as in cases of massive pulmonary embolism and right heart failure.

The apical 4-chamber window is best viewed with patients in left lateral decubitus positon but is often not possible in ICU patients due to hypotension, trauma, or critical illness. This window is obtained by placing the probe horizontally over the point of maximal impulse, generally under the left nipple. This view allowed to evaluate left and right ventricular function, valvular function, and atrial anatomy.

The subxyphoid long axis window is viewed with the probe placed in the epigastric area just underneath the xiphoid process and angled cranially pointing toward the left shoulder. This window can view all 4 chambers of the heart in the same plane as well as assess for pericardial effusion. It is used as part of the FAST examination and, therefore, is most commonly used as an initial evaluation by surgeons[1,2,8,11,20–25] (**Figs. 7** and **8**).

Inferior Vena Cava Long Axis Views

There is enough literature to prove or disprove the usefulness of the IVC size and variation for fluid status management. This is a dynamic measurement; I changes with the intrathoracic pressure so the size of the vessel and collapsibility have to be taken into clinical context.

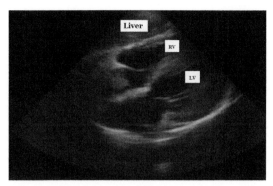

Fig. 7. The subcostal or subxyphoid view. The liver is located in the most superior part of the screen. LV, left ventricle; RV, right ventricle.

A flat IVC (collapsing >50% with respiratory variation) along with an empty heart (kissing ventricles) are diagnostic of hypovolemia in hypotensive patients.

Increased intrathoracic pressure can cause an increase IVC size even in the face of hypovolemia. Therefore, a full IVC cannot rule out hypovolemia, and other clinical parameters should be measured, such as urine output, strove volume variation, and so forth. IVC can be visualized in the subcostal view, right midclavicular line, or posterior midaxial line.[1,2,8,11,20–25]

Diagnostic Uses in Cardiac Ultrasound

Pericardial effusion/tamponade can be viewed in the subcostal, parasternal, and apical views. The size of effusion can be approximated by the distance between the pericardium and epicardial border and can be serous or hemorrhagic depending on history and clinical setting (**Fig. 9**). Pericardial tamponade occurs when the effusion causes a compression of the right ventricle, resulting in a decrease in cardiac filling and, therefore, cardiac output. This causes equilibration of pressures in the heart chambers.

Ultrasound can be useful in a hypotensive patient with concern for pulmonary embolism. Right ventricular enlargement with a thin ventricular wall, hemodynamic

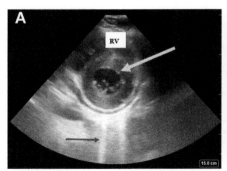
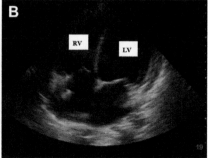

Fig. 8. (*A*) Parasternal short window. The blue arrow indicates the left ventricle. The red arrow shows comet tails emanating from the pericardium into the lung tissue. (*B*) An apical view. LV, left ventricle; RV, right ventricle.

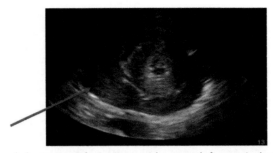

Fig. 9. A parasternal short view of a patient with severe left ventricular hypertrophy. The red arrow indicates the concentric pericardial effusion.

instability, and respiratory distress are highly suggestive of massive pulmonary embolism.

In the correct clinical scenario, trans thoracic echocardiogram (TTE) can be diagnostic of new myocardial ischemia. Signs include regional wall motion abnormalities, new-onset valvular disorders, intracardiac thrombus, and ventricular wall rupture.[1,2,8,11,20–25]

Furthermore, cardiac ultrasound can be used to guide resuscitation to euvolemia in critically ill patients.[15,23] An empty ventricle, hyperdynamic is diagnostic of hypovolemia, in contrast with a full heart with enlargement of the atria and dilation of the IVC, indicating a patient who is not fluid responsive. In some instances, excessive fluid resuscitation can lead to right-sided cardiac dysfunction. An example of a resuscitation protocol guided by ultrasound findings is shown in **Fig. 10**.

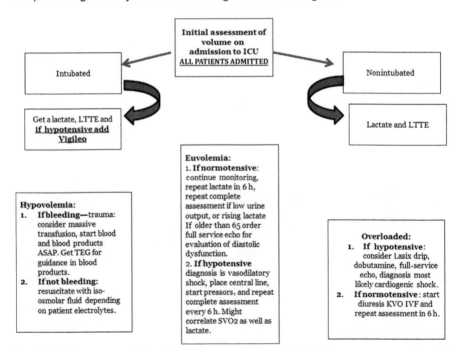

Fig. 10. Initial assessment of volume on admission to ICU. ASAP, as soon as possible; IVF, intravenous fluid; KVO, keep vein open; LTTE: limited transthoracic echocardiogram; PTS, patients; SVO₂, mixed venous O₂ saturation; TEG, thromboelastogram.

OTHER INNOVATIONS
Transesophageal Echocardiogram

The gold standard in cardiac imaging is TEE. Because the probe is in the esophagus, the images obtained are sharper and of much better quality than TTE.

TEE allows for visualization of the cardiac chambers, estimation of volume, and getting a sense for cardiac contractility and the overall function of the right and left ventricles.

TEE is more invasive than a transthoracic study; however, for surgeons this is not more difficult than performing an endoscopy at the bedside.

Smaller probes of easier placement have become available but these produce an image of lesser quality.

Some ultrasound machines used by emergency medicine physicians and surgeons have the capability to allow for TEE probes. These are additional tools in the armamentarium of intensivists, and acquiring expertise and credentialing should be available for physicians who treat these difficult patients.[26]

Transesophageal Doppler

Doppler ultrasound via a probe in the esophagus has been used to measure the blood velocity in the descending aorta. The blood velocity measurement in the descending aorta can be used to calculate stoke volume as a surrogate of intravascular volume.

The flexible probe that is placed in the esophagus has piezoelectric crystals that produce ultrasound images. The probe tip lies along the descending aorta. The velocity of the red blood cells is obtained and converted to flow, using an algorithm. Factors, such as age, gender, weight, and height, are taken into account.

To clarify, this method does not produce 2-D ultrasound images; therefore, the diameter of the descending aorta is not measured but calculated using patient characteristics as well as not having cardiac images to evaluate. It is use merely for volume calculation.[27]

SUMMARY

The use of ultrasound as a tool to guide therapy in acutely ill patients has been well defined. A few decades ago, the FAST examination was introduced to evaluate for free fluid in the abdominal cavity. In the acute trauma setting, free fluid in most cases is attributable to blood outside of the intravascular space. Blood in the abdominal cavity in the presence of hypotension is an absolute indication for operative exploration. Furthermore, the FAST examination was extended to the pleura to visualize intrapleural fluid and diagnose pneumothorax. Cardiac ultrasound has been shown useful to guide therapy in hypotension.

Because the ultrasound machine is portable, all these anatomic evaluations can be moved to wherever a patient in need is. Therefore, the use of this tool has been extended from the initial phase of resuscitation in the emergency department to the ICU.

In more stable situations, acute care surgeons can also use ultrasound to assist in procedures, evaluate for DVT, and evaluate other intra-abdominal organs.

Other innovations to treat deteriorating patients include transesophageal Doppler and TEE. Physicians who treat these sick patents need to be informed of the uses and applications of these tools to benefit critically ill patients.[2,9,26,28–33]

REFERENCES

1. 9th WINFOCUS World Congress on Ultrasound in Emergency and Critical Care. Crit Ultrasound J 2013;6(Suppl 1):A1–32.

2. Ferrada P. Image-based resuscitation of the hypotensive patient with cardiac ultrasound: an evidence-based review. J Trauma Acute Care Surg 2016;80(3): 511–8.

3. Wang G, Ji X, Xu Y, et al. Lung ultrasound: a promising tool to monitor ventilator-associated pneumonia in critically ill patients. Crit Care 2016;20(1):320.

4. Henwood PC, Mackenzie DC, Liteplo AS, et al. Point-of-care ultrasound use, accuracy, and impact on clinical decision making in Rwanda Hospitals. J Ultrasound Med 2017;36(6):1189–94.

5. Mongodi S, Bouhemad B, Orlando A, et al. Modified lung ultrasound score for assessing and monitoring pulmonary aeration. Ultraschall Med 2017. [Epub ahead of print].

6. Calamai I, Greco M, Bertolini G, et al, Italian Group for the Evaluation of Interventions in Intensive Care Medicine (GiViTI). Current adoption of lung ultrasound in Intensive Care Units: an Italian multi-centre survey. Minerva Anestesiol 2017; 83(7):720–7.

7. Montorfano MA, Pla F, Vera L, et al. Point-of-care ultrasound and Doppler ultrasound evaluation of vascular injuries in penetrating and blunt trauma. Crit Ultrasound J 2017;9(1):5.

8. Narasimhan M, Koenig SJ, Mayo PH. Advanced echocardiography for the critical care physician: part 1. Chest 2014;145(1):129–34.

9. Shiloh AL, Savel RH, Paulin LM, et al. Ultrasound-guided catheterization of the radial artery: a systematic review and meta-analysis of randomized controlled trials. Chest 2011;139(3):524–9.

10. Sobolev M, Slovut DP, Lee Chang A, et al. Ultrasound-guided catheterization of the femoral artery: a systematic review and meta-analysis of randomized controlled trials. J Invasive Cardiol 2015;27(7):318–23.

11. Via G, Breitkreutz R, Price S, et al. Detailed echocardiography (echo) protocols for the critical patient. J Trauma 2009;66(2):589–90 [author reply: 91].

12. Chenaitia H, Abrous K, Louis F, et al. Relevance of sonography for retroperitoneal hematoma. Am J Emerg Med 2011;29(7):827–8.

13. Rozycki GS, Knudson MM, Shackford SR, et al. Surgeon-performed bedside organ assessment with sonography after trauma (BOAST): a pilot study from the WTA Multicenter Group. J Trauma 2005;59(6):1356–64.

14. Rozycki GS, Ochsner MG, Feliciano DV, et al. Early detection of hemoperitoneum by ultrasound examination of the right upper quadrant: a multicenter study. J Trauma 1998;45(5):878–83.

15. Miri M, Goharani R, Sistanizad M. Deep vein thrombosis among intensive care unit patients; an epidemiologic study. Emergency 2017;5(1):e13.

16. Hoffman T, Du Plessis M, Prekupec MP, et al. Ultrasound-guided central venous catheterization: a review of the relevant anatomy, technique, complications, and anatomical variations. Clin Anat 2017;30(2):237–50.

17. Rabindranath KS, Kumar E, Shail R, et al. Use of real-time ultrasound guidance for the placement of hemodialysis catheters: a systematic review and meta-analysis of randomized controlled trials. Am J Kidney Dis 2011;58(6):964–70.

18. Lichtenstein DA, Menu Y. A bedside ultrasound sign ruling out pneumothorax in the critically ill. Chest 1995;108(5):1345–8.

19. Chen SW, Fu W, Liu J, et al. Routine application of lung ultrasonography in the neonatal intensive care unit. Medicine 2017;96(2):e5826.

20. Acar Y, Tezel O, Salman N, et al. 12th WINFOCUS world congress on ultrasound in emergency and critical care. Crit Ultrasound J 2016;8(Suppl 1):12.

21. Amini R, Stolz LA, Hernandez NC, et al. Sonography and hypotension: a change to critical problem solving in undergraduate medical education. Adv Med Educ Pract 2016;7:7–13.
22. Ferrada P, Evans D, Parker S, et al. 4107 limited echocardiogram examinations performed by intensivists: a surgeon-driven multidisciplinary program. Am Surg 2017;83(1):78–81.
23. Ferrada P, Vanguri P, Anand RJ, et al. A, B, C, D, echo: limited transthoracic echocardiogram is a useful tool to guide therapy for hypotension in the trauma bay–a pilot study. J Trauma Acute Care Surg 2013;74(1):220–3.
24. Ferrada P, Wolfe L, Anand RJ, et al. Use of limited transthoracic echocardiography in patients with traumatic cardiac arrest decreases the rate of nontherapeutic thoracotomy and hospital costs. J Ultrasound Med 2014;33(10):1829–32.
25. Price S, Via G, Sloth E, et al. Echocardiography practice, training and accreditation in the intensive care: document for the World Interactive Network Focused on Critical Ultrasound (WINFOCUS). Cardiovasc Ultrasound 2008;6:49.
26. Held JM, Litt J, Kennedy JD, et al. Surgeon-performed hemodynamic transesophageal echocardiography in the burn intensive care unit. J Burn Care Res 2016;37(1):e63–8.
27. Atlas G, Brealey D, Dhar S, et al. Additional hemodynamic measurements with an esophageal Doppler monitor: a preliminary report of compliance, force, kinetic energy, and afterload in the clinical setting. J Clin Monit Comput 2012;26(6):473–82.
28. Warnakulasuriya SR, Davies SJ, Wilson RJ, et al. Comparison of esophageal Doppler and plethysmographic variability index to guide intraoperative fluid therapy for low-risk patients undergoing colorectal surgery. J Clin Anesth 2016;34:600–8.
29. Spencer KT, Kimura BJ, Korcarz CE, et al. Focused cardiac ultrasound: recommendations from the American Society of Echocardiography. J Am Soc Echocardiogr 2013;26(6):567–81.
30. Rozycki GS, Ballard RB, Feliciano DV, et al. Surgeon-performed ultrasound for the assessment of truncal injuries: lessons learned from 1540 patients. Ann Surg 1998;228(4):557–67.
31. Ball CG, Williams BH, Wyrzykowski AD, et al. A caveat to the performance of pericardial ultrasound in patients with penetrating cardiac wounds. J Trauma 2009;67(5):1123–4.
32. Abdulrahman Y, Musthafa S, Hakim SY, et al. Utility of extended FAST in blunt chest trauma: is it the time to be used in the ATLS algorithm? World J Surg 2015;39(1):172–8.
33. Brass P, Hellmich M, Kolodziej L, et al. Ultrasound guidance versus anatomical landmarks for subclavian or femoral vein catheterization. Cochrane Database Syst Rev 2015;1:CD011447.

Sepsis and Septic Shock Strategies

Bracken A. Armstrong, MD*, Richard D. Betzold, MD, Addison K. May, MD

KEYWORDS

- Sepsis • Septic shock • Resuscitation • Goal-directed therapy • Critical care

KEY POINTS

- Three therapeutic principles most substantially improve organ dysfunction and survival in sepsis: (1) early, appropriate antimicrobial therapy; (2) restoration of adequate cellular perfusion; and (3) timely source control.
- The new definitions of sepsis and septic shock reflect the inadequate sensitivity, specify, and lack of prognostication of systemic inflammatory response syndrome criteria. Sequential (sepsis-related) organ failure assessment more effectively prognosticates in sepsis and critical illness.
- Inadequate cellular perfusion accelerates injury and reestablishing perfusion limits injury. The best methods to assess perfusion, target therapy, and reestablish adequate perfusion remain controversial.
- Multiple organ systems are affected by sepsis and septic shock and an evidence-based multipronged approach to systems-based therapy in critical illness results in improve outcomes.

INTRODUCTION

Sepsis and septic shock are syndromes of immense clinical importance. Suspected sepsis accounts for more than half a million emergency department visits annually in the United States.[1] Between 2003 and 2007, there was a 71% increase in the number of hospitalizations for sepsis and a 57% increase in hospital costs.[2] In 2013, sepsis was the most expensive reason for hospitalization, accounting for more than $23.7 billion (6.2%) of total US hospital costs and was the second most common reason for hospitalization, accounting for 3.6% of stays.[3] Of those admitted, 50% are treated in the intensive care unit (ICU) representing 10% of all ICU admissions. Surgical patients in particular account for nearly one-third of sepsis cases in the United States.[4] The mortality of sepsis has been reported to be declining from 45% in 1993 to 37% in

The authors have nothing to disclose.
Division of Trauma and Surgical Critical Care, Department of Surgery, Vanderbilt University Medical Center, 1211 21st Ave S Medical Arts Building 404, Nashville, TN 37212, USA
* Corresponding author.
E-mail address: bracken.a.armstrong@vanderbilt.edu

2003, 29% in 2007, and to as low as 18.4% in 2012.[2,5,6] Despite this trend, in another recent examination of 2 large complementary hospital cohorts from 2010 to 2012, sepsis was found to have a mortality range of 34% to 56% and most of those patients were identified to have sepsis at admission.[7] These data emphasize that sepsis mortality remains significant. Although there has been a vast amount of research directed toward improving outcomes in sepsis, 3 therapeutic principles most substantially improve organ dysfunction and survival in sepsis: (1) early, appropriate antimicrobial therapy; (2) restoration of adequate cellular perfusion; and (3) timely source control. Thus, survival is dependent on early recognition and rapid treatment. In the article to follow, the authors summarize recent changes in defining sepsis, highlight pathophysiologic rationale for current therapeutic strategies, and discuss therapeutic approaches to improve outcome.

DEFINITIONS

For more than 2 decades, sepsis had been defined by a combination of the systemic inflammatory response syndrome (SIRS) and the presence of infection (**Fig. 1**).[8,9] The inadequate sensitivity and specificity of SIRS combined with the latest information regarding sepsis pathobiology prompted a recent revised data-driven definition of sepsis and septic shock: the Third International Consensus Definitions for Sepsis and Septic Shock (Sepsis-3) (**Fig. 2**).[10] Sepsis is now defined as life-threatening organ dysfunction caused by a dysregulated host response to infection. Organ dysfunction can be identified as an acute change in the total Sequential (Sepsis-related) Organ Failure Assessment (SOFA) score ≥ 2 points consequent to the infection.[11-13] The term "severe sepsis" was removed from the definitions and deemed redundant. Septic shock is a subset of sepsis in which underlying circulatory,

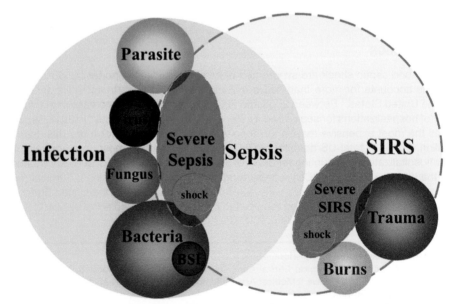

Fig. 1. Early conceptual view of the definition of SIRS, sepsis, severe sepsis, and septic shock whereby infection induces an inflammatory SIRS response. BSI, Blood Stream Infection. (*Adapted from* Bone RC, Balk RA, Cerra FB, et al. Definitions for sepsis and organ failure and guidelines for the use of innovative therapies in sepsis. Chest 1992;101:1645; with permission.)

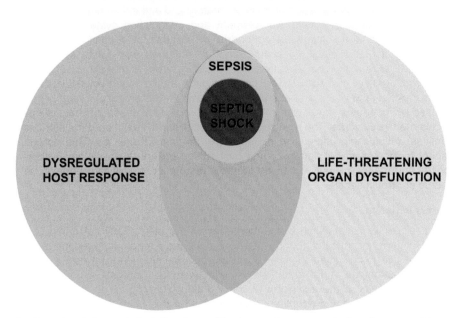

Fig. 2. In Sepsis-3, sepsis is defined as a life-threatening organ dysfunction caused by a dysregulated host response to infection and the term "severe sepsis" has been removed. (*From* Delano MJ, Ward PA. The immune system's role in sepsis progression, resolution, and long-term outcome. Immunol Rev 2016;274:332; with permission.)

cellular, and metabolic abnormalities are associated with a greater risk of mortality than sepsis alone. Septic shock in adults can be identified using clinical criteria of hypotension requiring vasopressor therapy to maintain a mean blood pressure of 65 mm Hg or greater and having a serum lactate level greater than 2 mmol/L, after adequate fluid resuscitation.[14]

The chronologic assessment of organ dysfunction using SOFA has shown to be useful in the prognostication of critically ill patients.[15] SIRS does not prognosticate well in severe sepsis.[16] SIRS criteria has been argued to be overly sensitive and not sufficiently specific, increasing the number of patients diagnosed with sepsis over the years but capturing a larger but less severely ill group of patients.[4,17] In particular, fever and leukocytosis are frequently not present in patients who prove to be infected with organ dysfunction.[18] The SIRS model also implied that sepsis followed a linear trajectory from SIRS to severe sepsis and then septic shock, when in fact it often does not. It has been reported that 68% to 93% of patients admitted to the ICU will meet SIRS criteria[19–21] and that almost half of patients hospitalized in regular wards will meet SIRS criteria at some time during their stay.[22] Using SOFA, the recently revised definitions are aimed to facilitate earlier recognition and more timely management of patients with sepsis, or at risk of developing sepsis, and identifying those with higher prognostic probability of mortality or poor outcome.

PATHOPHYSIOLOGY

Sepsis is an incompletely understood, nonlinear pathophysiologic process involving the activation and dysregulation of proinflammatory and anti-inflammatory responses of the innate immune system, complement and coagulation systems, metabolic changes, hormonal alterations, mitochondrial dysfunction (cytopathic hypoxia), and epithelial and microcirculatory dysfunction.[23–31] Although each of these systems may be characterized as adaptive, their dysregulated activation creates self-reinforcing organ injury through a final common pathway of profound oxidative cellular stress.[32] Although in sepsis, bacterial products initiate this series of events, shock-induced hypoperfusion and cellular hypoxia and products released by host cell injury accelerate the cascade. The resulting degree of cellular dysfunction demonstrates a nonlinear relationship, increasing exponentially as time progresses. This nonlinear aspect to increasing cellular injury and dysfunction provide a physiologic rationale for the importance of early antibiotic therapy, restoration of cellular perfusion, and source control in sepsis.

Process Initiation

Infection results in activation of the innate immune system. Early activation of the innate immune response occurs by interaction of pattern recognition receptors (predominately a group called toll-like receptors) on the cell surface of tissue macrophages, leukocytes, and endothelium with various microbial products. This interaction results in the activation of transcription factors such as nuclear factor (NF)-κβ that regulate the production of numerous cytokines, chemokines, acute phase proteins, adhesion molecules, receptors, and enzymes involved in the host immune response.[24,26,29] Once activated, the innate immune cells kill bacteria through numerous oxidative pathways.

Propagation to Sepsis

Most commonly, the immune response successfully controls infectious insults without a progression to systemic process. However, at times, the magnitude of the infectious insult produces a much more profound systemic activation. As the magnitude increases, activation of nitric oxide synthase leads to excessive nitric oxide production, increasing oxidative stress, loss of vascular resistance, and resulting distributive shock. Hypoxia, hypoperfusion, and oxidative stress results in the proteolytic cleavage of xanthine dehydrogenase (involved in ATP handling through purine metabolism) to xanthine oxidase. Although xanthine dehydrogenase catalyzes the conversion of hypoxanthine to xanthine and the production of nicotinamide adenine dinucleotide (NADH), xanthine oxidase catalyzes the conversion of hypoxanthine to xanthine with the production of the oxidative species superoxide. Excess superoxide and nitric oxide interact to form other potent oxidative species, such as peroxynitrite that directly injure cellular structures such as DNA, mitochondrial cytochromes, signaling proteins, and cellular and mitochondrial membranes. Oxidative injury of mitochondria further accelerates the process, limiting the ability to use oxygen by the cytochrome system to generate ATP (**Fig. 3**).[31,32]

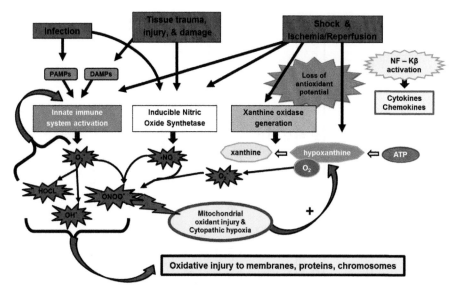

Fig. 3. A simplified model of oxidant stress in sepsis that leads to organ dysfunction. DAMPs, danger-associated molecular patterns; HOCl, hydrochlorous acid; NF-Kβ, nuclear factor; NO, nitric oxide; O_2-, superoxide anion; OH–, hydroxyl anion; ONOO–, peroxynitrite; PAMPs, pathogen-associated molecular patterns.

Organ Dysfunction and Sepsis

The cellular alterations produced by sepsis results in numerous alterations to the host's normal homeostasis, including immune dysregulation; metabolic changes; hormonal alterations; coagulation activation; and mitochondrial, epithelial, and microvascular dysfunction.[23–31] The cumulative effects of dysregulation and cellular injury produce significant organ dysfunction, including central nervous system injury (delirium), lung injury (acute respiratory distress syndrome), cardiovascular dysfunction, acute kidney injury, ileus, and hepatic dysfunction.

DIAGNOSIS

There is no gold standard diagnostic tool in sepsis. The early manifestations of sepsis are not specific or particularly sensitive. However, to limit organ dysfunction and reduce mortality, early recognition is paramount. In patients at risk, a high index of suspicion should be maintained. In patients suspected of possible infection and sepsis, a detailed history, physical examination, appropriate imaging, and laboratory data are all important in establishing the presence of sepsis and its source. There is a fairly strong association between declining organ function and the presence of and outcome from sepsis in patients at risk. This association led to the definition in Sepsis-3 of a change in SOFA score ≥ 2 from baseline in a patient with infection is used to define and diagnose sepsis (**Table 1**). This has been further evaluated and associated with an in-hospital mortality greater than 10% with a predictive value that appears best for patients in the ICU.[13,33]

Sepsis-3 also introduced and validated the concept of the quick SOFA (qSOFA) score as an alert that a non-ICU patient may be deteriorating and may require ICU admission or further workup for sepsis. The Sepsis-3 investigators emphasized

Table 1
Sequential (Sepsis-Related) Organ Function Assessment (SOFA) score

System/Score	0	1	2	3	4
Respiration: Pao_2/Fio_2, mm Hg (kPa)	≥400 (53.3)	<400 (53.3)	<300 (40)	<200 (26.7) with respiratory support	<100 (13.3) with respiratory support
Coagulation: Platelets × $10^3/\mu L$	≥150	<150	<100	<50	<20
Liver: Bilirubin, mg/dL (μmol/L)	<1.2 (20)	<1.2–1.9 (20–32)	2.0–5.9 (33–101)	6.0–11.9 (102–204)	>12.0 (204)
Cardiovascular	MAP ≥70 mm Hg	MAP <70 mm Hg	Dopamine <5 or dobutamine (any dose)[b]	Dopamine 5.1–15 or epinephrine ≤0.1, or norepinephrine ≤0.1	Dopamine >15 or epinephrine. >0.1, or norepinephrine >0.1
Central nervous system: Glasgow coma scale score	15	13–14	10–12	6–9	<6
Renal: Creatinine mg/dL (μmol/L); Urine output, mL/d	<1.2 (110)	1.2–1.9 (110–170)	2.0–3.4 (171–299)	3.5–4.9 (300–440); <500	>5.0 (440): <200

[b] Vasoactive agents are given for at least 1 h and units are μg/kg min.

From Vincent JL, Moreno R, Takala J, et al. Working group on sepsis-related problems of the European Society of Intensive Care Medicine. The SOFA (Sepsis-related Organ Failure Assessment) score to describe organ dysfunction/failure. Intensive Care Med 1996;22(7):708; with permission.

that although qSOFA is not part of the definition of sepsis, it is a simple scoring system that can be done at the bedside in the ward or emergency department without requiring laboratory data, to identify patients who are at risk of developing a poor outcome (death or ICU stay ≥3 days), and who may benefit from more frequent observations, targeted interventions, or transfer to higher levels of care (**Fig. 4**).[10,34] Recent studies have confirmed that using qSOFA outside the ICU has near equivalent[35,36] or greater[37] prognostic accuracy for in-hospital mortality than SIRS or severe sepsis, but another recent study determined that early warning scores (National Early Warning Score [NEWS] and Modified Early Warning Score) perform even more accurately than qSOFA or SIRS.[38] The NEWS is the mandated tool to identify patients outside the ICU at high risk of clinical deterioration in the United Kingdom.[39–42] The early warning scores, like SIRS, have been partly criticized for being overly sensitive[43,44] and qSOFA has been partly criticized for being too specific and not being sensitive enough, possibly capturing patients too late into their clinical decline.[45–47]

In summary, without a gold standard diagnostic tool for sepsis, our recommendation is to foremost, use a high index of suspicion in patients at risk and clinical judgment to recognize infection, early organ dysfunction, and clinical deterioration. Patients with new organ system dysfunction who are at risk should undergo rapid evaluation and if sepsis is confirmed, early appropriate antimicrobial therapy, resuscitation, and source control as achieving these 3 goals is associated with improved outcomes.[48–50]

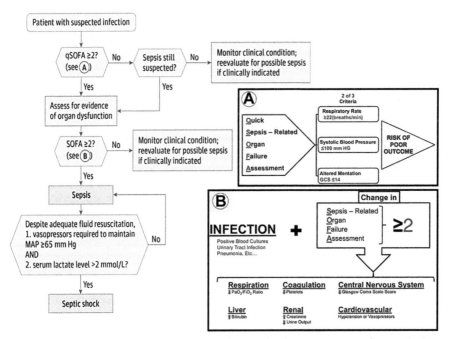

Fig. 4. Identification of patients with sepsis and septic shock using qSOFA and SOFA. (*Adapted from* Singer, Deutschman CS, Seymor CW, et al. The Third International Consensus Definitions for Sepsis and Septic Shock (Sepsis-3). JAMA 2016;315(8):808; and Delano MJ, Ward PA. The immune system's role in sepsis progression, resolution, and long-term outcome. Immunol Rev 2016; 274:332; with permission.)

INITIAL MANAGEMENT: SOURCE CONTROL AND ANTIBIOTIC THERAPY

All discussions of sepsis would be remiss without mentioning the critical concepts of source control and antibiotic therapy, possibly the 2 most important pillars in the treatment of sepsis. The literature is replete with publications about both topics, and representative literature is discussed here.

We recommend early and aggressive source control to remove the infectious nidus and prevent further progression of organ dysfunction. It may be intuitive to most surgeons that the early control of infectious source results in a strong positive impact on patient outcomes. However, data clearly quantifying the impact are somewhat complex. The 2 most common clinical settings in which surgeons are involved in source control are in the treatment of peritonitis and soft tissue infections. A detailed discussion regarding the approach to source control is beyond the scope of this review, although we will discuss the issue of timing. In one prospective study examining the timing to source control in patients with peritonitis and septic shock, Azuhata and colleagues[51] demonstrated that time to initiation of surgery was an independent predictor of survival by multiple logistic regression analysis. In their study cohort, those who had abdominal source control within 2 hours had a 98% 60-day survival, whereas there were no survivors in the group that waited more than 6 hours for initiation of surgery. For source control in necrotizing soft tissue infections, delay in debridement of more than 24 hours has clear deleterious effects on mortality.[52–54]

The second critical pillar in the treatment of sepsis is antibiotic treatment, and both the timing and appropriateness of antibiotic therapy. We recommend that antibiotic agents targeting the most likely pathogens suspected should be initiated as soon as the diagnosis of sepsis and septic shock is reasonably certain. Appropriate cultures should be obtained before antimicrobial therapy is initiated as long as obtaining said cultures does not delay starting the antimicrobials, this should include 2 sets of blood cultures.[55,56] Appropriate cultures before antimicrobial therapy is associated with improved outcomes.[57,58] Although the influence of timing and appropriateness of antibiotic therapy may be altered by other factors, such as the severity of disease and timing and appropriateness of source control, there is a huge body of literature supporting the critical role of this pillar. The influence of timing of antibiotic treatment in patients with severe sepsis and septic shock on outcome was investigated by Ferrer and colleagues[59] in retrospective analysis of 28,150 patients in the Surviving Sepsis Campaign's database. The adjusted in-hospital mortality odds ratio increased significantly with every hour that antibiotic treatment was delayed after 2 hours from when screening criteria were fulfilled, increasing to an odds ratio of 1.52 at 6 hours. Their findings are consistent with numerous other studies of patients with sepsis and shock.[49,60–63] However, as the time window for the introduction of therapy is compressed and variability of patient populations and severity of illness increases in studies, the significance of early antibiotic therapy is more difficult to establish. In a meta-analysis of studies examining 2 separate time windows for therapy, either (1) less than or greater than 3 hours from triage in the emergency department and/or (2) less than or greater than 1 hour from recognition of severe sepsis/septic shock, odds ratios favored earlier therapy, but both confidence intervals crossed 1.[64]

Appropriate empiric coverage of the pathogens involved is also of significant importance. Many studies have demonstrated roughly a 50% reduction in mortality with appropriate versus inappropriate empiric antibiotics.[65–73] In a retrospective analysis of more than 5700 patients admitted to 22 different institutions with septic shock, Kumar and colleagues[68] showed a fivefold increase in hospital mortality for those patients who had inappropriate antibiotic therapy. Thus, an understanding of the most likely pathogens involved in the clinical infection, local sensitivity patterns for likely pathogens, and the presence of various risk factors for the involvement of resistant bacteria is of significant importance if one is to achieve appropriate empiric therapeutic coverage. Risk factors for resistance include antibiotic exposure and acquisition of infection within a health care setting. For example, in gram-negative sepsis, recent antibiotic exposure was associated with a hospital mortality of 51% compared with 34% in those patients who had no recent exposure.[74] In a study of hospital-acquired intra-abdominal infections, 3 agents were required to adequately empirically cover most pathogens and inadequate coverage was an independent predictor of mortality.[71]

Although appropriate and timely antibiotic therapy likely substantially improves outcome in patients with sepsis and septic shock, unnecessary antibiotic exposure contributes to the risk of subsequent antibiotic-resistant infections, may actually increase the risk of all subsequent infectious complications, and likely increases the risk of adverse events due to antibiotics.[67,75–87] Two strategies, in particular, have been advocated to limit unnecessary antibiotic exposure: (1) de-escalation and (2) limiting treatment duration to what can be supported by literature. Broad empiric antibiotic therapy is required in many settings to adequately cover most likely pathogens. Thus, with appropriate culture data, including bacterial species identification and sensitivities, some agents may prove to be unnecessary. To limit antibiotic exposure and its added risk of the development of resistance, de-escalation of therapy is advocated. However, limited data exist to support enhanced clinical outcome for the specific infectious event.[88]

Limiting antibiotic duration to a period that is supported by prospective data also limits unnecessary antibiotic therapy. Until relatively recently, the duration of antibiotic therapy has been driven by empiric observations and an assumed requirement for resolution of inflammatory symptoms and not prospective data. However, good prospective randomized data now exist for both intra-abdominal infection and pneumonia. In both settings, shorter durations of antibiotic therapy have shown to be equivalent to longer courses in multiple disease processes. In the randomized Study to Optimize Peritoneal Infection Therapy (STOP-IT) trial for intra-abdominal infections, 4 days of therapy after source control was equivalent to any longer courses based on resolution of clinical signs of inflammation.[89] Similarly, 8 days of treatment for ventilator-associated pneumonia was equivalent to longer courses of therapy.[86] Persistence of organ dysfunction and signs of infection in the setting of adequate antibiotic therapy should prompt an evaluation of adequate source control or a change in pathogens rather than simply extending therapy.[90,91]

INITIAL MANAGEMENT: RESUSCITATION

The Surviving Sepsis Campaign (SSC) guidelines were first published in 2004, with revisions in 2008 and 2012.[92–96] In March 2017, the fourth revision of the SSC guidelines were published jointly in *Critical Care Medicine* and *Intensive Care Medicine*.[97,98] The updated guideline included 55 international experts representing 25 international organizations involved in the care of sepsis and provides 93 recommendations overall and 18 "best practice recommendations" on the early management of sepsis and septic shock incorporating literature searches through July 2016. Compliance with the implementation of previous iterations of the SSC guidelines and resuscitation bundles into clinical practice have been associated with decreased mortality that is sustained and improves with the time of compliance.[50,99,100] Many of the management strategies discussed in this article are based on these evidence-based consensus guidelines.

Sepsis and septic shock are considered medical emergencies, and initial resuscitation of a patient should occur immediately.[97,98] The landmark study by Rivers and colleagues[48] showed that more rapidly achieving targeted endpoints of resuscitation during the first 6 hours of resuscitation of patients with severe sepsis and septic shock was associated with improved outcome. It is currently recommended that initial resuscitation from sepsis-induced hypoperfusion includes at least 30 mL/kg of intravenous crystalloid fluid given within the first 3 hours (**Fig. 5**),[97,98,101,102] which is associated in the literature with good outcomes as shown in the ARISE, ProCESS, and ProMISe trials.[103–105] Following initial fluid resuscitation, additional fluids should be guided by frequent reassessment of hemodynamic status and evaluation of fluid responsiveness. One of the most significant changes to the new SSC guidelines include recommending the use of dynamic (eg, sequential bedside echocardiography and vena cava ultrasound, pulse or stroke volume variations induced by mechanical ventilation or passive leg raise test) over static variables (intravascular pressures or volumes, such as central venous pressure) to predict volume responsiveness. Central venous pressure (CVP) has been shown in a multiple studies to be a good indicator of preload but to not predict fluid responsiveness.[106–108]

Monnet and colleagues[109] recently published an excellent review for the prediction of fluid responsiveness that includes dynamic variables. A clinician's armamentarium

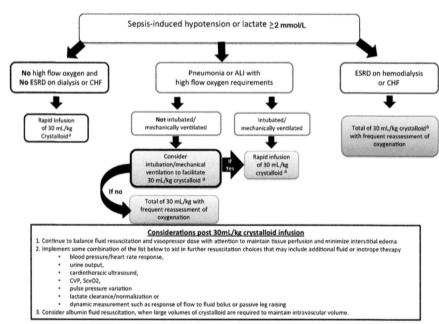

Fig. 5. A proposed application of fluid resuscitation in adult septic shock involving administration of 30 mL/kg of intravenous crystalloid for sepsis-induced hypotension with examples of reassessment tools to assess fluid responsiveness, following that initial fluid infusion. [a] Administer 30 mL/kg crystalloid within first 3 hours. ALI, acute lung injury; CHF, congestive heart failure; CVP, central venous pressure; ESRD, end-stage renal disease; ScvO2, superior vena cava oxygen saturation. (*Adapted from* Dellinger RP, Schorr CA, Levy MM. A users' guide to the 2016 Surviving Sepsis Guidelines. Intensive Care Med 2017;3:300; with permission.)

for assessing fluid responsiveness can include the following: pulse pressure variations/stroke volume variations (median threshold of 12%),[110–112] inferior vena cava diameter variations (distensibility index threshold of 18%, which discriminates fluid responders and nonresponders with 90% sensitivity and 90% specificity),[113] superior vena cava diameter variations (collapse >36% discriminates fluid responders and nonresponders with 90% sensitivity and 100% specificity),[114] passive leg raising (pooled sensitivity of 85% and specificity of 91% when used to measure cardiac output continuously in real time),[115–117] end-expiratory occlusion test (expiratory hold on the ventilator for at minimum 15 seconds, with threshold for increase in cardiac output >5%),[118] "mini"-fluid challenge of 100 mL of colloid (change in the velocity time integral of the left ventricular outflow tract measured with echocardiography, threshold of 10% increase),[119] and "conventional" fluid challenge of 500 mL of crystalloid.[120,121] Monnet and colleagues[109] emphasize to not hold fluids in cases of clear-cut hypovolemic shock and the early phases of septic shock (when fluid has not yet been administered) if waiting for tests of fluid responsiveness, and that fluid should be administered only when it will increase cardiac output, at all times weighing the risks and benefits of volume overload.

EARLY GOAL-DIRECTED THERAPY VERSUS STANDARD THERAPY

Previous resuscitation goals in the SSC guidelines[92–96] were based on early goal-directed therapy (EGDT), which is derived largely from the results of the previously mentioned pivotal trial by Rivers and colleagues,[48] which showed an absolute reduction in mortality of 16% in patients with severe sepsis and septic shock who received goal-directed therapy over standard therapy. EGDT (**Fig. 6**) includes identification of high-risk patients, proper cultures, source control, appropriate antibiotics, and early insertion of a central venous catheter to measure central venous oxygen saturation (ScVO$_2$) with therapy titrated to CVP 8 to 12, mean arterial pressure (MAP) $\geq$65 using vasopressors as necessary, urine output $\geq$0.5 mL/kg per hour, and ScVO$_2$ $\geq$70% within the first 6 hours of resuscitation. It also includes using inotropes and transfusing red blood cells (RBCs) (for a goal hematocrit $\geq$30%) to restore oxygen delivery to meet ScVO$_2$ goals. Standard therapy resuscitated to a CVP of 8 to 12 but did not use ScVO$_2$ monitoring.[48] A meta-analyses of randomized control trials by Gu and colleagues[122] showed a significant survival benefit with EGDT in the subgroup that received early intervention within 6 hours.

Despite these data, concerns with strict adherence to EGDT include the external validity of a single-center experience, and costs, risks, resources, compliance, and the complexity of implementation of EGDT-based sepsis bundles.[123–126] With these concerns in mind, more than a decade after Rivers and colleagues[48] and the first version of the SSC guidelines,[92] the ARISE,[103] ProCESS,[104] and ProMISe[105] trials aimed to compare EGDT with standard therapy: they showed equivalent survival between the two. Yet, in all 3 studies, patients had early risk stratification of high-risk patients using SIRS, lactate screening, early antibiotics, and more than 30 mL/kg of intravenous fluid before randomization, and then reported impressively low sepsis mortality rates for all treatment groups compared with multiple previous observational studies.[127] These revelations imply that the standard treatment of sepsis has changed dramatically via the influence of the SSC guidelines,[92–96] the trial by Rivers and colleagues[48] advocating EGDT, and data showing that delay of appropriate antibiotic administration increases mortality,[49,59,68] as sepsis mortality has progressively decreased since the adoption of these landmark publications.[6] Multiple systemic reviews and meta-analyses that include the data from ARISE, ProCESS, and ProMISe suggest that EGDT still has utility, as it shows no clinical harm, but strict adherence to EGDT may increase vasopressor use and ICU admission, and they suggest that alternative strategies may provide equal reduction in mortality.[97,98,127–132]

It may be inappropriate to entirely abandon EGDT, as there remains evidence for positive outcomes when obtaining certain goal-directed resuscitation endpoints. This warrants a discussion on the evidence for monitoring and optimizing CVP, hemoglobin, ScVO$_2$, lactic acid, and MAP in managing sepsis and septic shock. Knowing these data points can define the hemodynamic phenotype of each patient, which may help optimize and individualize clinical decisions. Recently proposed by Rivers and colleagues,[133] each hemodynamic phenotype, defined by lactic acid level, central

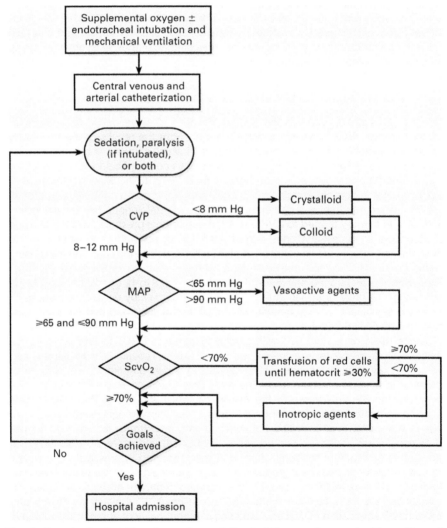

Fig. 6. The classic algorithm for early goal-directed therapy for sepsis. (*From* Rivers E, Nguyen B, Havstad S, et al. Early goal-directed therapy in the treatment of severe sepsis and septic shock. N Engl J Med 2001;345:1371; with permission.)

venous or mixed venous oxygen saturation, and MAP has a predicted, evidence-based mortality that is dependent on the subtypes of hemodynamic derangement and their associated treatment options (**Fig. 7**).[127]

CENTRAL VENOUS PRESSURE

We recommend that CVP alone, as previously discussed, should not be used to guide fluid responsiveness,[106–108,134,135] but the general use of CVP in the treatment of severe sepsis and septic shock has been associated with improved outcomes and can be considered "essential for the measurement of the volume state, the performance of

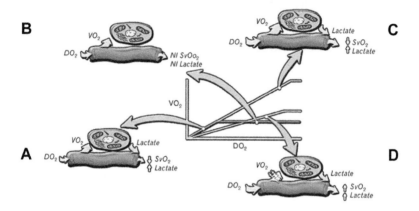

Stage	Haemodynamic Derangements	Lactate	SvO$_2$/ScvO$_2$	MAP	Mortality (%)	Treatment and Comments
A	Hypovolaemia, vasodilatation, myocardial suppression, increased metabolic demands	Normal ↑	↓	↓ Normal	15% (142) 23% (165) 21% (183) 24.9% (184) 35.2% (185) (cryptic shock)	Volume, vasopressors, correct anaemia, inotropic therapy, mechanical ventilation
B	Resuscitated, compensated and vasodilatory	Normal - ↑	Normal	↓ Normal	19.0% (183) 20% (186) 7.7% (187) 11.8% (188) 21% (143)	Hyperdynamic, vasopressors, low-dose corticosteroids
C	Continued DO$_2$ dependency, increased metabolic demands	↑	↓	↓	37.9% (188) 40% (143) 42.9% (187) 48% (184) 51% (142)	Decrease VO$_2$ and further augmentation of DO$_2$
D	Microcirculatory or OER defections and impairment of VO$_2$ Decreased VO$_2$ (dysoxic)	↑	↑	↓	34% (143) 40% (142) 41.7% (188) 52.3% (189) 60.3% (185)	Microcirculatory rescue, source control

Fig. 7. Proposed hemodynamic phenotypes of sepsis and septic shock. DO$_2$, systemic oxygen delivery; OER, oxygen extraction ratio; VO$_2$, systemic oxygen demands. (From Rivers EP, Yataco AC, Jaehne AK, et al. Oxygen extraction and perfusion markers in severe sepsis and septic shock: diagnostic, therapeutic and outcome implications. Curr Opin Crit Care 2015;21:383; with permission.)

the heart and the systemic vascular resistance."[135–137] CVP can be helpful in identifying a specific type of shock, but we recommend using it in conjunction with other variables. Previous SSC guidelines recommended a CVP goal of 8 to 12 mm Hg.[95,96] The updated guidelines no longer give a CVP goal, and instead recommend using dynamic measures (such as sequential echocardiography) over static variables to assess fluid responsiveness.[97,98]

HEMOGLOBIN

We recommend that hemoglobin levels be optimized and individualized based on patient characteristics and oxygen delivery needs. Elevating hemoglobin levels via transfusion may improve oxygen delivery if cardiac output is unchanged. In the setting of persistent hypoperfusion, previous SSC guidelines aimed for a hematocrit greater than 30% for a goal $ScVO_2$ greater than 70% in the first 6 hours.[95,96] The new SSC recommendation is to perform RBC transfusion for hemoglobin levels less than 7.0 g/dL in adults without myocardial ischemia, severe hypoxemia, or acute hemorrhage.[97,98] This is supported by the Transfusion Requirements in Septic Shock (TRISS) trial, which showed no significant difference in 90-day mortality for a transfusion threshold of 7 g/dL versus 9 g/dL in patients with septic shock admitted to the ICU.[138] At long-term follow-up, the TRISS study population showed no difference in mortality rate or health-related quality of life at 1 year.[139] Additionally, in the ProCESS trial, the EGDT group received RBC transfusion for hemoglobin less than 10 g/dL when $ScVO_2$ was less than 70% after initial resuscitation and the standard therapy group received transfusion for hemoglobin less than 7.5 g/dL, there was no significant difference in 60-day in-hospital mortality and 90-day mortality.[104] Of note, the median low level of hemoglobin in the TRISS trial was 8.5 g/dL, the highest lactate level was approximately 2.5 mmol/L, and lowest SCVO2 was approximately 70% in both the ProCESS and TRISS trials, which may indicate their patients had adequate oxygen delivery at baseline. A recent meta-analysis that included mainly observational studies and one randomized controlled trial (RCT) (the TRISS trial), concluded that restrictive RBC transfusion in sepsis has neither benefit nor harm compared with liberal transfusion strategies.[140]

CENTRAL VENOUS OXYGEN SATURATION

We recommend early and sequential ScVO2 monitoring with a goal of normalization if a central venous catheter is in place. $ScVO_2$ represents the balance between oxygen delivery and oxygen consumption as measured by the venous blood returning to the heart. A low $ScVO_2$ is a common finding in sepsis and has been used in EGDT as a measure of inappropriate tissue oxygenation.[48,95,96] A low $ScVO_2$ may indicate a decrease in oxygen delivery (macrocirculatory failure), an increase in oxygen extraction, or both. An $ScVO_2$ less than 70% on ICU admission is associated with a 10.4% increase in 28-day mortality (37.8% vs 27.4%).[141] If $ScVO_2$ remains less than 70% within the first 6 hours of resuscitation, the mortality rate has been reported to increase by 19% (40% for hypoxia vs 21% in patients with normoxia).[142] Yet even if macrocirculatory flow is optimized in sepsis, microcirculatory (distributive) flow is often disrupted,[30,143–147] and in addition mitochondrial dysfunction (cytopathic hypoxia) also occurs.[31,148–153] In other words, oxygen supply may be prevalent, but the tissue never sees it or the tissue cannot use it adequately, which results in an elevated $ScVO_2$. An $ScVO_2 \geq 90\%$ within the first 6 hours of resuscitation increases mortality rate by 13% (34% for hyperoxia vs 21% for normoxia).[142] In the EGDT trial by Rivers and colleagues,[48] initial ScVO2 was 49%, whereas in ARISE, ProCESS, and ProMISe, it was 72.7%, 71.0%, and 70.1%, respectively.[103–105] This is another example of the dissimilarity in the initial patient characteristics and level of sickness compared with the trial by Rivers and colleagues. As a result, recent reviews call into question how many patients in ARISE, ProCESS, and ProMISe required actual intervention to optimize their ScVO2.[127,128]

LACTIC ACID

We recommend early and sequential lactic acid monitoring with a goal of lactic acid level normalization. The previous and current SSC guidelines recommend targeting resuscitation to normalize lactate in patients with elevated lactate levels.[95–98] Traditionally, an elevated lactate level in the shock state has been thought to be a marker of tissue hypoperfusion and secondary anaerobic metabolism.[154] Lactate "clearance" was popularized in the study by Nguyen and colleagues[155] in 2004 that showed that patients with severe sepsis and septic shock with a higher percentage decrease in lactate levels after 6 hours of emergency department intervention had improved mortality, and presumed that lactate normalization was a marker for resolution of global tissue hypoxia. Additional studies in 2010 by Jones and colleagues[156] and Jansen and colleagues,[157] followed by a recent meta-analysis of RCTs, confirmed that the use of lactate "clearance" as a goal to guide early resuscitation therapy was associated with a reduction in the risk of death in adults with sepsis.[158]

Hyperlactatemia has been confirmed to be a marker of illness severity, is a strong predictor of mortality in sepsis, and the estimated mortality reduction from lactate screening approaches 11%.[159–165] Yet it is no longer clear that an elevated serum lactate is a direct measure of tissue hypoperfusion. Hyperlactatemia in sepsis also may be an adaptive response to stress explained by increased aerobic glycolysis, which facilitates improved metabolic efficiency through lactic oxidation.[166–168] Regardless of the mechanism of production, evidence suggests that lactate level reduction of at least 10% at a minimum of 2 hours after resuscitation is an appropriate way to evaluate initial response to the resuscitation and that the addition of lactate level normalization to sepsis bundles is associated with improved mortality.[155,156,169]

MEAN ARTERIAL PRESSURE

We agree with the current SSC guidelines that recommend an initial target MAP of 65 mm Hg in patients with septic shock requiring vasopressors, if fluid resuscitation of 30 mL/kg fails to achieve that goal.[97,98] MAP drives global tissue macrocirculatory perfusion and has variable effects on the microcirculation.[170–173] There is ongoing interest in validation of microcirculatory monitoring measures to improve organ perfusion and tissue oxygenation.[174] Prolonged hypotension in the first 6 hours of resuscitation with an MAP less than 65 mm Hg is one of the most powerful predictors of mortality in septic shock and each hour delay in initiating norepinephrine to reach goal MAP is associated with a 5.3% increase in mortality.[175,176] In one retrospective review of 2849 patients with septic shock who survived to 24 hours, Waechter and colleagues[177] concluded that the focus of the first hour of resuscitation should be aggressive fluid administration and to start vasopressors after the first hour, as the lowest mortality rates were when vasopressors were started between 1 and 6 hours after onset of septic shock.

Higher MAP targets also have been studied, including a large randomized clinical trial of 776 patients by Asfar and colleagues[178] that showed no difference in 28-day or 90-day mortality targeting an MAP of 65 to 70 mm Hg versus 80 to 85 mm Hg, but showed significantly increased rates of cardiac arrhythmia in the higher MAP target group. Other studies have shown that titration of norepinephrine to achieve

MAPs from 65 to 85 mm Hg resulted in an increases in cardiac index but did not change urinary output, arterial lactate levels, or oxygen consumption.[171,179] In Asfar and colleagues,[178] a subgroup of patients with chronic hypertension had lower rates of serum creatinine doubling and decreased need for renal replacement therapy when targeting an MAP of 80 to 85 mm Hg. Recent consensus guidelines recommend targeting an MAP higher than 65 mm Hg in septic patients with a history of hypertension "who improve" with higher blood pressure.[134]

SUMMARY: RESUSCITATION STRATEGY

It is clear that early quantitative resuscitation strategies impact a mortality reduction in sepsis and this has been validated in meta-analyses.[122,180] EGDT still has utility, and the benefit is especially evident in populations of septic patients with predicted high mortality (>40%).[181] It is important to understand the utilization and evidence for CVP, hemoglobin, $ScVO_2$, lactic acid, and MAP to optimize patient outcomes in sepsis and septic shock. We advocate a strategy of resuscitation and hemodynamic monitoring that closely align with expert consensus guidelines.[97,98,134] This also should include frequent measurement of heart rate, blood pressure, body temperature, and physical examination, including capillary refill, urine output, and mental status, with liberal use of a central venous catheter, arterial line, and dynamic measures (preferably sequential bedside echocardiography and vena cava ultrasound) over static variables to predict fluid responsiveness, and in complex patients or patients with refractory shock with right ventricular dysfunction: pulmonary artery catheterization.[134] We encourage an awareness of the unique and dynamic hemodynamic phenotype of each patient and recommend individualizing treatment as appropriate (see **Fig. 7**).[133,141,142,164,182–188]

SYSTEMS-BASED THERAPY
Septic Encephalopathy and Delirium

Septic encephalopathy is a transient and reversible brain dysfunction that affects 30% to 70% of patients with septses.[189,190] It results from inflammatory, ischemic, and neurotoxic processes and is characterized by altered mental status that can range from delirium to coma.[191–193] Delirium is a disturbance and change in baseline attention and awareness, and a change in cognition, which develops over a short period and fluctuates.[194] Delirium is associated with increased ICU and hospital stay, increased cost of care, increased mortality, incomplete recovery, and increased rates of cognitive impairment and decline following ICU care.[195–201] The Society of Critical Care Medicine recognizes delirium as a serious public health problem and recommends routine monitoring of delirium in adult ICU patients.[202] The Confusion Assessment Method for the Intensive Care Unit (CAM-ICU) is a validated and reliable tool to diagnose delirium and is more sensitive than physician assessment. Delirium is defined as a response to verbal stimulation with eye opening (Richmond Agitation-Sedation Scale score −3 to +4) and a positive CAM-ICU.[203,204] Recognizing delirium is the first step toward intervention and may offer insights for possible prevention.

Ultimately, the 3 previously mentioned therapeutic principles that most substantially improve organ dysfunction and survival in sepsis, (1) early, appropriate antimicrobial therapy, (2) restoration of adequate cellular perfusion, and (3) timely source control, still apply to prevent and manage septic encephalopathy and delirium. In addition, we recommend implementation and adherence to an ICU liberation model involving the ABCDEF (Awakening and Breathing Coordination, Choice of drugs, Delirium monitoring and management, Early mobility, and Family engagement) bundle, which is an evidence-based guide to improve and renormalize cognitive, emotional, and physical capacity and prevent a disability known as "the post–intensive care syndrome" (**Fig. 8**).[205,206] In a recent large study, ABCDEF bundle compliance was independently associated with improved survival and more days free of delirium in critically ill patients.[207]

Septic Cardiomyopathy and Inotropic Therapy

Sepsis-induced myocardial dysfunction is common, especially in septic shock, and occurs in 20% to 50% of septic patients overall.[208–211] Adequate fluid resuscitation to restore ventricular filling pressures and adequate MAP (restoration of adequate cellular perfusion), along with early, appropriate antimicrobial therapy and timely source control remain the mainstays of management. The pathophysiology and clinical importance of septic myocardial dysfunction is complex, evolving, and not yet fully elucidated.[212–214] Diastolic dysfunction is more common than systolic dysfunction. Systolic dysfunction does not appear to increase mortality in septic patients and there remains conflicting data on the effects of diastolic dysfunction. Decreases in ejection fraction are reversible, with full recovery usually in 7 to 10 days in survivors.[209,214–219] An elevated troponin level is also common in sepsis, even in the absence of coronary artery disease, and in fact does identify patients at higher risk of death.[220,221]

ICU Liberation: ABCDEF Bundle

Symptoms Pain, Agitation, Delirium Guidelines	**Monitoring** Tools	**Care** ABCDEF Bundle	**Done**
Pain	Critical-Care Pain Observation Tool (CPOT) NRS Numeric Rating Scale BPS Behavioral Pain Scale	A: Assess, Prevent and Manage Pain	☐
Agitation	Richmond Agitation-Sedation Scale (RASS) Sedation-Agitation Scale (SAS)	B: Both Spontaneous Awakening Trials (SAT) and Spontaneous Breathing Trials (SBT) C: Choice of Analgesia and Sedation	☐ ☐
Delirium	Confusion Assessment Method for the Intensive Care Unit (CAM-ICU) Intensive Care Delirium Screening Checklist (ICDSC)	D: Delirium: Assess, Prevent and Manage E: Early Mobility and Exercise F: Family Engagement and Empowerment	☐ ☐ ☐

Fig. 8. ICU liberation model involving the ABCDEF for use as a rounding checklist. (*From* Ely EW. The ABCDEF bundle: science and philosophy of how ICU liberation serves patients and families. Crit Care Med 2017;45(2):324; with permission.)

A subset of patients may have a complex hemodynamic picture requiring either invasive or noninvasive cardiac output monitoring. Patients with persistently low measured cardiac output despite adequate left ventricular filling pressures (volume resuscitated) may benefit from inotropic therapy if that will also improve oxygen delivery and improve tissue perfusion. The current recommended first-line inotrope is dobutamine and it was the inotrope of choice used in the EGDT studies.[48,97,98,103–105] Yet there remains no randomized clinical trial data to support this recommendation. Raising cardiac output to "supranormal" levels has not been shown to improve outcomes and is not recommended.[222–224]

Atrial Fibrillation

Atrial fibrillation is an independent predictor of mortality in critically ill patients, and we recommend appropriate workup and treatment. In one study, the development of any atrial fibrillation during the first 4 days in the ICU was associated with a 62% increased risk of in-hospital mortality.[225] New-onset atrial fibrillation is a common complication in sepsis, occurring in up to 23% of patients and is also independently associated with poor outcomes (prolonged length of stay and increased mortality). Developing atrial fibrillation during sepsis is associated with a twofold increase in cumulative ICU mortality and a 50% increase in daily risk of death in the ICU.[226,227] Failure to restore a normal sinus rhythm in atrial fibrillation in septic patients may be associated with increased in-hospital mortality.[228] Beta blockers may have beneficial effects in septic patients,[229] and in one study of patients who were septic with atrial fibrillation, intravenous beta blocker treatment was associated with lower mortality as compared with intravenous calcium channel blockers, digoxin, and amiodarone.[230] Patients are commonly anticoagulated for atrial fibrillation to reduce the risk of ischemic stroke. In one study in patients with atrial fibrillation during sepsis, parenteral anticoagulation was associated with higher bleeding rates but not reduced risk of ischemic stroke.[231] Despite the possible applications of these studies, there currently is not enough evidence to recommend an individualized approach to atrial fibrillation in sepsis and septic shock beyond consensus guideline evidence and management.[232–234]

Vasoactive Agents

We recommend norepinephrine as the first-line vasoactive agent in septic shock. There are multiple choices of vasoactive agents to choose from for restoring perfusion pressure in septic shock, including norepinephrine, dopamine, epinephrine, vasopressin, and phenylephrine. Prolonged hypotension and a delay in starting vasopressor therapy is associated with increased mortality, as previously iterated in our discussion on MAP goals. The users' guide to the 2016 SSC guidelines provides an exceptional flow diagram for vasopressor use in adult septic shock (**Fig. 9**).[101,102]

The 2012 and 2016 recommendation from the SSC guidelines is to use norepinephrine as the first-choice vasopressor and to target an MAP of 65 mm Hg.[95–98] Older recommendations were for norepinephrine or dopamine as the first-line agent.[92,93] This recommendation subsequently changed as evidence showed that dopamine was associated with greater or equivocal mortality and a higher incidence of arrhythmias compared with norepinephrine in patients with septic shock.[95–98,235–238] Dopamine has not been shown to provide renal protection.[237] It is currently recommended to use dopamine only in highly selected patients as an alternative to norepinephrine in those with low risk of tachyarrhythmias and absolute or relative bradycardia.[97,98]

A relative vasopressin deficiency may exist in septic shock.[239,240] The Vasopressin and Septic Shock Trial (VASST) showed the addition of low-dose vasopressin to norepinephrine infusion was safe, and suggested it may decrease mortality in patients

Vasopressor Use for Adult Septic Shock
(with guidance for steroid administration)

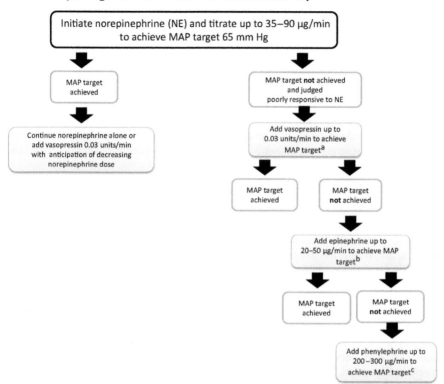

Fig. 9. A guide for vasopressor use for adult septic shock based on the 2016 Surviving Sepsis Campaign guidelines. IV, intravenous. [a] Consider IV steroid administration. [b] Administer IV steroids. [c] SSC guidelines are silent on phenylephrine. Notes: (1) Consider dopamine as niche vasopressor in the presence of sinus bradycardia. (2) Consider phenylephrine when serious tachyarrhythmias occur with norepinephrine or epinephrine. (3) Evidence based medicine does not allow the firm establishment of upper dose ranges of norepinephrine, epinephrine and phenylephrine and the dose ranges expressed in this figure are based on the authors interpretation of the literature that does exist and personal preference/experience. Maximum doses in any individual patient should be considered based on physiologic response and side effects. (*From* Dellinger RP, Schorr CA, Levy MM. A users' guide to the 2016 Surviving Sepsis Guidelines. Intensive Care Med 2017;3:301; with permission.)

with less severe forms of septic shock (patients with lower lactate levels, lower initial rates of norepinephrine infusion [5–15 μg/min], or if the patient was on only a single vasoactive agent at the time of vasopressin initiation) and for those who also received corticosteroids.[241–243] Vasopressin and corticosteroids may have a synergistic effect on maintaining MAP.[244] There may be a decreased need for renal replacement therapy when using vasopressin.[245] It is recommended in the current SSC guidelines to add vasopressin (up to 0.03 U/min) or epinephrine if an MAP ≥65 mm Hg is not achieved alone with norepinephrine. Vasopressin at 0.03 U/min can also be added to decrease the overall norepinephrine dosage.[97,98] The evidence behind these recommendations is weak and vasopressin was recently rebranded, increasing its average wholesale price by 50-fold, which may limit its utilization in some centers.[246]

Epinephrine was compared with norepinephrine infusion for critically ill patients requiring vasopressors (most of whom had sepsis) in one RCT and showed no difference in the time to achieving MAP goal, vasopressor-free days, or mortality. Epinephrine is associated with tachycardia and metabolic effects (lactic acidosis), which required stoppage of epinephrine in 12.9% in one study's patient population.[247] Another RCT compared epinephrine infusion with norepinephrine plus dobutamine for septic shock and showed no difference in time to achieving MAP goal, time to vasopressor withdrawal, SOFA score time course (resolution of organ dysfunction), or short-term and long-term mortality.[222] Last, data on phenylephrine for septic shock is relatively scarce, and the conclusions on its safety and efficacy in septic shock cannot currently be drawn.[248–250] Interestingly, when the United States experienced a norepinephrine shortage in 2011, phenylephrine was the most common vasopressor used as a replacement, and septic shock mortality increased during that time frame.[251]

Respiratory Failure and Ventilator Management

Essential to the management of the septic critically ill patient is an understanding of ventilator management. Established techniques for ventilated patients in the setting of acute respiratory distress syndrome (ARDS) are discussed first, followed by adjunct methods, and finally, the use of extracorporeal membrane oxygenation (ECMO). Other modes of ventilation, such as high-frequency ventilation, airway pressure release ventilation, and noninvasive ventilation strategies, are well described but this section is limited to techniques with proven mortality benefit in ARDS.

The ARDS Definition Task Force updated the categorization of ARDS with the objective of creating stages of ARDS that could be predictive of mortality. Instead of using changing nomenclature based on oxygenation parameters, they described ARDS on a continuum with worsening mortality as oxygenation worsened. Compared with the American-European Consensus Conference definition, the final Berlin Definition had better predictive validity for mortality.[252] The most widely accepted treatment for ARDS involves the utilization of lower tidal volumes to reduce lung injury and the subsequent inflammatory response. In a landmark study, which was terminated early due to clear mortality benefit, the death before discharge rate in the lower tidal volume group was 31% compared with 39.8% in the higher tidal volume group. Utilization of a 6 mL/kg of predicted body weight tidal volume was also associated with improvements in ventilator days, and more than a quarter of patients in each arm of the study were ventilated with a primary diagnosis of sepsis.[253] Previous and current SSC guidelines recommend a target tidal volume of 6 mL/kg predicted body weight in sepsis-induced ARDS and an upper limit goal for plateau pressures of 30 cm H_2O over higher plateau pressures with higher positive end-expiratory pressure (PEEP) over lower PEEP in patients with severe sepsis-induced ARDS.[95–98] A new recommendation is the use of lower tidal volumes over higher tidal volumes in patients with sepsis-induced respiratory failure without ARDS.[97,98] This new recommendation is based on recent studies that showed improved outcomes with low tidal volume ventilation in patients without ARDS, including decreased development of ARDS and decreased duration of mechanical ventilation, but no change in mortality.[254,255]

Prone positioning has shown to be beneficial in the setting of ARDS with low tidal volume settings. In a multicenter, prospective, randomized, controlled trial, Guerin and colleagues[256] showed that early prone positioning decreased 28-day mortality from 32% to 16% and 90-day mortality from 41.0% to 23.6%. Patients who had ARDS and Pao_2/Fio_2 less than 150 were placed in a prone position or standard supine position within the first 36 hours of intubation. The prone group was positioned for more than 16 consecutive hours each day until they met predefined oxygenation improvement requirements. The 2012 SSC guidelines recommended using prone over supine positioning in adult patients with sepsis-induced ARDS and a Pao_2/Fio_2 ratio less than 100.[95,96] This was changed to a Pao_2/Fio_2 ratio less than 150 in the newest guidelines.[97,98] A recent meta-analysis concluded there is a reduced mortality with prone compared with supine position for ARDS but is associated with an increase in pressure sores.[257]

Neuromuscular blockade in the setting of ARDS can improve gas-exchange, and Papazian and colleagues[258] further demonstrated a mortality benefit. In this multicenter, double-blind trial, patients with early ARDS and Pao_2/Fio_2 ratio less than 150 were randomized to high fixed dose cisatracurium besylate or placebo, with each group using low tidal volume ventilator settings: 28-day mortality improved from 33.3% to 23.7% in the neuromuscular blockade group and 90-day mortality improved from 40.7% to 31.6% with the addition of cisatracurium. This benefit was confined to the patients whose Pao_2/Fio_2 ratio was less than 120. Thus, these patients would be included in the moderate and severe Berlin stages of ARDS.[252] The most recent SSC guidelines give a weak recommendation for using neuromuscular blocking agents for $\leq$48 hours in adult patients with sepsis-induced ARDS and Pao_2/Fio_2 ratio less than 150.[97,98]

An evolving strategy in ARDS and sepsis is the use of ECMO. Peek and colleagues[259] published results of the CESAR trial in 2009, which was a multicenter trial comparing ECMO with conventional management. In their trial, the ECMO group had 63% 6-month survival compared with 47% in the conventional ventilator group. The conventional ventilator group included many patients who did not receive low tidal volume ventilation, so the true benefit of ECMO in the setting of current ARDS standard-of-care treatment remains to be seen.

Nutrition

Nutrition in the critically ill population is a complex issue that encompasses enteral options, parenteral options, and other supplements.[260] Robust caloric intake has been shown to improve the mortality of both the underweight and the overweight populations.[261] The preferred route for nutrition in the critically ill population is via enteral access. This becomes challenging in the setting of mechanical ventilation, where nutrition must come through means of enteric tubes. A randomized multicenter trial was conducted to determine whether trophic feeding was superior to full enteral feeding and the results showed no difference in mortality, infectious complications, or ventilator-free days between the groups.[262] Dispelling other common myths with regard to enteral nutrition, a recent systematic review showed no utility of measuring gastric residuals in the medical intensive care population. There was an increased association with aspiration in surgical patients with gastric residuals greater than 200 mL, so this must be considered when treating specific patient populations.[263] Acosta-Escribano and colleagues[264] helped solve another quandary in the area of enteral nutrition: transpyloric versus gastric feeding. In their prospective randomized study, they evaluated patients who received either transpyloric or gastric feeds. In their study, the transpyloric group had improved rates of pneumonia and had a higher total caloric intake, supporting the use of transpyloric feeding. This was further supported by a recent Cochrane review showing a 30% reduction in pneumonia rates in those patients who were fed past their pylorus.[265]

In those patients who cannot receive enteral nutrition, another option is parenteral nutrition. Parenteral nutrition carries many risks, including bloodstream-related infections, and the risk of such infections increases as the parenteral caloric intake increases.[266] Later initiation of parenteral nutrition therapy is actually associated with fewer complications, decreased ventilator days, and a cost savings with regard to early parenteral nutrition therapy.[267] When early enteral therapy is compared with early parenteral nutrition therapy, mortality was similar, but enteral nutrition had lower complication rates.[268] The current SSC guidelines recommend against the early administration of parenteral nutrition (based on no mortality benefit and increased cost and risk of infection) and to instead initiate intravenous glucose and advance enteral feeds as tolerated in the first 7 days in critically ill patients with sepsis or septic shock in whom early enteral feeding is not possible.[97,98]

Other supplements, such as glutamine, selenium, and other antioxidants, are being actively studied, but clear benefit to these supplements remains to be seen.[269–271] Clinical trials on omega-3 supplementation has not confirmed clinical benefit in patients who are critically ill or patients with ARDS.[272,273]

Fluid and Kidney Management

Discussions on the genitourinary system include the choice of fluids, acute kidney injury, fluid balance, diuresis, ultrafiltration, and the management of acidosis. Crystalloid and albumin are generally accepted as the resuscitation fluid of choice for sepsis and septic shock resuscitation. A systematic review and meta-analysis showed increased risk of death and increased need for renal replacement therapy when resuscitated with hydroxyethyl starches and their use is not recommended.[274,275] In a multicenter, randomized, double-blinded trial of ICU patients, the use of albumin was compared with saline for resuscitation. In the analysis, data on mortality, ventilator days, and total hospital stay were equivocal between the 2 groups. Albumin was found to be safe and equally as effective as 0.9% saline in the resuscitation.[276] The use of albumin was revisited in the severe sepsis population, and there was still no mortality benefit compared with crystalloid-based resuscitation at 28 or 90 days.[277] Yet in other meta-analyses of resuscitation in sepsis, albumin administration was found to have a mortality benefit compared with crystalloid resuscitation.[278,279] Correcting hypoalbuminemia (goal >3 g/dL) appears to decrease morbidity.[280] Currently, the expense of colloid limits its utilization, but the current SSC guidelines do make a weak recommendation to use albumin in addition to crystalloids in initial resuscitation when patients require "substantial" amounts of crystalloids to limit harmful fluid overload (see **Fig. 5**).[97,98,101,102]

Positive fluid balance is deleterious in the setting of sepsis and septic shock. In multiple analyses, late positive fluid balance was an independent risk factor for mortality.[281–284] Fluid should be restricted in the later stages of sepsis. Diuretics are widely used to reduce fluid overload. Unfortunately, the PICARD group showed a significant increase in both death and loss of renal recovery in patients who received diuretic therapy, thus diuretics should be used judiciously.[285] Improved net negative fluid balance and oxygenation occur when albumin is given concurrently with loop diuretics and this may protect against hypotension and need for vasopressors during diuresis.[286,287]

Metabolic acidosis is common in patients with sepsis or septic shock, and those who have a persistent metabolic acidosis are more often nonsurvivors than those patients who normalize.[288] Direct buffering of acidosis with bicarbonate has been more widely used, but in 1990, a prospective randomized study was performed showing that sodium bicarbonate had no positive effects on hemodynamics in patients with lactic acidosis.[289] This was further studied in 2009 in septic shock, and bicarbonate infusion had some benefit with regard to ICU length of stay and ventilator weaning, but there was no mortality benefit associated with its use.[290] Bicarbonate use is not recommended in patients with hypoperfusion-induced lactic acidemia with pH $\geq$7.15.[97,98]

Acute kidney injury (AKI) is a common insult in sepsis, and there is a wealth of information on the prevention and treatment of AKI.[291] An evolving practice is the use of renal replacement therapy (RRT). The degree of lactic acidosis at the initiation of RRT has not been shown to correlate with mortality.[292] In a multicenter randomized trial, Gaudry and colleagues[293] showed that there is no mortality benefit of initiating early RRT, although many of these patients were nonseptic. Current SSC guidelines recommend using RRT only in patients with definitive indications for dialysis and give a weak recommendation for using continuous RRT to facilitate management of fluid balance in hemodynamically unstable patients with sepses.[97,98] There currently appears to be no benefit of intermittent over continuous RRT with regard to hemodynamics or mortality.[294]

Corticosteroids

In those critical care patients in septic shock, the prevailing endocrine topics involve steroid use in adrenal suppression and glycemic control. Put simply, if you suspect adrenal suppression in patients with vasopressor requirements, then steroids can be given. In general, release of cortisol increases and cortisol metabolism decreases in periods of stress, whether that be infection, trauma, burns, or surgery.[295] The hypothalamic-pituitary-adrenal axis can be impaired during severe illness, and this can be manifested clinically. In those patients with hypotension refractory to vasopressor therapy, 200 mg of hydrocortisone in 24 hours can be given empirically or for those patients with a random cortisol level below 15 μg per deciliter. For intermediate cortisol levels, steroids also can be considered.[296] Although these guidelines are in place and are widely used, the utility of such treatment has come into question with the results of the CORTICUS trial,[297] the HYPRESS trial,[298] and a meta-analysis by Gibbison and colleagues,[299] which, in general, showed a shorter time to shock reversal with hydrocortisone use but no survival benefit.

Glycemic Control

Glycemic control without hypoglycemia improves outcomes and should be achieved if possible. The goal for an upper target should be $\leq$180 mg/dL via an arterial blood sample if possible, which is more accurate than point of care capillary blood glucose testing.[97,98,300] Hyperglycemia is widely associated with worse outcomes in the perioperative period in those patients with critical illness. Egi and colleagues[301] showed a 3.85 odds ratio of mortality in those nondiabetic ICU patients whose blood glucose exceeded 200 mg/dL. Moreover, the correction of hyperglycemia improves rates of infection, reoperation, anastomotic failure, and death in the general surgical population.[302] With this information, it follows that tight insulin control could improve patient outcomes even further. Van den Berghe and colleagues[303] showed improvements in both ICU survival as well as in-hospital survival if tight glucose control (target 80–110 mg/dL) was achieved. This was confuted by the NICE-SUGAR trial, which showed that intensive glucose control increased mortality among adults in the ICU.[304]

A meta-analysis by Griesdale and colleagues[305] showed intensive insulin therapy significantly increased the risk of hypoglycemia and conferred no overall mortality benefit among critically ill patients. However, patients in surgical ICUs appeared to benefit from intensive insulin therapy (relative risk 0.63, 95% confidence interval [CI] 0.44–0.91); patients in the other ICU settings did not (medical ICU: RR 1.0, 95% CI 0.78–1.28; mixed ICU: RR 0.99, 95% CI 0.86–1.12). Additional review of intensive insulin therapy (80–110 mg/dL) appeared beneficial in critically ill surgical patients but requires frequent measurement of glucose to avoid hypoglycemia.[306] As such, efforts should be mounted to tighten glucose control while preventing hypoglycemia. Balanced nutrition is protective from hypoglycemia and if there is no nutritional source, we recommend protective D10 W at 30 mL/h[307] Manual titration of insulin infusion therapy is prone to variability and it is difficult to measure compliance and we advocate a computerized protocol. This is supported by the results of Dortsch and colleagues[308] who compared a computerized insulin infusion titration protocol to a manual titration and showed significantly improved overall glucose control and significantly reduced hypoglycemic episodes with the computerized protocol.

SUMMARY

The new definitions of sepsis and septic shock reflect the inadequate sensitivity, specify and lack of prognostication of SIRS criteria.[10,16] SOFA more effectively prognosticates in sepsis and critical illness. Understanding the pathophysiology of sepsis improves understanding of why organ dysfunction occurs and offers opportunities for intervention. Three therapeutic principles most substantially improve organ dysfunction and survival in sepsis: (1) early, appropriate antimicrobial therapy; (2) restoration of adequate cellular perfusion; and (3) timely source control. Mortality from sepsis and septic shock has been greatly reduced over time from following these principles.[6] The timing and appropriateness of antibiotic therapy is vitally important. Antibiotic stewardship prevents resistance development and subsequent complex infections. It is clear that early quantitative resuscitation strategies impact a mortality reduction in sepsis and help define a hemodynamic phenotype of the patient.[133] Dynamic measures of fluid responsiveness should be used to help avoid unnecessary positive fluid balances, which result in poorer outcomes. We recommend ICU protocols that follow the models of the ABCDEF bundle[205–207] and follow the evidence-based SSC[97,98] and the European Society of Intensive Care Medicine[134] evidence-based expert consensus recommendations with regard to hemodynamic monitoring, fluid resuscitation, choice of vasoactive agents and inotropes, hydrocortisone use, and glycemic control without hypoglycemia.

REFERENCES

1. Wang HE, Shapiro NI, Angus DC, et al. National estimates of severe sepsis in United States emergency departments. Crit Care Med 2007;35(8):1928–36.
2. Lagu T, Rothberg MB, Shieh MS, et al. Hospitalizations, costs, outcomes of severe sepsis in the United States 2003 to 2007. Crit Care Med 2012;40:754–6 [Erratum appears in Crit Care Med 2012;40:2932].
3. Torio C, Moore B. National inpatient hospital costs: the most expensive conditions by payer, 2013. HCUP statistical brief #204. Rockville (MD): Agency for Healthcare Research and Quality; 2016.
4. Martin GS, Mannino DM, Eaton S, et al. The epidemiology of sepsis in the United States from 1979 through 2000. N Engl J Med 2003;348(16):1546–54.
5. Dombrovskiy VY, Martin AA, Sunderram J, et al. Rapid increase in hospitalization and mortality rates for severe sepsis in the United States: a trend analysis from 1993 to 2003. Crit Care Med 2007;35:1244–50.
6. Kaukonen JM, Bailey M, Suzuki S, et al. Mortality related to severe sepsis and septic shock among critically ill patients in Australia and New Zealand, 2000-2012. JAMA 2014;311(13):1308–16.
7. Liu V, Escobar GJ, Greene JD, et al. Hospital deaths in patients with sepsis from 2 independent cohorts. JAMA 2014;312(1):90–1.

8. Bone RC, Balk RA, Cerra FB, et al. Definitions for sepsis and organ failure and guidelines for the use of innovative therapies in sepsis. The ACCP/SCCM Consensus Conference Committee. American College of Chest Physicians/Society of Critical Care Medicine. Chest 1992;101:1644–55.

9. Levy MM, Fink MP, Marshal JC, et al. 2001 SCCM/ESICM/ACCP/ATS/SIS International Sepsis Definitions Conference. Crit Care Med 2003;31:1250–6.

10. Singer M, Deutschman CS, Seymor CW, et al. The Third International Consensus Definitions for Sepsis and Septic Shock (Sepsis-3). JAMA 2016;315(8):801–10.

11. Vincent JL, Moreno R, Takala J, et al, Working Group on Sepsis-Related Problems of the European Society of Intensive Care Medicine. The SOFA (Sepsis-related Organ Failure Assessment) score to describe organ dysfunction/failure. Intensive Care Med 1996;22(7):707–10.

12. Vincent JL, de Mendonca A, Cantraine F, et al. Use of the SOFA score to assess the incidence of organ dysfunction/failure in intensive care units: results of a multicenter, prospective study. Working Group on "Sepsis-Related Problems" of the European Society of Intensive Care Medicine. Crit Care Med 1998; 26(11):1793–800.

13. Seymour CW, Liu VX, Iwashyna TJ, et al. Assessment of clinical criteria for sepsis for the Third International Consensus Definitions for Sepsis and Septic Shock (Sepsis-3). JAMA 2016;315(8):762–74.

14. Shankar-Hari M, Phillips GS, Levy ML, et al. Developing a new definition and assessing new clinical criteria for septic shock for the Third International Consensus Definitions for Sepsis and Septic Shock (Sepsis-3). JAMA 2016; 315:775–87.

15. Ferreira FL, Bota DP, Bross A, et al. Serial evaluation of the SOFA score to predict outcome in critically ill patients. JAMA 2001;286(14):1754–8.

16. Kaukonen KM, Bailey M, Pilcher D, et al. Systemic inflammatory response syndrome criteria in defining sepsis. N Engl J Med 2015;372(17):1629–38.

17. Rhee C, Gohil S, Klompas M. Regulatory mandates for sepsis care-reasons for caution. N Engl J Med 2014;370(18):1673–6.

18. Crabtree TD, Pelletier SJ, Antevil JL, et al. Cohort study of fever and leukocytosis as diagnostic and prognostic indicators in infected surgical patients. World J Surg 2001;25:739–44.

19. Rangel-Frasto MS, Pittet D, Costigan M, et al. The natural history of the systemic inflammatory response syndrome (SIRS). A prospective study. JAMA 1995;273: 117–23.

20. Sprung CL, Sakr Y, Vincent JL, et al. An evaluation of systemic inflammatory response syndrome signs in the Sepsis Occurrence in Acutely Ill Patients (SOAP) study. Intensive Care Med 2006;32:421–7.

21. Dulhunty JM, Lipman J, Finfer S. Does severe non-infectious SIRS differ from severe sepsis? Results from a multi-centre Australian and New Zealand intensive care unit study. Intensive Care Med 2008;34:1654–61.

22. Churpek MM, Zadravecz FJ, Winslow C, et al. Incidence and prognosis value of the systemic inflammatory response syndrome and organ dysfunctions in ward patients. Am J Respir Crit Care Med 2015;192:958–64.

23. Hotchkiss RS, Monneret G, Payen D. Sepsis-induced immunosuppression: from cellular dysfunctions to immunotherapy. Nat Rev Immunol 2013;13(12):862–74.

24. Delano MJ, Ward PA. The immune system's role in sepsis progression, resolution, and long-term outcome. Immunol Rev 2016;274:330–53.

25. Angus DC, van der Poll T. Severe sepsis and septic shock. N Engl J Med 2013; 369(9):840–51.

26. Cinel I, Opal SM. Molecular biology of inflammation and sepsis: a primer. Crit Care Med 2009;37(1):291–304.

27. Deutschman CS, Tracey KJ. Sepsis: current dogma and new perspectives. Immunity 2014;40(4):463–75.

28. Singer M, De Santis V, Vitale D, et al. Multiorgan failure is an adaptive, endocrine mediated, metabolic response to overwhelming systemic inflammation. Lancet 2004;364(9433):545–8.

29. Nduka OO, Parillo JE. The pathophysiology of septic shock. Crit Care Clin 2009; 25:677–702.

30. Abraham E, Singer M. Mechanisms of sepsis-induced organ dysfunction. Crit Care Med 2007;35(10):2408–16.

31. Singer M. The role of mitochondrial dysfunction in sepsis-induced multi-organ failure. Virulence 2014;5(1):66–72.

32. Andrades ME, Morina A, Spasic S, et al. Bench-to-bedside review: sepsis—from the redox point of view. Crit Care 2011;15(230):1–12.

33. Raith EP, Udy AA, Baily M, et al. Prognostic accuracy of the SOFA score, SIRS criteria, and qSOFA score for in-hospital mortality among adults with suspected infection admitted to the intensive care unit. JAMA 2017;317(3):290–300.

34. Vincent JL, Martin GS, Levy MM. qSOFA does not replace SIRS in the definition of sepsis. Crit Care 2016;20:210.

35. April MD, Aguire J, Tannenbaum LI, et al. Sepsis clinical criteria in emergency department patients admitted to an intensive care unit: an external validation study of quick sequential organ failure assessment. J Emerg Med 2016;52(5): 622–31. Accessed March 10, 2017.

36. Williams JM, Greenslade JH, McKenzie JV, et al. Systemic inflammatory response syndrome, quick sequential organ dysfunction assessment, and organ dysfunction: insights from a prospective database of ED patients with infection. Chest 2017;151(3):586–96.

37. Freund Y, Lemachatti N, Krastinova E, et al. Prognostic accuracy of Sepsis-3 criteria for in-hospital mortality among patients with suspected infection presenting to the emergency department. JAMA 2017;317(3):301–8.

38. Churpek MM, Snyder AS, Han X, et al. qSOFA, SIRS, and early warning scores for detecting clinical deterioration in infected patients outside the ICU. Am J Respir Crit Care Med 2016;195(7):906–11. Accessed March 10, 2017.

39. Smith GB, Prytherch DR, Meredith P, et al. The ability of the national early warning score (NEWS) to discriminate patients at risk of early cardiac arrest, unanticipated intensive care unit admission and death. Resuscitation 2013;84: 465–70.

40. Royal College of Physicians. National early warning score (NEWS): standardising the assessment of acute illness severity in the NHS. London: Royal College of Physicians; 2012.

41. Jones DA, DeVita MA, Bellomo R. Rapid-response teams. N Engl J Med 2011; 365:139–46.

42. Smith ME, Chiovaro JC, O'Neil M, et al. Early warning system scores for clinical deterioration in hospitalized patients: a systematic review. Ann Am Thorac Soc 2014;11:1454–65.

43. Vincent JL. The challenge of early identification of the hospital patient at risk of septic complications. Ann Transl Med 2017;5(3):56.

44. McLymont N, Glover GW. Scoring systems for the characterization of sepsis and associated outcomes. Ann Transl Med 2016;4(24):527.

45. Simpson SQ. New sepsis criteria: a change we should not make. Chest 2016; 149:1117–8.

46. Cortes-Puch I, Hartog CS. Opening the debate on the new sepsis definition change is not necessarily progress: revision of the sepsis definition should be based on new scientific insights. Am J Respir Crit Care Med 2016;194(1):16–8.

47. Simpson SQ. Diagnosing sepsis: a step forward, and possibly a step back. Ann Transl Med 2017;5(3):55.

48. Rivers E, Nguyen B, Havstad S, et al, The Early Goal-Directed Therapy Collaborative Group. Early goal-directed therapy in the treatment of severe sepsis and septic shock. N Engl J Med 2001;345:1368–77.

49. Kumar A, Roberts D, Wood KE, et al. Duration of hypotension before initiation of effective antimicrobial therapy is the critical determinant of survival in human septic shock. Crit Care Med 2006;34:1589–96.

50. Levy MM, Dellinger RP, Townsend SR, et al. The Surviving Sepsis Campaign: results of an international guideline-based performance improvement program targeting severe sepsis. Intensive Care Med 2010;36:222–31.

51. Azuhata T, Kinoshita K, Kawano D, et al. Time from admission to initiation of surgery for source control is a critical determinant of survival in patients with gastrointestinal perforation with associated septic shock. Crit Care 2014;18:R87.

52. Wong CH, Chang HC, Pasupathy S, et al. Necrotizing fasciitis: clinical presentation, microbiology, and determinants of mortality. J Bone Joint Surg Am 2003; 85(8):1454–60.

53. Liu YM, Chi CY, Ho MW, et al. Microbiology and factors affecting mortality in necrotizing fasciitis. J Microbiol Immunol Infect 2005;38(6):430–5.

54. Golger A, Ching S, Goldsmith CH, et al. Mortality in patients with necrotizing fasciitis. Plast Reconstr Surg 2007;119(6):1803–7.

55. Zadroga R, Williams DN, Gottschall R, et al. Comparison of 2 blood culture media shows significant differences in bacterial recovery for patients on antimicrobial therapy. Clin Infect Dis 2013;56:790–7.

56. Weinstein MP, Reller LB, Murphy JR, et al. The clinical significance of positive blood cultures: a comprehensive analysis of 500 episodes of bacteremia and fungemia in adults. I. Laboratory and epidemiologic observations. Rev Infect Dis 1983;5:35–53.

57. Cardoso T, Carneiro AH, Ribeiro O, et al. Reducing mortality in severe sepsis with the implementation of a core 6-hour bundle: results from the Portuguese community-acquired sepsis study (SACiUCI study). Crit Care 2010;14:R83.

58. De Sousa AG, Fernandes Junior CJ, Santos GPD, et al. The impact of each action in the Surviving Sepsis Campaign measures on hospital mortality of patients with severe sepsis/septic chosk. Einstein 2008;6(3):323–7.

59. Ferrer R, Martin-Loeches I, Phillips G, et al. Empiric antibiotic treatment reduces mortality in severe sepsis and septic shock from the first hour: results from a guideline-based performance improvement program. Crit Care Med 2014; 42(8):1749–55.

60. Barie PS, Hydo LJ, Shou J, et al. Influence of antibiotic therapy on mortality of critical surgical illness caused or complicated by infection. Surg Infect (Larchmt) 2005;6(1):41–54.

61. Houck PM, Bratzler DW, Nsa W, et al. Timing of antibiotic administration and outcomes for Medicare patients hospitalized with community-acquired pneumonia. Arch Intern Med 2004;164(6):637–44.

62. Iregui M, Ward S, Sherman G, et al. Clinical importance of delays in the initiation of appropriate antibiotic treatment for ventilator-associated pneumonia. Chest 2002;122(1):262–8.

63. Meehan TP, Fine MJ, Krumholz HM, et al. Quality of care, process, and outcomes in elderly patients with pneumonia. JAMA 1997;278(23):2080–4.

64. Sterling SA, Miller WR, Pryor J, et al. The impact of timing of antibiotics on outcomes in severe sepsis and septic shock: a systematic review and meta-analysis. Crit Care Med 2015;43(9):1907–15.

65. Alvarez-Lerma F. Modification of empiric antibiotic treatment in patients with pneumonia acquired in the intensive care unit. ICU-Acquired Pneumonia Study Group. Intensive Care Med 1996;22(5):387–94.

66. Ibrahim EH, Sherman G, Ward S, et al. The influence of inadequate antimicrobial treatment of bloodstream infections on patient outcomes in the ICU setting. Chest 2000;118(1):146–55.

67. Kollef MH, Sherman G, Ward S, et al. Inadequate antimicrobial treatment of infections: a risk factor for hospital mortality among critically ill patients. Chest 1999;115(2):462–74.

68. Kumar A, Ellis P, Arabi Y, et al. Initiation of inappropriate antimicrobial therapy results in a fivefold reduction of survival in human septic shock. Chest 2009; 136(5):1237–48.

69. Leibovici L, Shraga I, Drucker M, et al. The benefit of appropriate empirical antibiotic treatment in patients with bloodstream infection. J Intern Med 1998; 244(5):379–86.

70. Luna CM, Vujacich P, Niederman MS, et al. Impact of BAL data on the therapy and outcome of ventilator-associated pneumonia. Chest 1997;111(3):676–85.

71. Montravers P, Gauzit R, Muller C, et al. Emergence of antibiotic-resistant bacteria in cases of peritonitis after intraabdominal surgery affects the efficacy of empirical antimicrobial therapy. Clin Infect Dis 1996;23(3):486–94.

72. Mosdell DM, Morris DM, Voltura A, et al. Antibiotic treatment for surgical peritonitis. Ann Surg 1991;214(5):543–9.

73. Paul M, Shani V, Muchtar E, et al. Systematic review and meta-analysis of the efficacy of appropriate empiric antibiotic therapy for sepsis. Antimicrob Agents Chemother 2010;54(11):4851–63.

74. Johnson MT, Reichley R, Hoppe-Bauer J, et al. Impact of previous antibiotic therapy on outcome of gram-negative severe sepsis. Crit Care Med 2011; 39(8):1859–65.

75. Dortch MJ, Fleming SB, Kauffmann RM, et al. Infection reduction strategies including antibiotic stewardship protocols in surgical and trauma intensive care units are associated with reduced resistant gram-negative healthcare-associated infections. Surg Infect (Larchmt) 2011;12(1):15–25.

76. Fabian TC, Croce MA, Payne LW, et al. Duration of antibiotic therapy for penetrating abdominal trauma: a prospective trial. Surgery 1992;112(4):788–94 [discussion: 794–5].

77. Namias N, Harvill S, Ball S, et al. Cost and morbidity associated with antibiotic prophylaxis in the ICU. J Am Coll Surg 1999;188(3):225–30.

78. Lotfi CJ, Cavalcanti Rde C, Costa e Silva AM, et al. Risk factors for surgical-site infections in head and neck cancer surgery. Otolaryngol Head Neck Surg 2008; 138(1):74–80.

79. Kollef MH, Silver P, Murphy DM, et al. The effect of late-onset ventilator-associated pneumonia in determining patient mortality. Chest 1995;108(6):1655–62.

80. Puzniak L, Teutsch S, Powderly W, et al. Has the epidemiology of nosocomial candidemia changed? Infect Control Hosp Epidemiol 2004;25(8):628–33.
81. Riccio LM, Popovsky KA, Hranjec T, et al. Association of excessive duration of antibiotic therapy for intra-abdominal infection with subsequent extra-abdominal infection and death: a study of 2,552 consecutive infections. Surg Infect (Larchmt) 2014;15(4):417–24.
82. Harbarth S, Samore MH, Lichtenberg D, et al. Prolonged antibiotic prophylaxis after cardiovascular surgery and its effect on surgical site infections and antimicrobial resistance. Circulation 2000;101(25):2916–21.
83. Velmahos GC, Toutouzas KG, Sarkisyan G, et al. Severe trauma is not an excuse for prolonged antibiotic prophylaxis. Arch Surg 2002;137(5):537–41 [discussion: 541–2].
84. May AK, Fleming SB, Carpenter RO, et al. Influence of broad-spectrum antibiotic prophylaxis on intracranial pressure monitor infections and subsequent infectious complications in head-injured patients. Surg Infect (Larchmt) 2006;7(5):409–17.
85. Trouillet JL, Chastre J, Vuagnat A, et al. Ventilator-associated pneumonia caused by potentially drug-resistant bacteria. Am J Respir Crit Care Med 1998;157(2):531–9.
86. Chastre J, Wolf M, Fagon JY, et al. Comparison of 8 vs 15 days of antibiotic therapy for ventilator-associated pneumonia in adults. JAMA 2003;290(19):2588–98.
87. Teshome B, Vouri S, Hampton N, et al. Duration of broad-spectrum antimicrobials in the critically ill and the development of new resistance. Crit Care Med 2016;44(12s):236.
88. Silva BNG, Andriolo RB, Atallah AN, et al. De-escalation of antimicrobial treatment for adults with sepsis, severe sepsis or septic shock. Cochrane Database Syst Rev 2013;(3):CD007934.
89. Sawyer RG, Claridge AB, Nathens OD, et al. Trial of short-course antimicrobial therapy for intraabdominal infection. N Engl J Med 2015;372:1996–2005.
90. Mazuski JE, Tessier JM, May AK, et al. The Surgical Infection Society revised guidelines on the management of intra-abdominal infection. Surg Infect (Larchmt) 2017;18(1):1–76.
91. Kalil AC, Metersky ML, Klompas M, et al. Management of adults with hospital-acquired and ventilator-associated pneumonia: 2016 clinical practice guidelines by the Infectious Diseases Society of America and the American Thoracic Society. Clin Infect Dis 2016;63(5):e61–111.
92. Dellinger RP, Carlet JM, Masur H, et al. Surviving sepsis campaign management guidelines committee: surviving sepsis campaign guidelines for management of severe sepsis and septic shock. Crit Care Med 2004;32:858–73.
93. Dellinger RP, Levy MM, Carlet JM, et al, International Surviving Sepsis Campaign Guidelines Committee, American Association of Critical-Care Nurses, American College of Chest Physicians, American College of Emergency Physicians, Canadian Critical Care Society, European Society of Clinical Microbiology and Infectious Diseases, European Society of Intensive Care Medicine; European Respiratory Society, International Sepsis Forum, Japanese Association for Acute Medicine, Japanese Society of Intensive Care medicine, Society of Critical Care Medicine, Society of Hospital Medicine, Surgical Infection Society, World Federation of Societies of Intensive and Critical Care Medicine. Surviving Sepsis Campaign: international guidelines for management of severe sepsis and septic shock: 2008. Crit Care Med 2008;36:296–327.

94. Dellinger RP, Levy MM, Carlet JM, et al, International Surviving Sepsis Campaign Guidelines Committee, American Association of Critical-Care Nurses, American College of Chest Physicians, American College of Emergency Physicians, Canadian Critical Care Society, European Society of Clinical Microbiology and Infectious Diseases, European Society of Intensive Care Medicine, European Respiratory Society, International Sepsis Forum, Japanese Association for Acute Medicine, Japanese Society of Intensive Care medicine, Society of Critical Care Medicine, Society of Hospital Medicine, Surgical Infection Society, World Federation of Societies of Intensive and Critical Care Medicine. Surviving Sepsis Campaign: international guidelines for management of severe sepsis and septic shock: 2008. Intensive Care Med 2008;34:17–60 [Erratum appears in Intensive Care Med 2008;34:783–5].

95. Dellinger RP, Levy MM, Rhodes A, et al. Surviving Sepsis Campaign Guidelines Committee including the Pediatric Subgroup: surviving sepsis campaign: international guidelines for management of severe sepsis and septic shock: 2012. Crit Care Med 2013;41:580–637.

96. Dellinger RP, Levy MM, Rhodes A, et al. Surviving Sepsis Campaign Guidelines Committee including the Pediatric Subgroup: surviving sepsis campaign: international guidelines for management of severe sepsis and septic shock: 2012. Intensive Care Med 2013;39:165–228.

97. Rhodes A, Evans LE, Alhazzani W, et al. Surviving Sepsis Campaign: international guidelines for management of sepsis and septic shock: 2016. Crit Care Med 2017;45(3):486–552.

98. Rhodes A, Evans LE, Alhazzani W, et al. Surviving Sepsis Campaign: international guidelines for management of sepsis and septic shock: 2016. Intensive Care Med 2017;43:304–77.

99. Levy MM, Rhodes A, Phillips GS, et al. Surviving Sepsis Campaign: Association between performance metrics and outcomes in a 7.5 year study. Crit Care Med 2015;43(3):3–12.

100. Rhodes A, Phillips G, Beale R, et al. The Surviving Sepsis Campaign bundles and outcome: results from the International Multicentre Prevalence Study on Sepsis (the IMPreSS study). Intensive Care Med 2015;41:1620–8.

101. Dellinger RP, Schorr CA, Levy MM. A users' guide to the 2016 surviving sepsis guidelines. Intensive Care Med 2017;3:299–303.

102. Dellinger RP, Schorr CA, Levy MM. A users' guide to the 2016 surviving sepsis guidelines. Crit Care Med 2017;45:381–5.

103. The ARISE Investigators and the ANZICS Clinical Trial Group, Peake SL, Delaney A, Bailey M, et al. Goal-directed resuscitation for patients with early septic shock. N Engl J Med 2014;371(16):1496–506.

104. The ProCESS Investigators, Yealy DM, Kellum JA, Huang DT, et al. A randomized trial of protocol-based care for early septic shock. N Engl J Med 2014;370(18):1683–93.

105. The ProMISe Investigators, Mouncey PR, Osborn TM, Power S, et al. Trial of early, goal-directed resuscitation for septic shock. N Engl J Med 2015;372: 1301–11.

106. Marik PE, Barma M, Vahid B. Does central venous pressure predict fluid responsiveness? A systemic review of the literature and the tale of seven mares. Chest 2008;134:172–8.

107. Marik PE, Cavallazzi R. Does the central venous pressure predict fluid responsiveness? An updated meta-analysis and a plea for some common sense. Crit Care Med 2013;41:1774–81.

108. Bentzer P, Griesdale DE, Boyd J, et al. Will this hemodynamically unstable patient respond to a bolus of intravenous fluids? JAMA 2016;316:1298–309.
109. Monnet X, Marik PE, Teboul JL. Prediction of fluid responsiveness: an update. Ann Intensive Care 2016;6(111):1–11.
110. Michard F, Boussat S, Chemla D, et al. Relation between respiratory changes in arterial pulse pressure and fluid responsiveness in septic patients with acute circulatory failure. Am J Respir Crit Care Med 2000;162:134–8.
111. Yang X, Du B. Does pulse pressure variation predict fluid responsiveness in critically ill patients? A systematic review and meta-analysis. Crit Care 2014;18:650.
112. Marik PE, Cavallazzi R, Vasu T, et al. Dynamic changes in arterial waveform derived variables and fluid responsiveness in mechanically ventilated patients: a systemic review of the literature. Crit Care Med 2009;37:2642–7.
113. Barbier C, Loubieres Y, Schmit C, et al. Respiratory changes in inferior vena diameter are helpful in predicting fluid responsiveness in ventilated septic patients. Intensive Care Med 2004;30:1740–6.
114. Viellard-Baron A, Chergui K, Rabiller A, et al. Superior vena cava collapsibility as a gauge of volume status in ventilated septic patients. Intensive Care Med 2004; 30:1734–9.
115. Monnet X, Rienzo M, Osman D, et al. Passive leg raising predicts fluid responsiveness in the critically ill. Crit Care Med 2006;34:1402–7.
116. Cherpanath TG, Hirsch A, Geerts BF, et al. Predicting fluid responsiveness by passive leg raising: a systematic review and meta-analysis of 23 clinical trials. Crit Care Med 2016;44:981–91.
117. Monnet X, Marik P, Teboul JL. Passive leg raising for predicting fluid responsiveness: a systematic review and meta-analysis. Intensive Care Med 2016;42(12): 1935–47.
118. Monnet X, Osman D, Ridel C, et al. Predicting volume responsiveness by using the end-expiratory occlusion in mechanically ventilated intensive care unit patients. Crit Care Med 2009;37:951–6.
119. Muller L, Toumi M, Bousquet PJ, et al. An increase in aortic blood flow after an infusion of 100 ml of colloid over 1 minute can predict fluid responsiveness: the Mini Fluid Challenge Study. Anesthesiology 2011;115:541–7.
120. Vincent JL, Weil MH. Fluid challenge revisited. Crit Care Med 2006;34:1333–7.
121. Cecconi M, Hofer C, Teboul JL, et al. Fluid challenges in intensive care: the FENICE study, a global inception cohort study. Intensive Care Med 2015;41: 1529–37.
122. Gu WJ, Wang F, Bakker J, et al. The effect of goal-directed therapy on mortality in patients with sepsis-earlier is better: a meta-analysis of randomized control trials. Crit Care 2014;18:570.
123. Ho BC, Bellom R, McGain F, et al. The incidence and outcome of septic shock patients in the absence of early goal-directed therapy. Crit Care 2006;10:R80.
124. Chapman M, Gattas D, Suntharalingam G. Why is early goal-directed therapy successful—is it the technology? Crit Care 2005;9:307–8.
125. Jones AE. Unbundling early sepsis resuscitation. Ann Emerg Med 2014;63(6): 654–5.
126. Lewis RJ. Disassembling goal-directed therapy for sepsis. JAMA 2010;303(8): 777–9.
127. Nguyen HB, Jaehne AK, Jayaprakash N, et al. Early goal-directed therapy in severe sepsis and septic shock: insights and comparisons to ProCESS, ProMISe, and ARISE. Crit Care 2016;20:160.

128. Yu H, Chi D, Wang S, et al. Effect of early goal-directed therapy on mortality in patients with severe sepsis or septic shock: a meta-analysis of randomized controlled trials. BMJ Open 2016;6:e008330.

129. Gupta RG, Hartigan SM, Kashiouris MG, et al. Early goal-directed resuscitation of patients with septic shock: current evidence and future directions. Crit Care 2015;19:286.

130. Angus DC, Barnato AE, Bell D, et al. A systematic review and meta-analysis of early goal-directed therapy for septic shock: the ARISE, ProCESS and ProMISe Investigators. Intensive Care Med 2015;41:1549–60.

131. Coccolin F, Sartelli M, Catena F, et al. Early goal-directed treatment versus standard care in the management of early septic shock: meta-analysis of randomized trials. J Trauma Acute Care Surg 2016;81(5):971–8.

132. Park SK, Shin SR, Hur M, et al. The effect of early goal-directed therapy for treatment of severe sepsis or septic shock: a systemic review and meta-analysis. J Crit Care 2017;38:115–22.

133. Rivers EP, Yataco AC, Jaehne AK, et al. Oxygen extraction and perfusion markers in severe sepsis and septic shock: diagnostic, therapeutic and outcome implications. Curr Opin Crit Care 2015;21:381–7.

134. Cecconi M, De Backer D, Antonelli M, et al. Consensus on circulatory shock and hemodynamic monitoring. Task force of the European Society of Intensive Care Medicine. Intensive Care Med 2014;40:1795–815.

135. Eskesen TG, Wetterslev M, Perner A. Systematic review including re-analysis of 1148 individual data sets of central venous pressure as a predictor of fluid responsiveness. Intensive Care Med 2016;42:324–32.

136. Walkey AJ, Wiener RS, Lindenauer PK. Utilization patterns and outcomes associated with central venous catheter in septic shock: a population based study. Crit Care Med 2013;41:1450–7.

137. Sondergaard S, Parkin G, Aneman A. Central venous pressure: soon an outcome-associated matter. Curr Opin Anaesthesiol 2016;29:179–85.

138. Holst LB, Haase N, Wetterslev J, et al, The TRISS Trial Group and the Scandinavian Critical Care Trials Group. Lower versus higher hemoglobin threshold for transfusion in septic shock. N Engl J Med 2014;371:1381–91.

139. Rygard SL, Holst LB, Wetterslev J, et al, The TRISS Trial Group and the Scandanvian Critical Care Trials Group. Long-term outcomes in patients with septic shock transfused at lower versus a higher haemoglobin threshold: the TRISS randomized, multicenter clinical trial. Intensive Care Med 2016;42:1685–94.

140. Dupuis C, Sonneville R, Adrie C, et al. Impact of transfusion on patients with sepsis admitted to the intensive care unit: a systematic review and meta-analysis. Ann Intensive Care 2017;7(5):1–13.

141. Boulain T, Garot D, Vignon P, et al. Prevalence of low central venous oxygen saturation in the first hours of intensive care unit admission and associated mortality in septic shock patients: a prospective multicentre study. Crit Care 2014; 18(6):609.

142. Pope JV, Jones AE, Gaieski DF, et al. Multicenter study of central venous oxygen saturation (ScVO2) as a predictor of mortality in patients with sepsis. Ann Emerg Med 2010;55(1):40–6.

143. De Backer D, Creteur J, Preiser JC, et al. Microvascular blood flow is altered in patients with sepsis. Am J Respir Care Med 2002;166:98–104.

144. Spronk PE, Ince C, Gardien MJ, et al. Nitroglycerin in septic shock after intravascular volume resuscitation. Lancet 2002;360:1395–6.

145. Spronk PE, Zandstra DF, Ince C. Bench-to-bedside review: sepsis is a disease of the microcirculation. Crit Care 2004;8(6):462–8.
146. Sakr YL, Dubois MJ, De Backer D, et al. Persistent microcirculatory alterations are associated with organ failure and death in patients with septic shock. Crit Care Med 2004;32:1825–31.
147. Trzeciak S, Dellinger RP, Parrillo JE, et al. Early microcirculatory perfusion derangements in patients with severe sepsis and septic shock: relationship to hemodynamics, oxygen transport, and survival. Ann Emerg Med 2007;49(1): 88–98.e2.
148. Brealey D, Brand M, Hargreaves I, et al. Association between mitochondrial dysfunction and severity and outcome of septic shock. Lancet 2002;360: 219–23.
149. Fink MP. Bench-to-bedside review: cytopathic hypoxia. Crit Care 2002;6:491–9.
150. Crouser ED. Mitochondrial dysfunction in septic shock and multiple organ dysfunction syndrome. Mitochondrion 2004;4:729–41.
151. Protti A, Singer M. Bench-to-bedside review: potential strategies to protect or reverse mitochondrial dysfunction in sepsis-induced organ failure. Crit Care 2006;10(228):1–7.
152. Levy RJ. Mitochondrial dysfunction, bioenergetics impairment, and metabolic down-regulation in sepsis. Shock 2007;28(1):24–8.
153. Ruggieri AJ, Levy RJ, Deutschman CS. Mitochondrial dysfunction and resuscitation in sepsis. Crit Care Clin 2010;26:567–75.
154. Mizock BA, Falk JL. Lactic acidosis in critical illness. Crit Care Med 1992;20: 80–93.
155. Nguyen BH, Rivers EP, Knoblich BP, et al. Early lactate clearance is associated with improved outcome in severe sepsis and septic shock. Crit Care Med 2004; 32(8):1637–42.
156. Jones AE, Shapiro NI, Trzeciak S, et al. Lactate clearance vs central venous oxygen saturation as goals of early sepsis therapy: a randomized clinical trial. JAMA 2010;303:739–46.
157. Jansen TC, van Bommel J, Schoonderbeek FJ, et al. Early lactate-guided therapy in intensive care unit patients: a multicenter, open-label, randomized control trial. Am J Respir Crit Care Med 2010;182:752–61.
158. Gu WJ, Zhang Z, Bakker J. Early lactate clearance-guided therapy in patients with sepsis: a meta-analysis with trial sequential analysis of randomized controlled trials. Intensive Care Med 2015;41:1862–3.
159. Bakker J, Gris P, Coffernils M, et al. Serial blood lactate levels can predict the development of multiple organ failure following septic shock. Am J Surg 1996; 171:221–6.
160. Shapiro NI, Howell MD, Talmor D, et al. Serum lactate as a predictor of mortality in emergency department patients with infection. Ann Emerg Med 2005;45: 524–8.
161. Mikkelsen ME, Miltiades AN, Gaieski DF, et al. Serum lactate is associated with mortality in severe sepsis independent of organ failure and shock. Crit Care Med 2009;37(5):1670–7.
162. Arnold RC, Shapiro NI, Jones AE, et al. Multi-center study of early lactate clearance as a determinant of survival in patients with presumed sepsis. Shock 2009; 32:36–9.
163. Puskarich MA, Trzeciak S, Shapiro N, et al. Prognostic value and agreement of achieving lactate clearance or central venous oxygen saturation goals during early sepsis resuscitation. Acad Emerg Med 2012;19(3):252–8.

164. Casserly B, Phillips GS, Schorr C, et al. Lactate measurements in sepsis-induced tissue hypoperfusion: results from the Surviving Sepsis Campaign database. Crit Care Med 2015;43:567–73.

165. Chertoff J, Chisum M, Simmons L, et al. Prognostic utility of plasma lactate measured between 24 and 48 h after initiation of early goal-directed therapy in the management of sepsis, severe sepsis, and septic shock. J Intensive Care 2016;4(13):1–8.

166. Gladden LB. Lactate metabolism: a new paradigm for the third millennium. J Physiol 2004;558(1):5–30.

167. Levy B. Lactate and the shock state: the metabolic view. Curr Opin Crit Care 2006;12:315–21.

168. Garcia-Alvarez M, Marik P, Bellomo R. Sepsis-associated hyperlactatemia. Crit Care 2014;18(503):1–11.

169. Nguyen HB, Kuan WS, Batech M, et al, The ATLAS (Asia Network to Regulate Sepsis care) Investigators. Outcome effectiveness of the severe sepsis resuscitation bundle with addition of lactate clearance as a bundle item: a multi-national evaluation. Crit Care 2011;15(R229):1–10.

170. Dubin A, O Pozo M, Casabella CA, et al. Increasing arterial blood pressure with norepinephrine does not improve microcirculatory blood flow: a prospective study. Crit Care 2009;13(R92):1–8.

171. LeDoux D, Astiz ME, Carpati CM, et al. Effects of perfusion pressure on tissue perfusion in septic shock. Crit Care Med 2000;28(8):2729–32.

172. Thooft A, Favory R, Salgado DR, et al. Effects of changes in arterial pressure on organ perfusion during septic shock. Crit Care 2011;15(R222):1–8.

173. Xu JY, Ma SQ, Pan C, et al. A high mean arterial pressure target is associated with improved microcirculation in septic shock patients with previous hypertension: a prospective open label study. Crit Care 2015;19(130):1–8.

174. Ince C. Hemodynamic coherence and the rationale for monitoring the microcirculation. Crit Care 2015;19(S8):1–13.

175. Varpula M, Tallgren M, Saukkonen K, et al. Hemodynamic variables related to outcome in septic shock. Intensive Care Med 2005;31:1066–71.

176. Bai X, Yu W, Ji W, et al. Early versus delayed administration of norepinephrine in patients with septic shock. Crit Care 2014;18(532):1–8.

177. Waechter J, Kumar A, Lapinsky S, et al, The Cooperative Antimicrobial Therapy of Septic Shock Database Research Group. Interaction between fluids and vasoactive agents on mortality in septic shock: a multicenter, observational study. Crit Care Med 2014;42(10):2158–68.

178. Asfar P, Meziani F, Hamel JF, et al, The SEPSISPAM Investigators. High versus low blood-pressure target in patients with septic shock. N Engl J Med 2014; 370(17):1583–651.

179. Bourgoin A, Leone M, Delmas A, et al. Increasing mean arterial pressure in patients with septic shock: effects on oxygen variables and renal function. Crit Care Med 2005;33(4):780–6.

180. Jones AE, Brown MD, Trzeciak S, et al, On Behalf of the Emergency Medicine Shock Research Network Investigators. The effect of quantitative resuscitation strategy on mortality in patients with sepsis: a meta-analysis. Crit Care Med 2008;36(10):2734–9.

181. Simpson SQ, Gaines M, Hussein Y, et al. Early goal-directed therapy for severe sepsis and septic shock: a living systematic review. J Crit Care 2016;36:43–8.

182. Puskarich MA, Trzeciak S, Shapiro NI, et al. Outcomes of patients undergoing early sepsis resuscitation for cryptic shock compared with overt shock. Resuscitation 2011;82:1289–93.

183. Cannon CM, Holthaus CV, Zubrow MT, et al. The GENESIS project (GEN-earlized Early Sepsis Intervnetion Strategies): a multicenter quality improvement collaborative. J Intensive Care Med 2013;28:355–68.

184. Ranzani OT, Monteiro MB, Ferreira EM, et al. Reclassifying the spectrum of septic patients using lactate: severe sepsis, cryptic shock, vasoplegic shock and dysoxic shock. Rev Bras Ter Intensiva 2013;25:270–8.

185. Dugas AF, Mackenhauer J, Salciccioli JD, et al. Prevalence and characteristics of nonlactate and lactate expressors in septic shock. J Crit Care 2012;27: 344–50.

186. Hernandez G, Castro R, Romero CI, et al. Persistent sepsis-induced hypotension without hyperlactatemia: is it really septic shock? J Crit Care 2011;26: 435.e9-14.

187. Park JS, Kim SJ, Lee SW, et al. Initial low oxygen extraction ratio is related to severe organ dysfunction and high in-hospital mortality in severe sepsis and septic shock patients. J Emerg Med 2015;49(3):261–7.

188. Thomas-Rueddel DO, Poidinger B, Weiss M, et al. Hyperlactatemia is an independent predictor of mortality and denotes distinct subtypes of severe sepsis and septic shock. J Crit Care 2015;30:439.

189. Eidelman LA, Putterman D, Putterman C, et al. The spectrum of septic encephalopathy. Definitions, etiologies, and mortalities. JAMA 1996;275:470–3.

190. Ebersoldt M, Sharshar T, Annane D. Sepsis-associated delirium. Intensive Care Med 2007;33:941–50.

191. Heming N, Mazeraud A, Verdonk F, et al. Neuroanatomy of sepsis-associated encephalopathy. Crit Care 2017;21(65):1–6.

192. Tauber S, Eiffert H, Bruck W, et al. Septic encephalopathy and septic encephalitis. Expert Rev Anti Infect Ther 2017;15(2):121–32.

193. Tsuruta R, Oda Y. A clinical perspective of sepsis-associated delirium. J Intensive Care 2016;4(18):1–7.

194. American Psychiatric Association. Diagnostic and statistical manual of mental disorders. 5th edition. Arlington (VA): American Psychiatric Publishing; 2013.

195. Ely EW, Shintani A, Truman B, et al. Delirium as a predictor of mortality in mechanically ventilated patients in the intensive care unit. JAMA 2004;291: 1753–62.

196. McCusker J, Cole M, Abrahamowicz M, et al. Delirium predicts 12-month mortality. Arch Intern Med 2002;162(4):457–63.

197. Leslie D, Zhang Y, Holford T, et al. Premature death associated with delirium at 1-year follow-up. Arch Intern Med 2005;165(14):1657–62.

198. Milbrandt EB, Deppen S, Harrison PL, et al. Costs associated with delirium in mechanically ventilated patients. Crit Care Med 2004;32:955–62.

199. Andrew M, Freter S, Rockwood K. Incomplete functional recovery after delirium in elderly people: a prospective cohort study. BMC Geriatr 2005;5:5.

200. Girard TD, Jackson JC, Pandharipande PP, et al. Delirium as a predictor of long-term cognitive impairment in survivors of critical illness. Crit Care Med 2010;38: 1513–20.

201. Pandharipande PP, Girard TD, Jackson JC, et al. Long-term cognitive impairment after critical illness. N Engl J Med 2013;369:1306–16.

202. Barr J, Fraser GL, Puntillo K, et al. Clinical practice guidelines for the management of pain, agitation, and delirium in adult patients in the intensive care unit. Crit Care Med 2013;41:263–306.

203. Ely EW, Inouye SK, Bernard GR, et al. Delirium in mechanically ventilated patients: validity and reliability of the confusion assessment method for the intensive care unit (CAM-ICU). JAMA 2001;286:2703–10.

204. van Eijk MM, van Marum RJ, Klijn IA, et al. Comparison of delirium assessment tools in a mixed intensive care unit. Crit Care Med 2009;37:1881–5.

205. Ely EW. The ABCDEF bundle: science and philosophy of how ICU liberation serves patients and families. Crit Care Med 2017;45(2):321–30.

206. Marra A, Ely EW, Pandharipande PP, et al. The ABCDEF bundle in critical care. Crit Care Clin 2017;33(2):225–43.

207. Barnes-Daly MA, Phillips G, Ely EW. Improving hospital survival and reducing brain dysfunction at seven California community hospitals: implementing PAD guidelines via the ABCDEF bundle in 6,064 patients. Crit Care Med 2017; 45(2):171–8.

208. Bouhemad B, Nicolas-Robin A, Arbelot C, et al. Isolated and reversible impairment of ventricular relaxation in patients with septic shock. Crit Care Med 2015; 41:1004–13.

209. Gonzalez C, Begot E, Dalmay F, et al. Prognostic impact of left ventricular diastolic function in patients with septic shock. Ann Intensive Care 2016;6(36):1–8.

210. Calvin JE, Driedger AA, Sibbald WJ. An assessment of myocardial function in human sepsis utilizing ECG gated cardiac scintigraphy. Chest 1981;80:579–86.

211. Parker MM, Shelhamer JH, Bacharach SL, et al. Profound but reversible myocardial depression in patients with septic shock. Ann Intern Med 1984;100:483–90.

212. Rudiger A, Singer M. Mechanisms of sepsis-induced cardiac dysfunction. Crit Care Med 2007;35(6):1599–608.

213. Suffredini AF, Fromm RE, Parker MM, et al. The cardiovascular response of normal humans to the administration of endotoxin. N Engl J Med 1989;321: 280–7.

214. Landesberg G, Levin PD, Gilon D, et al. Myocardial dysfunction in severe sepsis and septic shock: no correlation with inflammatory cytokines in real-life clinical setting. Chest 2015;148(1):93–102.

215. Sanfilippo F, Corredor C, Fletcher N, et al. Diastolic dysfunction and mortality in septic patients: a systematic review and meta-analysis. Intensive Care Med 2015;41:1004–13.

216. Landesberg G, Gilon D, Meroz Y, et al. Diastolic dysfunction and mortality in severe sepsis and septic shock. Eur Heart J 2012;33:895–903.

217. Sevilla Berrios RA, O'Horo JC, Velagapudi V, et al. Correlation of left ventricular systolic dysfunction determined by low ejection fraction and 30-day mortality in patients with severe sepsis and septic shock: a systematic review and meta-analysis. J Crit Care 2014;29:495–9.

218. Pulido JN, Afessa B, Masaki M, et al. Clinical spectrum, frequency, and significance of myocardial dysfunction in severe sepsis and septic shock. Mayo Clin Proc 2012;87(7):620–8.

219. Huang SJ, Nalos M, McLean AS. Is early ventricular dysfunction or dilation associated with lower mortality rate in adult severe sepsis and septic shock? A meta-analysis. Crit Care 2013;17(R96):1–13.

220. Bessiere F, Khenifer S, Dubourg J, et al. Prognostic value of troponins in sepsis: a meta-analysis. Intensive Care Med 2013;39:1181–9.

221. Maeder M, Fehr T, Rickli H, et al. Sepsis-associated myocardial dysfunction: diagnostic and prognostic impact of cardiac troponins and natriuretic peptides. Chest 2006;129(5):1349–66.

222. Annane D, Vignon P, Renault A, et al, The CATS Study Group. Norepinephrine plus dobutamine versus epinephrine alone for management of septic shock: a randomised trial. Lancet 2007;370:676–84.

223. Hayes MA, Timmins AC, Yau EH, et al. Elevation of systemic oxygen delivery in the treatment of critically ill patients. N Engl J Med 1994;330:1717–22.

224. Vincent JL. The International Sepsis Forum's frontiers in sepsis: high cardiac output should be maintained in severe sepsis. Crit Care 2003;7(4):276–8.

225. Shaver CM, Chen W, Janz DR, et al. Atrial fibrillation is an independent predictor of mortality in critically ill patients. Crit Care Med 2015;43(10):2104–11.

226. Kuipers S, Klein Klouwenberg PMC, Cremer OL. Incidence, risk factors and outcomes of new-onset atrial fibrillation in patients with sepsis: a systematic review. Crit Care 2014;18(6):1–9.

227. Klein Klouwenberg PMC, Frencken JF, Kuipers S, et al. Incidence, predictors, and outcomes of new-onset atrial fibrillation in critically ill patients with sepsis: a cohort study. Am J Respir Care Med 2017;195(2):205–11.

228. Liu WC, Lin WY, Lin SC, et al. Prognostic impact of restored sinus rhythm in patients with sepsis and new-onset atrial fibrillation. Crit Care 2016;20(373):1–9.

229. Morelli A, Ertmer C, Westphal M, et al. Effect of heart rate control with esmolol on hemodynamic and clinical outcomes in patients with septic shock: a randomized clinical trial. JAMA 2013;310:1683–91.

230. Walkey AJ, Evans SR, Winter MR, et al. Practice patterns and outcomes of treatments for atrial fibrillation during sepsis: a propensity-matched cohort study. Chest 2016;149(1):74–83.

231. Walkey AJ, Quin EK, Winter MR, et al. Practice patterns and outcomes associated with use of anticoagulation among patients with atrial fibrillation during sepsis. JAMA Cardiol 2016;1(6):682–90.

232. January CT, Wann LS, Alpert JS, et al, The ACC/AHA Task Force Members. 2014 AHA/ACC/HRS guideline for the management of patients with atrial fibrillation: executive summary: a report of the American College of Cardiology/American Heart Association Task Force on practice guidelines and the Heart Rhythm Society. Circulation 2014;130(23):2071–104.

233. Heidenreich PA, Solis P, Estes NA 3rd, et al. 2016 ACC/AHA clinical performance and quality measures for adults with atrial fibrillation or atrial flutter: a report of the American College of Cardiology/American Heart Association Task Force on Performance Measures. J Am Coll Cardiol 2016;68(5):525–68.

234. Barnett AS, Lewis WR, Field ME, et al. Quality of evidence underlying the American Heart Association/American College of Cardiology/Heart Rhythm Society guidelines on the management of atrial fibrillation. JAMA Cardiol 2017;2(3):319–23.

235. De Backer D, Aldecoa C, Njimi H, et al. Dopamine versus norepinephrine in the treatment of septic shock: a meta-analysis. Crit Care Med 2012;40(3):725–30.

236. Gamper G, Havel C, Arrich J, et al. Vasopressors for hypotensive shock. Cochrane Database Syst Rev 2016;(2):CD003709.

237. De Backer D, Biston P, Devriendt J, et al, SOAP II Investigators. Comparison of dopamine and norepinephrine in the treatment of shock. N Engl J Med 2010;362(9):779–89.

238. Avni T, Lador A, Lev S, et al. Vasopressors for the treatment of septic shock: systematic review and meta-analysis. PLoS One 2015;10(8):e0129305.

239. Landry DW, Levin HR, Gallant EM, et al. Vasopressin deficiency contributes to the vasodilation of septic shock. Circulation 1997;95:1122–5.

240. Sharshar T, Blanchard A, Paillard M, et al. Circulating vasopressin levels in septic shock. Crit Care Med 2003;31:1752–8.

241. Russel JA, Walley KR, Singer J, et al, The VASST Investigators. Vasopressin versus norepinephrine infusion in patients with septic shock. N Engl J Med 2008;358:877–87.

242. Russell JA, Walley KR, Gordon AC, et al. Interaction of vasopressin infusion, corticosteroid treatment, and mortality of septic shock. Crit Care Med 2009; 37:811–8.

243. Russell JA. Bench-to-bedside review: vasopressin in the management of septic shock. Crit Care 2011;15(226):1–19.

244. Gordon AC, Mason AJ, Perkins GD, et al. The interaction of vasopressin and corticosteroids in septic shock: a pilot randomized controlled trial. Crit Care Med 2014;42:1325–33.

245. Gordon AC, Mason AJ, Thirunavukkarasu N, et al, The VANISH Investigators. Effect of early vasopressin vs norepinephrine on kidney failure in patients with septic shock: the VANISH randomized clinical trial. JAMA 2016;316(5):509–18.

246. Curtis N, Corapi J, Roberts R, et al. Rebranding of generic parenteral vasopressin: effect on clinician practices and perceptions. Am J Health Syst Pharm 2017;74(3):105–6.

247. Myburgh JA, Higgins A, Jovanovska A, et al, The CAT Study Investigators. A comparison of epinephrine and norepinephrine in critically ill patients. Intensive Care Med 2008;34:2226–34.

248. Morelli A, Ertmer C, Rehberg S, et al. Phenylephrine versus norepinephrine for initial hemodynamic support of patients with septic shock: a randomized, controlled trial. Crit Care 2008;12(R143):1–11.

249. Morelli A, Lange M, Ertmer C, et al. Short-term effects of phenylephrine on systemic and regional hemodynamics in patients with septic shock: a crossover pilot study. Shock 2008;29:446–51.

250. Gregory JS, Bonfiglio MF, Dasta JF, et al. Experience with phenylephrine as a component of the pharmacologic support of septic shock. Crit Care Med 1991;19(11):1395–400.

251. Vail E, Gershengorn HB, Hua M, et al. Association between US norepinephrine shortage and mortality among patients with septic shock. JAMA 2017;317(14): 1433–42.

252. ARDS Definition Task force, Ranieri VM, Rubenfeld GD, Thompson BT, et al. Acute respiratory distress syndrome: the Berlin definition. JAMA 2012; 307(23):2526–33.

253. Acute Respiratory Distress Syndrome Network, Brower RG, Matthay MA, Morris A, et al. Ventilation with lower tidal volumes as compared with traditional tidal volumes for acute lung injury and the acute respiratory distress syndrome. N Engl J Med 2000;342(18):1301–8.

254. Futier E, Constantin JM, Paugam-Burtz C, et al, IMPROVE Study Group. A trial of intraoperative low-tidal volume ventilation in abdominal surgery. N Engl J Med 2013;369:428–37.

255. Pinheiro de Oliveira R, Hetzel MP, dos Anjos Silva M, et al. Mechanical ventilation with high tidal volume induces inflammation in patients without lung disease. Crit Care 2010;14(2):R39.

256. Guerin C, Reignier J, Richard JC, et al. Prone positioning in severe acute respiratory distress syndrome. N Engl J Med 2013;368(23):2159–68.

257. Beitler JR, Shaeif S, Montesi SB, et al. Prone positioning reduces mortality from acute respiratory distress syndrome in the low tidal volume era: a meta-analysis. Intensive Care Med 2014;40:332–41.

258. Papazian L, Forel JM, Gacouin A, et al. Neuromuscular blockers in early acute respiratory distress syndrome. N Engl J Med 2010;363(12):1107–16.

259. Peek GJ, Mugford M, Tiruvoipati R, et al. Efficacy and economic assessment of conventional ventilatory support versus extracorporeal membrane oxygenation for severe adult respiratory failure (CESAR): a multicenter randomized controlled trial. Lancet 2009;374:1351–63.

260. Casaer MP, Van den Berghe G. Nutrition in the acute phase of critical illness. N Engl J Med 2014;370(23):1227–36.

261. Alberda C, Gramlich L, Jones N, et al. The relationship between nutritional intake and clinical outcomes in critically ill patients: results of an international multi-center observational study. Intensive Care Med 2009;35:1728–37.

262. National Heart, Lung, and Blood Institute Acute Respiratory Distress Syndrome (ARDS) Clinical Trials Network, Rice TW, Wheeler AP, Thompson BT, et al. Initial trophic vs full enteral feeding in patients with acute lung injury. JAMA 2012; 307(8):795–803.

263. Kuppinger DD, Rittler P, Hartl WH, et al. Use of gastric residual volume to guide enteral nutrition in critically ill patients: a brief systematic review of clinical studies. Nutrition 2013;29(9):1075–9.

264. Acosta-Escribano J, Fernandez-Vivas M, Carmona TG, et al. Gastric versus transpyloric feeding in severe traumatic brain injury: a prospective, randomized trial. Intensive Care Med 2010;36:1532–9.

265. Alkhawaja S, Martin C, Butler RJ, et al. Post-pyloric versus gastric tube feeding for preventing pneumonia and improving nutritional outcomes in critically ill adults. Cochrane Database Syst Rev 2015;(8):CD008875.

266. Dissanaike S, Shelton M, Warner K, et al. The risk for bloodstream infections is associated with increased parenteral caloric intake in patients receiving parenteral nutrition. Crit Care 2007;11:R114.

267. Casaer M, Mesotten D, Hermans G, et al. Early versus late parenteral nutrition in critically ill adults. N Engl J Med 2011;365:506–17.

268. Peter JV, Moral JL, Phillips-Hughes J. A metaanalysis of treatment outcomes of early enteral versus early parenteral nutrition in hospitalized patients. Crit Care Med 2005;33(1):213–20.

269. Heyland D, Muscedere J, Wischmeyer PE, et al. A randomized trial of glutamine and antioxidants in critically ill patients. N Engl J Med 2013;368(16):1489–97.

270. Andrews PJ, Avenell A, Noble DW, et al. Randomised trial of glutamine, selenium, or both, to supplement parenteral nutrition for critically ill patients. BMJ 2011;342:d1542.

271. Pontes-Arruda A, Martins LF, de Lima SM, et al. Enteral nutrition with eicosapentaenoic acid, gamma-linolenic acid and antioxidants in the early treatment of sepsis: results from a multicenter, prospective, randomized, double-blinded, controlled study: the INTERSEPT Study. Crit Care 2011;15:R144.

272. Manzanares W, Dhaliwal R, Jurewitsch B, et al. Parenteral fish oil lipid emulsions in the critically ill: a systematic review and meta-analysis. JPEN J Parenter Enteral Nutr 2014;38:20–8.

273. Zhu D, Zhang Y, Li S, et al. Enteral omega-3 fatty acid supplementation in adult patients with acute respiratory distress syndrome: a systematic review of randomized controlled trials with meta-analysis and trial sequential analysis. Intensive Care Med 2014;40:504–12.

274. Rochwerg B, Alhazzani W, Sindi A, et al. Fluids in sepsis and septic shock group: fluid resuscitation in sepsis: a systematic review and network meta-analysis. Ann Intern Med 2014;161:347–55.

275. Haase N, Perner A, Hennings LI, et al. Hydroxyethyl starch 130/0.38–0.45 versus crystalloid or albumin in patients with sepsis: systematic review with meta-analysis and trial sequential analysis. BMJ 2013;346:f839.

276. Finfer S, Bellomo R, Boyce N, et al, The SAFE Study Investigators. A comparison of albumin and saline for fluid resuscitation in the intensive care unit. N Engl J Med 2004;350:2247–56.

277. Caironi P, Tognoni G, Masson S, et al, ALBIOS Study Investigators. Albumin replacement in patients with severe sepsis or septic shock. N Engl J Med 2014;370:1412–21.

278. Delaney AP, Dan A, McCaffrey J, et al. The role of albumin as a resuscitation fluid for patients with sepsis: a systematic review and meta-analysis. Crit Care Med 2011;39:386–91.

279. Rochwerg B, Alhazzani W, Sindi A, et al. Fluid resuscitation in sepsis: a systematic review and network meta-analysis. Ann Intern Med 2014;161:347–55.

280. Vincent JL, Navickis RJ, Wilkes MM. Morbidity in hospitalized patients receiving human albumin: a meta-analysis of randomized, controlled trials. Crit Care Med 2004;32:2029–38.

281. de Oliveira FS, Freitas FG, Ferreira EM, et al. Positive fluid balance as a prognostic factor for mortality and acute kidney injury in severe sepsis and septic shock. J Crit Care 2015;30:97–101.

282. Acheampong A, Vincent JL. A positive fluid balance is an independent prognostic factor in patients with sepsis. Crit Care 2015;19:251.

283. Malbrain ML, Marik PE, Witters I, et al. Fluid overload, de-resuscitation, and outcomes in critically ill or injured patients: a systemic review with suggestions for clinical practice. Anaesthesiol Intensive Ther 2014;46:361–80.

284. Boyd JH, Forbes J, Nakada TA, et al. Fluid resuscitation in septic shock: a positive fluid balance and elevated central venous pressure are associated with increased mortality. Crit Care Med 2011;39:259–65.

285. Mehta RL, Pascual MT, Soroko S, et al, PICARD Study Group. Diuretics, mortality, and nonrecovery of renal function in acute renal failure. JAMA 2002;288(20):2547–53.

286. Martin GS, Moss M, Wheeler AP, et al. A randomized, controlled trial of furosemide with or without albumin in hypoproteinemic patients with acute lung injury. Crit Care Med 2005;33:1681–7.

287. Uhlig C, Silva PL, Deckert S, et al. Albumin versus crystalloid solutions in patients with the acute respiratory distress syndrome: a systematic review and meta-analysis. Crit Care 2014;18:R10.

288. Noritomi DT, Soriano FG, Kellum JA, et al. Metabolic acidosis in patients with severe sepsis and septic shock: a longitudinal quantitative study. Crit Care Med 2009;37(10):2733–9.

289. Cooper DJ, Walley KR, Wiggs BR, et al. Bicarbonate does not improve hemodynamics in critically ill patients who have lactic acidosis. Ann Intern Med 1990;112:492–8.

290. El-Solh AA, Jaoude PA, Porhomayon J. Bicarbonate therapy in the treatment of septic shock: a second look. Intern Emerg Med 2010;5:341–7.

291. Honore PM, Jacobs R, Hendrickx I, et al. Prevention and treatment of sepsis-induced acute kidney injury: an update. Ann Intensive Care 2015;5(1):51.

292. De Corte W, Vuylsteke S, De Waele JJ, et al. Severe lactic acidosis in critically ill patients with acute kidney injury treated with renal replacement therapy. J Crit Care 2014;29(4):650–5.
293. Gaudry S, Hajage D, Schortgen F, et al. Initiation strategies for renal-replacement therapy in the intensive care unit. N Engl J Med 2016;375(2): 122–33.
294. Tonelli M, Manns B, Feller-Kopman D. Acute renal failure in the intensive care unit: a systematic review of the impact of dialytic modality on mortality and renal recovery. Am J Kidney Dis 2002;40:875–85.
295. Boonen E, Vervenne H, Meersseman P, et al. Reduced cortisol metabolism during critical illness. N Engl J Med 2013;368(18):1477–88.
296. Cooper MS, Stewart PM. Corticosteroid insufficiency in acutely ill patients. N Engl J Med 2003;348:727–34.
297. Sprung CL, Annane D, Keh D, et al. Hydrocortisone therapy for patients with septic shock. N Engl J Med 2008;358(2):111–24.
298. Keh D, Trips E, Marx G. Effect of hydrocortisone on development of shock among patients with severe sepsis. JAMA 2016;316(17):1775–85.
299. Gibbison B, Lopez-Lopez J, Higgins JP, et al. Corticosteroids in septic shock: a systematic review and network meta-analysis. Crit Care 2017;21:78.
300. Inoue S, Egi M, Kotani J, et al. Accuracy of blood-glucose measurements using glucose meters and arterial blood gas analyzers in critically ill adult patients: systematic review. Crit Care 2013;17:R48.
301. Egi M, Bellomo R, Stachowski E, et al. Intensive insulin therapy in postoperative intensive care unit patients: a decision analysis. Am J Respir Crit Care Med 2006;173(4):407–13.
302. Kwon S, Thompson R, Dellinger P, et al. Importance of perioperative glycemic control in general surgery: a report from the surgical care and outcomes assessment program. Ann Surg 2013;257(1):8–14.
303. Van den Berghe G, Wouters P, Weekers F, et al. Intensive insulin therapy in critically ill patients. N Engl J Med 2011;345(19):1359–67.
304. NICE-SUGAR Study Investigators, Finfer S, Chittock DR, Su SY, et al. Intensive versus conventional glucose control in critically ill patients. N Engl J Med 2009; 360(13):1283–97.
305. Griesdale DE, de Souza RJ, van Dam RM, et al. Intensive insulin therapy and mortality among critically ill patients: a meta-analysis including NICE-SUGAR study data. CMAJ 2009;180(8):821–7.
306. May AK, Kauffmann RM, Collier BR. The place for glycemic control in the surgical patient. Surg Infect (Larchmt) 2011;12(5):405–18.
307. Kauffmann RM, Hayes RM, Jenkins JM, et al. Provision of balanced nutrition protects against hypoglycemia in the critically ill surgical patient. JPEN J Parenter Enteral Nutr 2011;35(6):686–94.
308. Dortsch MJ, Mowery NT, Ozdas A, et al. A computerized insulin infusion titration protocol improves glucose control with less hypoglycemia compared to a manual titration protocol in a trauma intensive care unit. JPEN J Parenter Enteral Nutr 2008;32(1):18–27.

Ventilator Strategies for Chronic Obstructive Pulmonary Disease and Acute Respiratory Distress Syndrome

Nathan T. Mowery, MD

KEYWORDS

- Respiratory failure • Hypoxia • ARDS • COPD • APRV
- Airway pressure release ventilation • ALI • PEEP

KEY POINTS

- Identification of high-risk patients for pulmonary complications is an important part of determining outcomes.
- Low tidal volume ventilation is the only ventilator strategy that has been shown in prospective randomized trials to improve mortality in ARDS and COPD.
- Once COPD patients are intubated the minute ventilation should be titrated to Ph and not to the $Paco_2$.
- A restrictive fluid schedule that maintains perfusion but aims at keeping patients fluid neutral has been associated with shorter ICU and ventilator days in ARDS.
- In ARDS several studies show APRV to have physiologic benefits and to improve some measures of clinical outcome, such as oxygenation, use of sedation, hemodynamics, and respiratory mechanics. None have shown a survival benefit when compared with conventional lung protective ventilation.

INTRODUCTION

Worldwide 52 million people have been diagnosed with COPD. The incidence and the complications that it has caused are increasing.[1] In 1990 it was the 6th most common cause of death worldwide but is expected to be the third most common by the year 2020.[2] Patients with COPD often require respiratory support for a variety of reasons including exacerbations of the disease, complications related to other medical conditions and elective and emergent surgical interventions. In these surgical situations if the clinical situations allows the best time to optimize the patient to prevent complication is pre-operatively. When mechanical ventilation becomes necessary in this challenging population morbidity can be minimized with the application of evidence-based approaches.

The author has nothing to disclose.
Wake Forest Baptist Medical Center, Department of Surgery, Medical Center Boulevard, Winston-Salem, NC 27157, USA
E-mail address: nmowery@wakehealth.edu

Surg Clin N Am 97 (2017) 1381–1397
http://dx.doi.org/10.1016/j.suc.2017.07.006
0039-6109/17/© 2017 Elsevier Inc. All rights reserved.

surgical.theclinics.com

Acute respiratory distress syndrome (ARDS) is defined by the acute onset of hypoxemia and bilateral infiltrates after a trigger. The definition has changed over time to its current status. Although it only effects about 5% of mechanically ventilated patients, 75% of those present with a moderate or severe form.[3] Unlike COPD, the incidence of ARDS is decreasing secondary to the decrease in the numbers of triggers secondary to the institution of such interventions, such as limited resuscitations, early source control, restrictive transfusion strategies, ventilator care bundles, and lung-protective ventilation.[4]

This article discusses the basic concepts of mechanical ventilation in patients with COPD and ARDS, reviews predisposing factors to the development of complications, and discusses current strategies for the recognition and prevention of these adverse effects in the application of mechanical ventilation in this population.

PREDICTING PULMONARY COMPLICATIONS

Ventilator strategies can play a pivotal role in the deciding the outcome of patient once pulmonary complications have developed. The issue is that by far the best means to improve pulmonary-related morbidity is to prevent it from happening. A large part of that preventive piece is to recognize high-risk groups so that at the very least preparations can be made. Virtually all of the interventions described herein have been shown to be at least partially protective if instituted before pulmonary complications have developed. For example, low tidal volume ventilation is a proven ventilator strategy for the treatment of both COPD and ARDS, and has also been shown to minimize the risk of the development of ARDS. In high-risk patient populations, it would only stand to reason that strict adherence to low tidal volume protocols be observed.

The risk of postoperative pulmonary complications (PPCs) increases nearly up to 3-fold for patients with a moderate or severe systemic disease (American Society of Anesthesiology class III) and up to 5-fold in moribund patients (American Society of Anesthesiology class IV).[5] The individual risk does not only relate to a patient's comorbidities, but is also influenced by the type and/or duration of surgery, and it may also be modified by the corresponding type of anesthesia.[6] Therefore, an American Society of Anesthesiology class IV patient undergoing a short, low-risk procedure under regional anesthesia might have a lower risk of PPCs than a patient without comorbidities planned to undergo a long-lasting, high-risk surgical procedure under general anesthesia. Tailoring the type of anesthesia to the patient is an important step in avoiding PCC.

Active smokers have an increase in tracheobronchial secretions and a decrease in mucociliary clearance. They depend on coughing for the removal of secretions, and they may need longer weaning from mechanical ventilation on the intensive care unit (ICU).[7] Smoking is also associated with pulmonary and cardiac diseases. Smokers have been included in all studies on intraoperative lung-protective ventilation strategies. Whether smokers benefit more than nonsmokers from any specific ventilator settings remains unclear.[8,9]

Advanced age, specifically an age of greater than 65 years, approximately doubles the risk of PPC not only owing to "accumulating comorbid conditions,"[10] but as an independent predictor of outcome based on age-related changes in the lungs, which are summarized in **Table 1**.[2,11,12]

In an animal model of mechanical ventilation with high tidal volumes, older lungs developed more severe pulmonary injury than younger ones.[13] It seems that elderly patients are more vulnerable to high tidal volumes, and that, in turn, they may benefit more from lung-protective mechanical ventilation than younger ones.[14]

The development of PCC starts early in the patient's hospital course and the intra-operative ventilator settings have been shown to impact outcome in the elderly. Two trials so far specifically addressed this patient population and found at low tidal volume strategies intraoperatively lead to higher intraoperative pulmonary compliance, lower airway resistance, higher Pao_2/Fio_2 ratio, and higher $Paco_2$ levels in the intervention group.[8,15]

MANAGEMENT OF CHRONIC OBSTRUCTIVE PULMONARY DISEASE

Patients with COPD suffer from chronic inflammation of small airways and lung parenchyma, resulting in obstructive bronchiolitis, parenchymal destruction, and emphysema. Increased airway resistance and decreased elastic recoil lead to limited airflow and an impaired ability of the airways to remain open at the end of expiration. In turn, the collapse of airways at the end of expiration results in incomplete expiration, higher residual end-expiratory volume, hyperinflation, and auto–positive end-expiratory pressure (auto-PEEP). Progression of chronic inflammation and parenchymal destruction result in impaired gas exchange with hypoxemia and hypercapnia. In case of the need for ventilatory support for acute exacerbations, the use of noninvasive mechanical ventilation reduces mortality in patients with COPD.[9,10]

Patients with COPD planning to undergo elective surgery should be in a stable disease condition, and they should receive optimal individual medical treatment. In case of acute exacerbations, surgery should be postponed. However, even stable patients with COPD have an up to a 4-fold increased risk of PPC,[16,17] which is higher the worse the disease is. Absolute cutoff levels as contraindications for surgery[18] or predictors of the perioperative risk of patients with COPD are missing. Nevertheless, patients with an FEV_1 of greater than 60% are typically considered to be at low risk of PPC, even if they had planned to undergo lung resection.[19]

Physiologic Changes in Chronic Obstructive Pulmonary Disease Relevant to Mechanical Ventilation

Expiratory flow limitation is the principal physiologic alteration in COPD and is overcome by increasing the inspiratory flow and lung volume. Although the issue is expiratory, the compensation is inspiratory, and this, combined with high respiratory drive, leads to the development of inspiratory muscle fatigue, which is of central pathophysiologic importance in the development of acute respiratory failure in these patients.

The airflow obstruction, low elastic recoil, high ventilatory demand, and short expiratory time result in air trapping and consequent DH. In patients with COPD with acute respiratory failure, DH is the main factor explaining the increased intrathoracic pressure, increased work of breathing (WOB), ventilator dependency and weaning failure.[11,12]

Role of Noninvasive Positive-Pressure Ventilation in Treating Obstructive Pulmonary Disease Patients

Noninvasive positive-pressure ventilation (NPPV) has been accepted widely as the first choice in treating obstructive airway disease patients with respiratory failure. It provides a significant reduction in endotracheal intubation and thereby its complications (eg, ventilator-associated pneumonia, tracheal and laryngeal complications) if considered early in the course of the disease.[10,13,14]

Expiratory positive airway pressure applied offsets intrinsic PEEP resulting from expiratory airflow obstruction. Inspiratory positive airway pressure augments tidal volume for any given respiratory effort leading to less mechanical disadvantage, decreased respiratory rate, decreased WOB, and improvements in ventilation (generally reduced $Paco_2$).[20]

Indications for Invasive Mechanical Ventilation

Although NPPV is now considered the first choice for the treatment of selected patients experiencing COPD exacerbations, there are some patients for whom NPPV may not be suitable owing to the severity of their conditions.[9] Another requirement for continuing with NPPV is the patient maintains a level of alertness to protect their airway. Having a patient vomit with a tight-fitting NPPV mask in place can be a recipe for a poor outcome. The main goals of mechanical ventilation are to improve pulmonary gas exchange and to rest compromised respiratory muscles sufficiently to recover from the fatigued state.

Major criteria (any one of the following)[9,21]
- Respiratory arrest
- Loss of consciousness
- Psychomotor agitation requiring sedation
- Hemodynamic instability with a systolic blood pressure less than 70 or greater than 180 mm Hg
- Heart rate less than 50 beats/min with loss of alertness
- Gasping for air

Minor criteria (any two of the following)
- Respiratory rate >35 breath/min
- Worsening acidemia or pH <7.25
- Pao_2 less than 40 mm Hg or Pao_2/Fio_2 less than 200 mm Hg despite oxygen
- Decreasing level of consciousness

Choice of Ventilator Mode in Chronic Obstructive Pulmonary Disease

Accomplishing gas exchange and alleviating respiratory muscle fatigue may be accomplished using any mode available on the ventilator, but the choice may vary with the status of the patient with COPD. For the obtunded or postoperative patient, pressure-support ventilation may not be the first choice until the patient respiratory drive returns. Therefore, either assist-control or synchronized intermittent mandatory ventilation, with either volume or pressure targets, should be used. High inspiratory flow rates are preferred to reduce the inspiratory–expiratory ratio, thus allowing more time for expiration. If the patient's respiratory drive is still present after intubation, the use of pressure-support ventilation or of synchronized intermittent mandatory ventilation with a low rate is preferable, because this is less likely to induce or worsen any preexisting DH and auto-PEEP.[22]

Clinicians have to be aware of the patient's baseline condition after assuming control of the pulmonary dynamics of patients with COPD. The main hazard is overventilating the patient. There may be an impulse to increase the respiratory rate and tidal volumes in an attempt to "normalize" the blood gas of the patient with COPD. The higher expiratory flows to accomplish this increased minute volume may lead to additional air trapping. This in turn would lead to worsen hypercapnia and respiratory dyssynchrony. The increased intrathoracic pressure would also lead to decreased venous return and right-sided heart failure, exacerbating the situation.

Owing to the patients baseline metabolic compensation, if the $Paco_2$ is normalized to 40 mm Hg, acute alkalemia ensues. This alkalemia is a problem, because it prolongs mechanical ventilation by depressing the respiratory center and increasing respiratory muscle weakness. Continuing mechanical ventilation in this manner for 2 to 3 days would facilitate renal excretion of bicarbonate, thereby returning the acid–base status of the patient with COPD to normal. Unfortunately, when weaning is attempted, the patient is likely to develop acute respiratory acidosis or respiratory failure. To prevent this cycle, minute ventilation should be titrated to the pH and not to the $Paco_2$.

As we will see in the treatment of ARDS, the choice of low tidal volume ventilation is beneficial in the prevention overventilation. Low tidal volumes limit peak alveolar (plateau) pressure to less than 30 cm H_2O for patients with COPD.[23] With a lower tidal volume, the inspiratory–expiratory ratio is decreased, allowing longer expiration so that the hyperinflated COPD lung can empty. Consequently, this method is unlikely to induce alkalemia, cause or aggravate DH and auto-PEEP, or overdistend the alveolar lung units in the ventilated patient with COPD. Reducing respiratory rate and increasing inspiratory flow also increases expiratory time and facilitates emptying of the lung.

The Use of Positive End-Expiratory Pressure in Patients with Chronic Obstructive Pulmonary Disease

The balance in using PEEP in this patient population that already traps air (and causes intrinsic or auto-PEEP) is by applying to much PEEP and limiting expiratory flow (**Figs. 1** and **2**). To prevent this from occurring, external PEEP should be kept below 75% to 85% of auto-PEEP to avoid any worsening of hyperinflation or circulatory compromise.[16,24] Determination of dynamic pulmonary hyperinflation is, however, not easy to perform in an ICU. It requires insertion of an esophageal balloon and assessment of the abdominal muscles that can be recruited during expiration.[17] It has been shown, however, that changes in inspiratory capacity replicate that of hyperinflation, the greater the inspiratory capacity, the lower the end-expiratory lung volume assuming a constant total lung capacity.[18]

Diagnosis of Auto–positive End-Expiratory Pressure

Quantifying auto-PEEP is not a precise process. Auto-PEEP can vary among individual lung units owing to different degrees of obstruction; auto-PEEP is not uniformly distributed throughout the lung, but varies in direct proportion to the airway resistance present in a particular lung unit. A number of methods can be used to detect auto-PEEP in the mechanically ventilated patient. On some ventilators, a 2-second pause can be invoked after the end of expiration. This technique, however, is valid only if

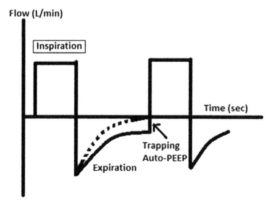

Fig. 1. Generation of auto–positive end-expiratory pressure (PEEP). (*From* Ahmed SM, Athar M. Mechanical ventilation in patients with chronic obstructive pulmonary disease and bronchial asthma. Indian J Anaesth 2015;59(9):589–98; with permission.)

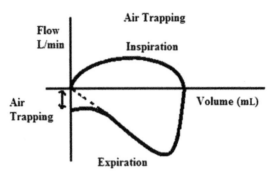

Fig. 2. Air trapping in a flow–volume loop. (*From* Ahmed SM, Athar M. Mechanical ventilation in patients with chronic obstructive pulmonary disease and bronchial asthma. Indian J Anaesth 2015;59(9):589–98; with permission.)

the patient is not breathing spontaneously. The auto-PEEP is then calculated by subtracting the external PEEP from the total PEEP.[19] This method limits the procedure's application to the heavily sedated, paralyzed, or physically exhausted patient with COPD. An esophageal balloon avoids this problem, but may not be readily available in all hospital ICUs. If the patient has a central venous pressure (CVP) line, auto-PEEP effects can be detected owing to the increased WOB reflected by greater changes in pleural pressure (which are transmitted to intrathoracic blood vessels and can be measured via CVP or pulmonary artery catheter). A large decrease in CVP during a spontaneous or assisted breath suggests that a high inspiratory threshold is needed to trigger the ventilator.

Diagnosis of Dynamic Hyperinflation

1. Slow filling of manual ventilator bag
2. Capnography trace not reaching plateau
3. Expiratory flow not reaching zero in flow-time–volume graph
4. Measure the intrinsic PEEP

Auto-PEEP can also be detected on ventilators equipped with graphic waveform monitoring. Although not readily quantifiable, auto-PEEP is easily recognized on the expiratory portion of the flow waveform. If expiratory flow does not return to zero before the next inspiration, auto-PEEP is present. For patients who are making spontaneous efforts to breathe, observing their respiratory efforts and the ventilators response is another useful technique, provided the ventilators sensitivity is set correctly (at -1 cm H_2O or on flow triggering). Because auto-PEEP increases the pressure gradient required to inhale, the patient's effort may not be able to trigger the ventilator; the result is a missed breath or cycle. Clinical signs associated with auto-PEEP (in patients making spontaneous efforts to breathe) include accessory muscle use, retractions, and increased ventilatory drive.

Management of Auto–positive End-Expiratory Pressure

The basic goal in the situation of auto-PEEP is to allowing more time for exhalation. This can be accomplished by reducing the respiratory rate or inspiratory–expiratory ratio (typically to 1:3–1:5) to allow more time for exhalation and reduce breath stacking. However, this pattern can result in low minute ventilation causing hypercapnia, hypoxia, or acidosis. This leads to increased pulmonary vascular resistance and worsened hemodynamic instability. If this is a concern, a higher inspiratory flow rate with high peak pressures can be used, but this places the patient at increased risk of barotrauma.

Application of Positive End-Expiratory Pressure

The use of external PEEP in ventilated patients with COPD has theoretic benefits by keeping small airways open during late exhalation, so potentially reducing intrinsic PEEP or auto-PEEP. Additionally, it has been seen that if external PEEP is kept below the intrinsic PEEP, no significant increase in alveolar pressure and cardiovascular compromise occurs.[25]

There are only 3 factors that determine auto-PEEP: (1) minute ventilation, (2) inspiratory–expiratory ratio, (3) expiratory time constants. Of the 3 factors, minute ventilation is the most important factor that causes DH. Hence, when ventilating patients with COPD, a smaller tidal volume, slow respiratory rate, and high peak flow should be used with an aim to target normal pH and not $Paco_2$ (permissive hypercapnia).

Strategies to Improve Pulmonary Gas Exchange

The hypoxemia of obstructive air diseases is basically due to 1 of the 3 general causes: shunt, ventilation–perfusion abnormalities, and diffusion defects. In general, individuals with acute exacerbations of COPD have a greater degree of ventilation defect (causing hypercapnia) than chronic patients, who mainly develop perfusion defect (causing hypoxia). Nonetheless, hypoxic vasoconstriction and collateral ventilation in chronic patients decrease the expected ventilation–perfusion abnormalities. Thus, managing the cause is of prime importance in the treatment of hypoxemia of COPD. Moreover, evidence shows beneficial effects of controlled breathing techniques such as active expiration, slow and deep breathing, pursed-lips breathing, relaxation therapy, specific body positions, and inspiratory muscle training.

Strategies to Rest Compromised Respiratory Muscles and Reduce the Work of Breathing

In patients with COPD they live in a state of compromised pulmonary mechanics coupled with a high respiratory drive. This combination leaves them teetering at the edge of their physiologic reserve. Recognition of the factors that contribute to their already increased work of breathing can help the clinician minimize these factors to optimize the patient (**Table 1**). Many of the interventions done to combat COPD have the goal of decreasing respiratory work load, increasing muscular strength and if needed providing mechanical ventilatory support.

Table 1
Factors affecting respiratory work of breathing

Obstructions to Inhalation	Respiratory Muscle Inhibitors	Ventilator Circuit Factors
Resistive load (bronchospasm)	Sedation causing depressed drive	Narrow endotracheal tube External PEEP
Parenchymal compliance (pulmonary edema, pneumonia, atelectasis)	Muscle weakness (electrolyte abnormalities, chronic atrophy)	Decreased trigger threshold of the ventilator
Chest wall compliance (obesity, pleural effusion, abdominal distention)		

Abbreviation: PEEP, positive end-expiratory pressure.

OUTCOMES IN PATIENTS WITH CHRONIC OBSTRUCTIVE PULMONARY DISEASE

Predicting PPCs remains a challenge for most of the researchers. Although many studies have attempted to predict PPCs, they were not specifically for patients with COPD. Patients with COPD are at an increased risk for PPCs. A recent review estimated the incidence of unadjusted PPCs as 18.2% in patients with COPD undergoing surgery.[5] Increasing severity of COPD confers greater risk, from 10% with mild to moderate disease to 23% in patients with severe disease.[26]

Evidence shows that history and physical examination are poor predictors of airway obstruction and its severity. However, the presence of history of a greater than 55 pack-year smoking, wheezing on auscultation, and patient self-reported wheezing can be considered predictive of airflow obstruction, defined as postbronchodilator forced expiratory volume 1 (FEV_1) or forced vital capacity of less than 0.70.[2] Spirometry is useful to identify airflow obstruction in symptomatic patients, but its usefulness in patients without respiratory symptoms is questionable. Smokers with normal spirometry have only a 4% risk of PPC.[27] Symptomatic patients with an FEV_1 of less than 60% predicted will benefit from inhaled treatments, but evidence does not support treating asymptomatic patients, regardless of the risk factors and airflow obstruction.[2] However, unlike in pulmonary resection, there is no cutoff value of FEV_1 or any other spirometric index to consider these patients unsuitable for surgery.

Arterial blood gas analyses are not indicated unless the patient's history suggests arterial hypoxemia or severe enough COPD that one suspects CO_2 retention. Then, the arterial blood gas should be used in essentially the same manner as one might use preoperative pulmonary function tests, that is, to look for reversible disease or to define the severity of the disease at its baseline. Defining baseline Pao_2 and $Paco_2$ is particularly important if one anticipates postoperatively ventilating a patient who has severe COPD.

Heliox

Heliox was introduced in 1934 for the treatment of airway obstruction.[28] Because airway turbulence depends on density, heliox (having a lower density) decreases the airway resistance and, therefore, the WOB, particularly in situations associated with upper airway obstruction. When used as a carrier, heliox has also been found to improve the deposition of aerosolized bronchodilators in the lung.[29] The percentage of oxygen in heliox should be at least 20% to prevent hypoxia, and no more than 40% for heliox to show a clinically significant effect.[29] It has been shown to reduce DH by 15%, which will probably place the respiratory muscles at a better mechanical advantage and decrease the WOB.[30] Indeed, a significant decline in VCO_2 was also noted, supporting a reduced WOB leading to small but significant decrease in the $Paco_2$.[31] However, owing to presence of conflicting literature, heliox therapy, which is costly and cumbersome, is not warranted for stable patients with COPD at rest with moderate to severe disease, but could be effective as an adjuvant therapy to enhance the efficacy of medical treatment. Thus, further research to identify the patients with COPD potentially able to benefit from this type of therapy is required.[31]

Corticosteroids

Short courses of systemic corticosteroids may provide important benefits in patients with exacerbations of COPD a more rapid increase in FEV_1, fewer withdrawals, and a significantly shorter duration of hospital stay.[32] This has to be balanced with the infectious complications and wound healing issues in the postoperative patient.

WEANING IN CHRONIC OBSTRUCTIVE PULMONARY DISEASE

Like all ventilator patients, an aggressive weaning policy is justified in patients with COPD because prolonged intubation is associated with a variety of poor outcomes. The first step is to address any offending agent that precipitated the COPD exacerbation. Marginal respiratory mechanics and continued presence of auto-PEEP make weaning difficult in patients with COPD. Hence, factors that increase resistance such as size, secretions, kinking of the tube, and the presence of elbow-shaped parts or a heat and moisture exchanger in the circuit have to be optimized to promote early weaning. Weaning can be done with a pressure support mode, along with spontaneous breathing trials. Sequential weaning (early extubation followed by NPPV) is found to be good alternative in patients showing failed spontaneous breathing trials.[33] In contrast, role of tracheostomy is uncertain, but owing to marginal respiratory mechanics, it is also expected to help in weaning.

Summary

Ventilatory support is a lifesaving procedure in acute exacerbations of COPD. The therapeutic goals are to improve gas exchange, rest fatigued respiratory muscles, and relieve respiratory distress. NPPV is regarded as the first line of treatment, whereas invasive ventilation is reserved for life-threatening respiratory failure. However, it can cause a considerable increase in morbidity and mortality if not used properly. Therefore, it is necessary to have a good understanding of pathophysiology, mechanics, and pattern of flow obstruction and DH to provide the most suitable ventilation to these patients. The ventilatory graphics (flow, pressure, and volume) of the most of the modern ventilators becomes a valuable tool in these situations and assist in early diagnosis and management of the patient's condition before it becomes clinically overt.

MANAGEMENT OF ACUTE RESPIRATORY DISTRESS SYNDROME

ARDS is a serious clinical problem with more than 200,000 cases annually[34] that is resistant to treatment once the syndrome is fully clinically established. ARDS has a mortality rate of 30% to 60% with significant costs of care and debilitating lifelong sequelae for survivors.[35] Despite decades of research only one therapeutic modality, low tidal volume ventilation has been demonstrated to modestly improve ARDS-related mortality (9%).[36] People with ARDS are by definition severely hypoxemic, and nearly all require invasive mechanical ventilation. Yet mechanical ventilation itself can further injure damaged lungs (so-called ventilator-induced lung injury); minimizing any additional damage while maintaining adequate gas exchange ("compatible with life") is the central goal of mechanical ventilation in ARDS and acute lung injury, its less severe form.

Benefits of Low Tidal Volume Ventilation in Acute Respiratory Distress Syndrome

Low tidal volume ventilation reduces the damaging, excessive stretch of lung tissue and alveoli (so-called volutrauma), and is the standard of care for people with ARDS requiring mechanical ventilation. The ARDSnet[36] is the largest clinical trial supporting this paradigm. Although it has been noted to have some design flaws (the control arm had a high 12 mL/kg volume given) and ethical concerns (informed consent issues), it has been the foundation that using low tidal volumes improves survival for people with ARDS. Taken together, the trials suggest that a strategy of low tidal volume ventilation (6–8 mL/kg ideal body weight) reduces absolute mortality by about 7% to 9%, as compared with using 12 mL/kg tidal volumes (approximately 42% mortality in control groups vs approximately 34% in the low tidal volume ventilation groups). This translates to a "number needed to treat" of between 11 and 15 people with ARDS to prevent 1 death by using low tidal volume ventilation.

How to Use Low Tidal Volume Ventilation in Acute Respiratory Distress Syndrome

The protocol from the ARMA trial can serve as a guide to performing low tidal volume ventilation for mechanically ventilated patients with ARDS:

- Start in any ventilator mode with initial tidal volumes of 8 mL/kg predicted body weight in kg, calculated by: [2.3 × (height in inches - 60) + 45.5 for women or + 50 for men].
- Set the respiratory rate up to 35 breaths/min to deliver the expected minute ventilation requirement (generally, 7–9 L/min).
- Set PEEP to at least 5 cm H_2O, and Fio_2 to maintain an arterial oxygen saturation (SaO_2) of 88% to 95% (Pao_2 55–80 mm Hg). Titrate Fio_2 to less than 70% when feasible.
- Over a period of less than 4 hours, reduce tidal volumes to 7 mL/kg, and then to 6 mL/kg.

Ventilator adjustments are then made with the primary goal of keeping plateau pressure (measured during an inspiratory hold of 0.5 seconds) less than 30 cm H_2O, and preferably as low as possible, while keeping blood gas parameters "compatible with life." High plateau pressures vastly elevate the risk for harmful alveolar distension (ie, ventilator-associated lung injury, volutrauma). If plateau pressures remain elevated after following the this protocol, further strategies should be tried:

- *Further reduce tidal volume,* to as low as 4 mL/kg by 1 mL/kg stepwise increments.
- *Sedate the patient* to minimize ventilator–patient dyssynchrony.
- *Consider other etiologies* for the increased plateau pressure besides the stiff, noncompliant lungs of ARDS.

Permissive Hypercapnia in Acute Respiratory Distress Syndrome

This single-minded focus on reducing plateau pressures derives from the likely survival benefit from low tidal volume ventilation and low plateau pressures observed in clinical trials. Achieving these low plateau pressures usually requires tidal volumes low enough to result in hypoventilation, with resulting increases in Pco_2 and respiratory acidemia that can be severe and, to the treating physician, anxiety provoking. This approach, "permissive hypercapnia," represents a paradigm shift from previous eras, in which achieving normal blood gas values was the main goal of mechanical ventilation. Mechanically ventilated patients with ARDS seem to tolerate very low blood pH and very high Pco_2s without any adverse sequelae:

- Current consensus suggests it is safe to allow pH to fall to at least 7.20.
- The actual Pco_2 is of little importance.
- When the pH falls below 7.20, many physicians choose to administer sodium bicarbonate, Carbicarb, or THAM (tris-hydroxymethyl amino-methane) to maintain blood pH between 7.15 and 7.20.
- However, it is unknown whether such correction of acidemia is helpful, harmful, or neither (good evidence is lacking for any of these hypotheses).

Conditions in which permissive hypercapnia for ARDS could theoretically be harmful include cerebral edema, mass lesions or seizures, active coronary artery disease, arrhythmias, hypovolemia, gastrointestinal bleeding, and possibly others. These are hypothetical harms based on pathophysiology and not outcomes data, and the harm of ventilator-induced lung injury and the benefits of a protective ventilator strategy in ARDS are real and known. The potential risks of hypercapnia in such patients must be weighed against the risks of ARDS, and therapy individualized.

Limitations in the Use of Plateau Pressure for Acute Respiratory Distress Syndrome

Patients with reduced chest wall compliance—most commonly owing to obesity—may have higher plateau pressures at baseline[37] and during ARDS than nonobese patients. It is possible that, in some obese patients, titrating tidal volumes to plateau pressures less than 30 cm H_2O may be inadequate[38] and result in worsened hypoventilation. There are no recommendations to treat obese patients with acute lung injury or ARDS differently than nonobese patients with regard to mechanical ventilation. Esophageal manometry is considered superior to plateau pressures through its measurement of transpulmonary pressure, considered a more precise measure of potentially injurious pressures in the lung. Because it is invasive and the probes are prone to migration, esophageal manometry is not widely used.

Prone Positioning in Acute Respiratory Distress Syndrome

Prone positioning improves gas exchange and has long been used as an adjunctive or salvage therapy for severe or refractory ARDS. Prone positioning is gaining credibility as a new standard of care for ARDS after a multicenter trial published in 2013, demonstrated a dramatic near 50% relative risk reduction, and a 17% absolute risk reduction for mortality. Patients were kept in prone position for 16 hours a day in that trial conducted at 27 European centers highly experienced with prone positioning for ARDS.[39] The benefits of prone positioning have not yet been replicated in a large US trial, but a metaanalysis of 6 randomized trials[40] also concluded prone positioning saves lives in ARDS when added to a lung-protective ventilatory strategy.

High Versus Low Positive End-Expiratory Pressure in Acute Respiratory Distress Syndrome

A strategy using higher PEEP along with low tidal volume ventilation should be considered for patients receiving mechanical ventilation for ARDS. This suggestion is based on a 2010 metaanalysis of 3 randomized trials (n = 2229)[41] testing higher versus lower PEEP in patients with acute lung injury or ARDS, in which ARDS patients receiving higher PEEP had a strong trend toward improved survival. High versus low PEEP was defined as a rolling definition as the hospital stay went on but a blunt cutoff would be 10 cm H_2O to define the 2 groups.

However, patients with milder acute lung injury (Pao_2/Fio_2 ratio >200) receiving higher PEEP had a strong trend toward harm in that same metaanalysis (27.2% in the higher PEEP group and 19.4% in the lower PEEP group). Higher PEEP can conceivably cause ventilator-induced lung injury by increasing plateau pressures, or cause pneumothorax or decreased cardiac output. The ARDSnet group investigated the adverse effects of high PEEP and did not find a correlation with poor outcomes. These investigator concluded that patients who received low tidal volumes and maintained plateau pressures less than 30 cm H_2O had similar outcomes whether high or low PEEP was used.[42]

Alternative and Rescue Ventilator Modes in Acute Respiratory Distress Syndrome

Some patients with severe ARDS develop severe hypoxemia or hypercarbia with acidemia despite optimal treatment with low tidal volume mechanical ventilation. In these situations, alternative, salvage or "rescue" ventilator strategies are often used. Their common goal is to maintain high airway pressures to maximize alveolar recruitment and oxygenation, while minimizing alveolar stretch or shear stress. The most commonly used alternative ventilatory strategies are high-frequency oscillatory ventilation (HFOV) or airway pressure release ventilation (APRV or "bilevel").

HFOV is not appropriate as a first-line treatment for ARDS.[43,44] There have been 2 randomized trials on the topic and neither was able to the show an improvement in outcomes. In contrast, the North American study showed 47% in the HFOV group died in-hospital, versus 35% receiving conventional low-tidal volume ventilation (relative risk for death with HFOV of 1.33; 95% CI, 1.09-1.64; $P = .005$). The trial was stopped for harm at this point, far short of its planned 1200 patient enrollment, when statistical analyses showed a near impossibility of equivalence or benefit from HFOV.[43] Both studies showed that HFOV patients required more sedation and more neuromuscular blockade to keep the patient on HFOV.

APRV maintains a sustained airway pressure over a large proportion of the respiratory cycle. Animal and clinical studies have demonstrated that, compared with conventional ventilation, APRV has beneficial effects on lung recruitment, oxygenation, end-organ blood flow, pulmonary vasoconstriction, and sedation requirements.[45,46] APRV has shown promise in both preventing the development on ARDS in animal models.[47] Adequate studies to show a mortality benefit when compared with low tidal volume ventilation have not yet been performed.

Extracorporeal membrane oxygenation

Extracorporeal membrane oxygenation (ECMO) has also become a more commonly used salvage therapy for ARDS, thanks to improvements in technology making it safer and more feasible to administer. The use of ECMO for the treatment of ARDS was introduced in the early 1970s with the aim of guaranteeing a protective ventilation, as an artificial lung may provide an adequate blood CO_2 removal and oxygenation, allowing to reduce mechanical ventilation. There remains 1 randomized trial (CESAR study) of patients with ARDS. In this study, patients referred to an ECMO center showed a higher 6-month survival rate (63% vs 47%) and no difference in quality of life and spirometric parameters compared with patients treated with conventional mechanical ventilation. There have been no additional studies since then validating ECMO and its use is limited to specialized centers.[48]

Pharmacologic Adjuncts to Ventilator Strategies

Treatment with inhaled nitric oxide as a rescue therapy for ARDS has shown significant improvement in oxygenation for a short period of 48 hours. However, no benefit in terms of survival has been demonstrated.[49] Because the clinical effect of inhaled nitric oxide is counterbalanced by its very high cost, other inhaled pharmacologic alternatives were explored. Specifically, inhaled prostaglandins have been increasingly used. A recently published study that compared inhaled epoprostenol versus inhaled nitric oxide in patients with refractory hypoxemia revealed similar efficacy and safety outcomes.[50] Randomized clinical studies assessing the effectiveness of inhaled prostaglandins in ARDS have rarely been performed. A Cochrane review was able to identify only 1 clinical trial, which included 14 critically ill children with ARDS. The investigators concluded there was no evidence to support or refute the use of inhaled prostoglandins.[51]

Beta-agonist infusions have been tried owing to the idea that they could decrease patients plateau pressures and pulmonary edema. A randomized trial showed they were found to be harmful to ARDS patients, likely owing to the associated arrhythmias.[52] Similarly, aerosolized beta-agonists have not shown improvements in outcomes.[53]

Chemical paralysis

To augment patient–ventilator synchrony and to reduce the oxygen consumption related to respiratory muscle activity, many clinicians decide to abolish any spontaneous respiratory effort by using neuromuscular blocking agents. An additional effect of neuromuscular blocking agents is the reduction of the negative increase in pleural pressure seen during spontaneous breathing, with the likely consequent reduction of stress and strain applied to the lung. It has been shown how patients with severe ARDS treated with an early, short course of neuromuscular blocking agents presented with lower mortality, reduced duration of mechanical ventilation, and fewer episodes of barotrauma. Patients with ARDS who were started on 48 hours of neuromuscular blockade within the first 48 hours of their symptoms had a significant mortality reduction 1.6% (95% CI, 25.2–38.8) in the cisatracurium group and 40.7% (95% CI, 33.5–48.4)[54]

Systemic corticosteroids

The central role of the inflammatory response in the pathogenesis of ARDS is the rationale behind the idea to use corticosteroids as a therapy in ARDS patient. Based on these concepts, several trials investigated corticosteroids use,[55,56] however, with heterogeneous results. Meduri and colleagues[55] in a study conducted in the early phase of ARDS demonstrated a decrease in ICU mortality rate; however, these findings could not be replicated in other studies.[56,57]

Volume Status

Noncardiogenic pulmonary edema is an important part of the ARDS picture. Intravenous fluid management is brought into question for the ability to worsen or improve the patient's gas exchange. Intravenous fluids are critical to maintain appropriate intravascular volume to assure hemodynamic stability; however, excessive fluid administration can worsen lung edema, further impairing gas exchange. Fluid management practices are quite variable and are often guided by philosophic approaches ranging from the very liberal or "wet" approach (prioritizes maximizing perfusion) to the very conservative or "dry" approach (prioritizes reductions in lung edema). The FACTT trial (Fluids and Catheters Treatment Trial) was performed by the ARDSnet group to try to identify the optimal approach in the ARDS setting. The investigators randomized 1000 patients to wet or dry groups with an additional factor of fluid management being guided by a CVP or a Swan Ganz catheter.[58] The wet group was approximately 1 L positive for the day, which coincided with other ARDSnet trials, suggesting that a liberal fluid strategy was the "normal" approach. The restrictive group was kept fluid neutral using diuretics. There was no difference in mortality among the groups. The 60-day mortality was 25.5% in the conservative group versus 28.4% in the liberal group ($P = .3005$; 95% CI for the difference, −2.6 to +8.4). The restrictive group had a significant improvement in ventilator parameters such as plateau pressure, and required less PEEP leading to fewer ventilator and ICU days.[59]

PREDICTING SURVIVAL AND OUTCOMES AFTER ACUTE RESPIRATORY DISTRESS SYNDROME

In a 2012 retrospective analysis in *JAMA*[60] including data from more than 4400 patients with ARDS enrolled in randomized trials, only the severity of hypoxemia (low Pao_2/Fio_2 ratio) was predictive of mortality. Commonly used clinical parameters of severity (static compliance, degree of PEEP, and extent of opacities on chest radiography) were not predictive of outcome. A "high-risk" patient profile with a 52% mortality was identified post hoc, composed of severe ARDS (Pao_2/Fio_2 ratio <100) with either a high corrected expired volume of 13 L/min or greater, or a low static compliance of less than 20 mL/cm H_2O. Reviews of ARDS outcomes[61] suggest that most people who survive ARDS recover pulmonary function, but may remain impaired for months or years in other domains, both physically[35] and psychologically.[62]

SUMMARY

Ventilatory support is a lifesaving procedure in acute exacerbation of COPD and ARDS. The goals of ventilator support between the 2 groups are the same, which is to maintain gas exchange and rest fatigued respiratory muscles. Titration of the ventilator setting may differ among the groups but low tidal volume ventilation has been shown to be beneficial in both groups. The use of adjunct interventions may help to improve patient outcomes in both groups.

REFERENCES

1. Available at: http://www.nhlbi.nih.gov/health/public/lung/other/copd_fact.htm.2006. COPD: fact sheet. Accessed August 19, 2017.
2. Mannino D. COPD: Epidemiology, preva- lence, morbidity and mortality, and disease heterogeneity. Chest 2002;121:121s–6s.
3. Esteban A, Ferguson ND, Meade MO, et al. Evolution of mechanical ventilation in response to clinical research. Am J Respir Crit Care Med 2008;177(2):170–7.
4. Umbrello M, Formenti P, Bolgiaghi L, et al. Current concepts of ARDS: a narrative review. Int J Mol Sci 2016;18(1) [pii:E64].
5. Smetana GW, Lawrence VA, Cornell JE, American College of Physicians. Preoperative pulmonary risk stratification for noncardiothoracic surgery: systematic review for the American College of Physicians. Ann Intern Med 2006;144(8): 581–95.
6. Smetana GW. Postoperative pulmonary complications: an update on risk assessment and reduction. Cleve Clin J Med 2009;76(Suppl 4):S60–5.
7. Bluman LG, Mosca L, Newman N, et al. Preoperative smoking habits and postoperative pulmonary complications. Chest 1998;113(4):883–9.
8. Ge Y, Yuan L, Jiang X, et al. Effect of lung protection mechanical ventilation on respiratory function in the elderly undergoing spinal fusion. Zhong Nan Da Xue Xue Bao Yi Xue Ban 2013;38(1):81–5 [in Chinese].
9. Brochard L, Mancebo J, Wysocki M, et al. Noninvasive ventilation for acute exacerbations of chronic obstructive pulmonary disease. N Engl J Med 1995;333(13): 817–22.
10. Girou E, Schortgen F, Delclaux C, et al. Association of noninvasive ventilation with nosocomial infections and survival in critically ill patients. JAMA 2000;284(18): 2361–7.
11. Coussa ML, Guérin C, Eissa NT, et al. Partitioning of work of breathing in mechanically ventilated COPD patients. J Appl Physiol (1985) 1993;75(4):1711–9.
12. Purro A, Appendini L, De Gaetano A, et al. Physiologic determinants of ventilator dependence in long-term mechanically ventilated patients. Am J Respir Crit Care Med 2000;161(4 Pt 1):1115–23.
13. Evans TW. International Consensus Conferences in Intensive Care Medicine: noninvasive positive pressure ventilation in acute respiratory failure. Organised jointly by the American Thoracic Society, the European Respiratory Society, the

European Society of Intensive Care Medicine, and the Societe de Reanimation de Langue Francaise, and approved by the ATS Board of Directors, December 2000. Intensive Care Med 2001;27(1):166–78.

14. Girou E, Brun-Buisson C, Taillé S, et al. Secular trends in nosocomial infections and mortality associated with noninvasive ventilation in patients with exacerbation of COPD and pulmonary edema. JAMA 2003;290(22):2985–91.

15. Weingarten TN, Whalen FX, Warner DO, et al. Comparison of two ventilatory strategies in elderly patients undergoing major abdominal surgery. Br J Anaesth 2010;104(1):16–22.

16. Ranieri VM, Giuliani R, Cinnella G, et al. Physiologic effects of positive end-expiratory pressure in patients with chronic obstructive pulmonary disease during acute ventilatory failure and controlled mechanical ventilation. Am Rev Respir Dis 1993;147(1):5–13.

17. Lessard MR, Lofaso F, Brochard L. Expiratory muscle activity increases intrinsic positive end-expiratory pressure independently of dynamic hyperinflation in mechanically ventilated patients. Am J Respir Crit Care Med 1995;151(2 Pt 1):562–9.

18. Yan S, Kaminski D, Sliwinski P. Reliability of inspiratory capacity for estimating end-expiratory lung volume changes during exercise in patients with chronic obstructive pulmonary disease. Am J Respir Crit Care Med 1997;156(1):55–9.

19. Reddy RM, Guntupalli KK. Review of ventilatory techniques to optimize mechanical ventilation in acute exacerbation of chronic obstructive pulmonary disease. Int J Chron Obstruct Pulmon Dis 2007;2(4):441–52.

20. Ambrosino N, Strambi S. New strategies to improve exercise tolerance in chronic obstructive pulmonary disease. Eur Respir J 2004;24(2):313–22.

21. Brochard L, Isabey D, Piquet J, et al. Reversal of acute exacerbations of chronic obstructive lung disease by inspiratory assistance with a face mask. N Engl J Med 1990;323(22):1523–30.

22. Tuxen DV, Lane S. The effects of ventilatory pattern on hyperinflation, airway pressures, and circulation in mechanical ventilation of patients with severe air-flow obstruction. Am Rev Respir Dis 1987;136(4):872–9.

23. Tuxen DV. Permissive hypercapnic ventilation. Am J Respir Crit Care Med 1994; 150(3):870–4.

24. Petrof BJ, Legaré M, Goldberg P, et al. Continuous positive airway pressure reduces work of breathing and dyspnea during weaning from mechanical ventilation in severe chronic obstructive pulmonary disease. Am Rev Respir Dis 1990; 141(2):281–9.

25. Jolliet P, Watremez C, Roeseler J, et al. Comparative effects of helium-oxygen and external positive end-expiratory pressure on respiratory mechanics, gas exchange, and ventilation-perfusion relationships in mechanically ventilated patients with chronic obstructive pulmonary disease. Intensive Care Med 2003; 29(9):1442–50.

26. Cook MW, Lisco SJ. Prevention of postoperative pulmonary complications. Int Anesthesiol Clin 2009;47(4):65–88.

27. Kroenke K, Lawrence VA, Theroux JF, et al. Postoperative complications after thoracic and major abdominal surgery in patients with and without obstructive lung disease. Chest 1993;104(5):1445–51.

28. Barach AL. Use of helium as a new therapeutic gas. Proc Soc Exp Biol Med 1934; 32:462–4.

29. Anderson M, Svartengren M, Bylin G, et al. Deposition in asthmatics of particles inhaled in air or in helium-oxygen. Am Rev Respir Dis 1993;147(3):524–8.

30. Swidwa DM, Montenegro HD, Goldman MD, et al. Helium-oxygen breathing in severe chronic obstructive pulmonary disease. Chest 1985;87(6):790–5.

31. Rodrigo G, Pollack C, Rodrigo C, et al. Heliox for treatment of exacerbations of chronic obstructive pulmonary disease. Cochrane Database Syst Rev 2002;(2):CD003571.

32. Davies L, Angus RM, Calverley PM. Oral corticosteroids in patients admitted to hospital with exacerbations of chronic obstructive pulmonary disease: a prospective randomised controlled trial. Lancet 1999;354(9177):456–60.

33. Glossop AJ, Shephard N, Bryden DC, et al. Non-invasive ventilation for weaning, avoiding reintubation after extubation and in the postoperative period: a meta-analysis. Br J Anaesth 2012;109(3):305–14.

34. Rubenfeld GD, Herridge MS. Epidemiology and outcomes of acute lung injury. Chest 2007;131(2):554–62.

35. Herridge MS, Tansey CM, Matté A, et al. Functional disability 5 years after acute respiratory distress syndrome. N Engl J Med 2011;364(14):1293–304.

36. The Acute Respiratory Distress Syndrome Network, Brower RG, Matthay MA, Morris A, et al. Ventilation with lower tidal volumes as compared with traditional tidal volumes for acute lung injury and the acute respiratory distress syndrome. N Engl J Med 2000;342(18):1301–8.

37. Sohl AE. Critical care management of the obese patient. New York: Wiley-Blackwell; 2012. p. 254.

38. Talmor D, Sarge T, O'Donnell CR, et al. Esophageal and transpulmonary pressures in acute respiratory failure. Crit Care Med 2006;34(5):1389–94.

39. Guerin C, Reignier J, Richard JC, et al. Prone positioning in severe acute respiratory distress syndrome. N Engl J Med 2013;368(23):2159–68.

40. Sud S, Friedrich JO, Adhikari NK, et al. Effect of prone positioning during mechanical ventilation on mortality among patients with acute respiratory distress syndrome: a systematic review and meta-analysis. CMAJ 2014;186(10):E381–90.

41. Briel M, Meade M, Mercat A, et al. Higher vs lower positive end-expiratory pressure in patients with acute lung injury and acute respiratory distress syndrome: systematic review and meta-analysis. JAMA 2010;303(9):865–73.

42. Brower RG, Lanken PN, MacIntyre N, et al. Higher versus lower positive end-expiratory pressures in patients with the acute respiratory distress syndrome. N Engl J Med 2004;351(4):327–36.

43. Ferguson ND, Cook DJ, Guyatt GH, et al. High-frequency oscillation in early acute respiratory distress syndrome. N Engl J Med 2013;368(9):795–805.

44. Young D, Lamb SE, Shah S, et al. High-frequency oscillation for acute respiratory distress syndrome. N Engl J Med 2013;368(9):806–13.

45. Putensen C, Zech S, Wrigge H, et al. Long-term effects of spontaneous breathing during ventilatory support in patients with acute lung injury. Am J Respir Crit Care Med 2001;164(1):43–9.

46. Falkenhain SK, Reilley TE, Gregory JS. Improvement in cardiac output during airway pressure release ventilation. Crit Care Med 1992;20(9):1358–60.

47. Roy S, Habashi N, Sadowitz B, et al. Early airway pressure release ventilation prevents ARDS-a novel preventive approach to lung injury. Shock 2013;39(1):28–38.

48. Peek GJ, Mugford M, Tiruvoipati R, et al. Efficacy and economic assessment of conventional ventilatory support versus extracorporeal membrane oxygenation for severe adult respiratory failure (CESAR): a multicentre randomised controlled trial. Lancet 2009;374(9698):1351–63.

49. Taylor RW, Zimmerman JL, Dellinger RP, et al. Low-dose inhaled nitric oxide in patients with acute lung injury: a randomized controlled trial. JAMA 2004;291(13): 1603–9.

50. Torbic H, Szumita PM, Anger KE, et al. Inhaled epoprostenol vs inhaled nitric oxide for refractory hypoxemia in critically ill patients. J Crit Care 2013;28(5):844–8.

51. Afshari A, Brok J, Møller AM, et al. Aerosolized prostacyclin for acute lung injury (ALI) and acute respiratory distress syndrome (ARDS). Cochrane Database Syst Rev 2010;(8):CD007733.

52. Gao Smith F, Perkins GD, Gates S, et al. Effect of intravenous beta-2 agonist treatment on clinical outcomes in acute respiratory distress syndrome (BALTI-2): a multicentre, randomised controlled trial. Lancet 2012;379(9812):229–35.

53. National Heart, Lung, and Blood Institute Acute Respiratory Distress Syndrome (ARDS) Clinical Trials Network, Matthay MA, Brower RG, Carson S, et al. Randomized, placebo-controlled clinical trial of an aerosolized beta(2)-agonist for treatment of acute lung injury. Am J Respir Crit Care Med 2011;184(5):561–8.

54. Papazian L, Forel JM, Gacouin A, et al. Neuromuscular blockers in early acute respiratory distress syndrome. N Engl J Med 2010;363(12):1107–16.

55. Meduri GU, Headley AS, Golden E, et al. Effect of prolonged methylprednisolone therapy in unresolving acute respiratory distress syndrome: a randomized controlled trial. JAMA 1998;280(2):159–65.

56. Steinberg KP, Hudson LD, Goodman RB, et al. Efficacy and safety of corticosteroids for persistent acute respiratory distress syndrome. N Engl J Med 2006; 354(16):1671–84.

57. Bernard GR, Luce JM, Sprung CL, et al. High-dose corticosteroids in patients with the adult respiratory distress syndrome. N Engl J Med 1987;317(25): 1565–70.

58. National Heart, Lung, and Blood Institute Acute Respiratory Distress Syndrome (ARDS) Clinical Trials Network, Wheeler AP, Bernard GR, Thompson BT, et al. Pulmonary-artery versus central venous catheter to guide treatment of acute lung injury. N Engl J Med 2006;354(21):2213–24.

59. National Heart, Lung, and Blood Institute Acute Respiratory Distress Syndrome (ARDS) Clinical Trials Network, Wiedemann HP, Wheeler AP, Bernard GR, et al. Comparison of two fluid-management strategies in acute lung injury. N Engl J Med 2006;354(24):2564–75.

60. ARDS Definition Task Force, Ranieri VM, Rubenfeld GD, Thompson BT, et al. Acute respiratory distress syndrome: the Berlin Definition. JAMA 2012;307(23): 2526–33.

61. Herridge MS. Recovery and long-term outcome in acute respiratory distress syndrome. Crit Care Clin 2011;27(3):685–704.

62. Adhikari NK, Tansey CM, McAndrews MP, et al. Self-reported depressive symptoms and memory complaints in survivors five years after ARDS. Chest 2011; 140(6):1484–93.

Acute Kidney Injury in the Critically Ill

Robert A. Maxwell, MD*, Christopher Michael Bell, MD

KEYWORDS

- Acute kidney injury • Acute tubular necrosis • Volume overload
- Indications for dialysis • Renal replacement therapy

KEY POINTS

- Acute kidney injury (AKI) occurs in up to 50% of postsurgical intensive care unit patients with reported mortalities from 15% to 80%, with more than 50% of cases being secondary to sepsis.
- Diuretics may be used to treat volume overload in patients with AKI but should not be given to treat or reverse AKI.
- All critically ill patients and patients with AKI should be considered at risk for contrast-induced nephropathy and should receive prophylaxis with volume loading and administration of N-acetyl cystine.
- Initiating renal replacement therapy (RRT) early when AKI is detected remains controversial; however, current guidelines recommend the standard indications to initiate RRT, which are volume overload, azotemia, electrolyte abnormalities, and acidosis.

INTRODUCTION AND DEFINITION

Acute kidney injury (AKI) is an often overlooked and unappreciated disease process that carries significant morbidity and mortality in up to half of critically ill patients. Mortalities range from 15% to 80% and the associated morbidity leads to a high resource and financial burden. The term AKI is a generic reference to a variety of underlying disease processes that can either result in acute tubular necrosis (ATN) caused by renal ischemia or interstitial nephritis resulting in damage to the interstitium surrounding the renal tubule caused by deposition of immune complexes that lead to decreased renal function.[1] Historically there was not a consensus on the clinical definition of AKI, but in 2012 the Kidney Disease and Improving Global Outcomes (KDIGO) work group combined the definitions for

Disclosure: The authors have nothing to disclose.
Department of Surgery, University of Tennessee College of Medicine, Chattanooga, Chattanooga, TN, USA
* Corresponding author. 979 East Third Street, Suite B401, Chattanooga, TN 37403.
E-mail address: Robert.maxwell@erlanger.org

AKI from the Acute Kidney Injury Network (AKIN) and the Risk Injury Failure Loss End Stage (RIFLE) system[2–4]:

- Increase in serum creatinine level by greater than or equal to 0.3 mg/dL ($\geq$26.5 µmol/L) within 48 hours
- Increase in serum creatinine level to greater than or equal to 1.5 times baseline within the previous 7 days
- Urine volume less than or equal to 0.5 mL/kg/h for 6 hours

The RIFLE system was simplified to 3 clinical stages depicting the degree of renal injury (**Table 1**). The rationale for the staging system has evolved from a plethora of data showing that the risk of death and need for renal replacement therapy (RRT) depend on quantitative changes in urine output and creatinine level.[4] Throughout this article, wherever the KDIGO work group has defined level of evidence for a recommendation in its guidelines, the grade is included parenthetically based on the Grading of Recommendations Assessment, Development and Evaluation guidelines for evaluating the quality of scientific publications[5] (**Table 2**).

Although creatinine level and urine output are the most readily available ways to assess renal function, several limitations need to be appreciated in clinical practice. Patients with sepsis, liver failure, or sarcopenia may have reduced creatinine production, which may result in falsely increased calculations of glomerular filtration rate (GFR).[6–8] Major increases in protein catabolism associated with large burns, rhabdomyolysis, or major trauma can lead to increased creatinine production, which can falsely decrease GFR calculations.[6,9] Creatinine is equally distributed throughout all fluid compartments so its concentration varies according to total body water. Therefore, using creatinine as the determinant of renal function in acute volume overload can lead to delays in the recognition of AKI until new steady states are reached.[10] In an intensive care unit (ICU) population, Liu and colleagues[11] showed that a simple formula:

Corrected creatinine = serum creatinine $\times$ (1 + current total body water/baseline total body water)

where total body water = 60% $\times$ patient's weight could correct for changes in fluid balance and that many patients with normal serum creatinine levels met the definition of AKI when creatinine level was corrected for the volume of distribution. The patients with corrected creatinine levels who went from normal to meeting the definition for AKI after correction had significantly higher mortality than those patients who did not have significant changes in their corrected serum creatinine levels (31% mortality vs 12%, $P<.001$).[11]

Urine output alone can be a poor predictor of AKI. Some patients maintain adequate urine output up to the point of anuria and some patients are oliguric secondary to

Table 1
Kidney Disease and Improving Global Outcomes acute kidney injury guidelines

Stage	Serum Creatinine	Urine Output
1	1.5–1.9 times baseline or >0.3 mg/dL increase	<0.5 mL/kg/h for 6–12 h
2	2.0–2.9 times baseline	<0.5 mL/kg/h for >12 h
3	3 times baseline or >4.0 mg/dL or initiation of RRT or in patients <18 y old a decrease in eGFR <35 mL/min/1.73 m^2	<0.3 mL/kg/h for >24 h or anuria >12 h

Abbreviation: eGFR, estimated glomerular filtration rate.

Table 2
Levels of evidence

Grade		Implications
Level 1: recommended		• Most patients should receive the recommended course of action • The recommendation can be evaluated as a candidate for developing a policy or a performance measure
Level 2: suggested		• Different choices are appropriate for different patients. Each patient needs help to arrive at a management decision consistent with clinicians' values and preferences

Grade	Quality of Evidence	Meaning
A	High	Further research is very unlikely to change clinicians' confidence in the estimate of effect • Several high-quality studies with consistent results • In special cases: 1 large, high-quality multicenter trial
B	Moderate	Further research is likely to have an important impact on confidence in the estimate of effect and may change the estimate • One high-quality study • Several studies with some limitations
C	Low	Further research is very likely to have an important impact on confidence in the estimate of effect and is likely to change the estimate • One or more studies with severe limitations
D	Very low	Any estimate of effect is very uncertain • Expert opinion • No direct research evidence • One or more studies with very severe limitations

Data from Grade Working Group. Available from: http://www.gradeworkinggroup.org/. Accessed Feburary 13, 2017.

hypovolemia, response to general anesthetic, and stress of trauma but do not have sustained AKI.[12–15] Ralib and colleagues[16] showed that AKI and increased mortality can be predicted by oliguria for just 6 hours and not the 12-hour period stated in the present KDIGO guidelines. Prowle and colleagues[15] found that oliguria occurred frequently in critically ill patients but only 10% went on to develop AKI, whereas hemodynamic instability and increased vasopressor use was a significant risk factor. In addition, the European Renal Best Practices Work Group recommends using ideal body weight in determining weight-based urine output, thus potentially reducing the overdiagnosis of AKI and unnecessary fluid administration.[1] Diagnosis of AKI is therefore subject to the interpretation of multiple patient-specific conditions and, despite certain limitations, creatinine and urine output are the best clinical markers at this time for monitoring renal function.[13]

CAUSES AND CAUSE OF ACUTE KIDNEY INJURY

Critically ill patients with AKI may have several causative factors that should all be determined by starting with a careful review of the history, medical record, and physical examination. Sepsis, major surgery (particularly coronary artery bypass surgery), and uncompensated heart failure are the most common causes of AKI in the ICU, with sepsis accounting for more than 50% of cases. Trauma, hemorrhagic pancreatitis, and hypovolemia are other causes (**Table 3**).[17,18] Another frequent contributing cause

Table 3
Causes of acute kidney injury in surgical intensive care units

Major Causes	Contributing Factors
Sepsis	CIN
Postoperative (CABG, major vascular)	CKD
Trauma	Nephrotoxic drugs
Hemorrhage	CHF
Pancreatitis	Liver disease
Cardiorenal syndrome	Cancer
	Blood transfusion
	Volume overload
	Diabetes mellitus

Abbreviations: CABG, coronary artery bypass graft; CHF, congestive heart failure; CIN, contrast-induced nephropathy; CKD, chronic kidney disease.

is exposure to nephrotoxic drugs and intravenous contrast dye. A list of possible causes and potentiating factors should be identified and corrective actions undertaken in a timely fashion.

Drugs are the primary or associated cause of AKI in up to 25% of ICU patients and can affect the kidney in all phases of urine production.[19] Twenty-two percent of the top 100 drugs used in an adult ICU at a tertiary care center were considered potentially nephrotoxic.[20] Intensivists should be aware of these potential risks and have a good understanding of the nephrotoxic drugs (**Table 4**). Current and past medication lists should be reviewed and any potentially nephrotoxic drugs should be replaced or

Table 4
Common nephrotoxic medications

Drug Classification	Nephrotoxicity Risk
Prerenal Failure	
Diuretics	Excessive diuresis depletes extracellular volume
Antihypertensive peripheral vasodilators	Decreases systemic vascular resistance
NSAIDs, COX-2 inhibitors, anesthetics	Increased renal vascular resistance
ACE inhibitor, ARB	Decreases transcapillary pressure
Renal Failure	
Amphotericin B, iodinated contrast agents, antiretrovirals, cocaine	ATN
Antibiotics (penicillins, vancomycin, ciprofloxacin, macrolides, sulfonamides) NSAIDs, omeprazole, phenytoin, cimetidine, ranitidine, diuretics	Acute interstitial nephritis
NSAIDs, ampicillin, lithium, hydralazine, heroin	Acute glomerulonephritis
Postrenal Failure	
Acyclovir, methotrexate, sulfonamides, triamterene, ephedrine	Tubular precipitation
Anticholinergics	Bladder obstruction

Abbreviations: ACE, angiotensin-converting enzyme; ARB, angiotensin receptor blocker; COX-2, cycloxygenase-2; NSAID, nonsteroidal antiinflammatory drug.

eliminated. The comorbidities that most notably increase the risk for drug-induced nephrotoxicity are chronic kidney disease (CKD), cirrhosis and liver failure, acute or chronic left heart failure, pulmonary artery hypertension with/without right heart failure, and malignancy. In addition, several major surgical procedures, such as cardiac surgery, aortic surgery, and major intra-abdominal surgery, enhance the risk of nephrotoxic drugs as well as the risk of AKI.[21]

On a microvascular level the basic underlying mechanism causing renal ischemia, cellular injury, and ATN is similar regardless of the type of precipitating event. Impaired renal blood flow secondary to hypotension, shock, and loss of autoregulation within the nephron causes imbalances in oxygen delivery, nutrient delivery, and metabolic demand, particularly within the renal tubule. The outer renal medulla maintains a low oxygen tension under normal physiologic conditions because of the countercurrent exchange mechanism that occurs as part of normal tubular resorptive function. This normally low oxygen tension in the outer renal medulla makes this area at highest risk to ischemic injury.[22] Hypoxic injury leads to structural damage to tubular cells, which subsequently forms casts that obstruct tubules and cause back-leak of filtrate.[22,23] Edema formation can further contribute to reduced blood flow and diffusion, further complicating the situation.

WORK-UP

The work-up of AKI in most patients should include serum and urine chemistries, urinalysis, and possibly renal ultrasonography. Urinalysis can be helpful in finding treatable causes such as interstitial nephritis (eosinophilia), pyelonephritis (pyuria and nitrites), and glomerulonephritis (hematuria and proteinuria).[24] In post–cardiac surgical patients a simple urine dipstick test positive for protein can be a predictor of postoperative AKI.[25] Urine microscopy can differentiate ATN from the presence of renal tubular cells or granular casts versus the presence of epithelial cells, which may indicate a normal finding.[26] A moderate or large number of epithelial cells could indicate infection, inflammation, or malignancy. Increased number of epithelial cells may prompt a cytologic analysis by the laboratory (**Table 5**).

Table 5
Urine microscopy findings and associated diagnosis

Microscopic Finding	Significance
Epithelial cells	Small amount: normal Moderate to large amount: consider cytologic analysis
Renal tubular cells	ATN
Granular casts	ATN, significant renal disease
Dysmorphic RBCs	Glomerular disease
Nondysmorphic RBCs	Nonglomerular bleeding from anywhere in urinary tract system
Red cell casts	Glomerular disease
Leukocytes	Inflammation of urinary tract
White cell casts	Renal infection
Hyaline casts	Any renal disease
Muddy brown casts	Necrotic tubular cells indicating ATN
Bacteria	Urinary tract infection

Abbreviation: RBC, red blood cells.

Historically, evaluation of patients with AKI includes determining potential prerenal, renal, and postrenal causes. A prerenal state indicates decreased preload and that fluid resuscitation is necessary. An important distinction emerges between prerenal AKI, which implies that the creatinine level will normalize within 72 hours after appropriate hydration and stabilization compared with those patients who develop sustained evidence of renal injury, known as intrinsic AKI (creatinine level increase after 72 hours).[27–31] Clinically, patients with fractional excretion of sodium (FE_{Na}) less than 1% have been classified as having prerenal AKI, implying that they have preserved the ability to resorb sodium from the tubule and should recover if further insult is avoided (**Table 6**).[32]

However, patients with prerenal AKI do have evidence of parenchymal injury, shown by increased levels of serum biomarkers of renal injury (**Table 7**). Patients with increased creatinine levels and prerenal AKI ($FE_{Na}<1\%$) are considered part of a continuum of AKI and do not just have a hydration deficit.[33] Judicious fluid replacement in this setting is essential to improving patient outcomes. Overly aggressive fluid resuscitation leads to increased morbidity, ICU length of stay, and mortality.[11,34] In light of concerns over the definition of prerenal and intrinsic AKI, the Acute Dialysis Quality Initiative (ADQI) work group has proposed that a new classification scheme be used to differentiate between functional AKI and kidney damage in lieu of prerenal, intrinsic, and postrenal states based on increased levels of certain renal injury biomarkers.[35] However, until these biomarkers become readily available laboratory tests, they have little practical clinical utility.

FE_{Na} and fractional excretion of urea (FE_{Urea}) can both be helpful in evaluating renal function. During volume contraction, normal functioning kidneys concentrate the urine, resulting in an increase of urine osmoles and decreased urine sodium and urea levels. The end result is an FE_{Na} of less than 1% or FE_{Urea} less than 35% as the body attempts to conserve water. A FE_{Na} greater than 1% or FE_{Urea} greater than 35% indicates renal tubular injury and ATN.[36–38] When evaluating a patient who has recently received loop diuretics (eg, furosemide), the FE_{Na} may be falsely increased by more than 1%, despite the volume status. The interpretation of FE_{Na} is erroneous under these conditions because furosemide is a natriuretic, blocking resorption of sodium in the ascending loop of Henle. However, loop diuretics do not affect urea excretion in the tubule so FE_{Urea} can therefore be substituted for FE_{Na}.[36] FE_{Na} or FE_{Urea} is a good starting point in the differentiation of prerenal AKI from intrinsic AKI and their values can be factored into the global assessment (see **Table 6**). However, taken independently, neither has proved to be a reliable indicator of volume status or fluid responsiveness. As such, additional determinations of volume status by means other than fractional excretion, such as echocardiography or pulmonary artery catheter, are necessary in critically ill patients with AKI.[39,40]

Table 6 Diagnostic thresholds for acute kidney injury			
	Prerenal	**Intrinsic**	**Postrenal**
FE_{Na} (%)	<1	>1	>4
U_{Na} (mmol/L)	<20	>40	>40
FE_{Urea}	<35%	>50%	N/A

Abbreviations: FE_{Urea}, fractionated excretion of urea; U_{Na}, urine sodium level.

Table 7
Comparison of the most common biomarkers of acute kidney injury diagnosis

Biomarker	Site of Injury	Disadvantage	Benefits
NGAL	Tubular Injury	Upregulated in sepsis 3 different types	Well studied
CyC	GFR/tubular Injury	No specific reference range	Not affected by age, gender, muscle mass, or diet
IL-18	Tubular injury	Upregulated in sepsis	Stronger predictor in patients with baseline eGFR <60 mL/min/1.73 m² Better in children and adolescents
TIMP-2/IGFBP7	Cell cycle arrest		Strong negative predictive value

Abbreviations: CyC, cystatin C; IGFBP7, insulinlike growth factor binding protein 7; NGAL, neutrophil gelatinase-associated lipocalin; TIMP-2, tissue inhibitor of metalloproteinases-2.

$$FE_{Na}\% = 100 \times (Serum_{Cr} \times Urine_{Na})/(Serum_{Na} \times Urine_{Cr})$$

$$FE_{Urea}\% = 100 \times (Serum_{Cr} \times Urine_{Urea})/(Serum_{Urea} \times Urine_{Cr})$$

In addition, the urine osmolality can be useful if differentiating prerenal disease from ATN. In ATN the kidney loses its ability to concentrate urine, resulting in urine osmolalities less than 350 mOsmol/kg. In a prerenal disease, hypovolemia stimulates antidiuretic hormone secretion and the resulting urine osmolality is usually more than 500 mOsmol/kg.[41] However, lower values similar to those in ATN may be seen in prerenal disease and are interpreted with caution, especially in the setting of glycosuria, metabolic alkalosis, bicarbonaturia, salt-wasting disorders, or CKD.[42]

Postrenal causes of AKI can be further evaluated with bladder ultrasonography to exclude the simple possibility of urinary retention, bladder outlet obstruction, and neurogenic bladder. A formal renal ultrasonography scan may be useful when there is ureteral obstruction from malignancy or bladder outlet abnormalities, or when the history reveals postsurgical exploration of the retroperitoneum or pelvis.[43] If there is no clinical suspicion of ureteral obstruction, a formal renal ultrasonography scan is likely to be a low-yield study.[44] Intensivist-performed Doppler studies may have a place in determining renal perfusion in the ICU, but until further parameters are developed the role of clinician-driven bedside ultrasonography has yet to be defined.[45]

BIOMARKERS IN ACUTE KIDNEY INJURY

Translational research focusing on biomarkers of kidney injury, such as neutrophil gelatinase-associated lipocalin (NGAL), cystatin C (CyC), interleukin-18 (IL-18), tissue inhibitor of metalloproteinases-2 (TIMP-2), and insulinlike growth factor binding protein 7(IGFBP7), have shown promise in screening for AKI before creatinine level increases, determining the degree of renal injury and the location of injury within the nephron (glomerulus vs tubule) (see **Table 7**). NGAL is a lipocalin protein that is covalently bound to gelatinase from neutrophils and immediately following AKI NGAL is massively upregulated in the distal part of the nephron, specifically the thick ascending limb of Henle loop, distal tubule, and collecting duct. This process leads to increased urinary and plasma NGAL levels.[46,47] A meta-analysis conducted in 2009 by Haase and colleagues[48] showed plasma NGAL/urine NGAL and urine

NGAL alone to be predictors of the severity of AKI, need for RRT, and mortality. In cardiac surgery patients, levels of plasma NGAL and IL-18 correlated with progression of AKI.[49] IL-18 is a cytokine that induces interferon gamma and T-cell activation, and has been shown to be a reliable marker of ATN.[50,51] In a meta-analysis, urinary IL-18 was found to be a useful biomarker of AKI in cardiac surgery patients, ICU patients, and pediatric patients.[52] CyC is an unbound protein produced by all nucleated cells that is filtered greater than 99% by the glomeruli.[53] In contrast with serum creatinine, it is not affected by age, gender, diet, or muscle mass.[54] Serum CyC has been shown to be a good biomarker in the prediction of AKI, whereas urinary CyC excretion has only moderate diagnostic value. Patients with serum CyC levels less than 0.8 mg/L are less likely to develop AKI after renal insult, whereas those with levels greater than 2.04 mg/L are at increased risk of developing AKI. Patients with high CyC levels can be targeted for early intervention.[55] Urine TIMP/IGFBP7 are biomarkers expressed in the very early phase of renal tubular epithelial cell damage.[56] Meersch and colleagues[57] showed that urine TIMP/IGFBP7 levels in post–cardiac bypass surgery patients were increased 4 hours postoperatively in patients who went on to develop AKI. A significant decrease in the urinary TIMP/IGFBP7 level predicted recovery of renal function. At present AKI biomarkers are not commercially available and therefore their use in everyday clinical practice is not common. As technology improves the availability of assays, the use of biomarkers is likely to become relevant in the treatment of patients with AKI.

Chawla and colleagues[58] reported the use of a furosemide stress test (FST) as an alternative to serum biomarkers in the assessment of moderate to severe AKI. Following a dose of 1 to 1.5 mg/kg of furosemide, less than 200 mL over 2 hours indicated progression to severe AKI and need for RRT.[58] FST outperformed NGAL, IL-18, and TIMP-2/IGFBP7 in identifying patients with severe AKI and need for RRT, showing the utility of this simple test in the assessment of AKI.[59]

Flechet and colleagues[60] reported on an online prognostic calculator (AKIPredictor. com) that uses demographics, comorbidities, and baseline and laboratory values 24 hours after ICU admission to compute the likelihood of AKI.[60]

PREVENTION OF ACUTE KIDNEY INJURY

Early recognition and prevention of further injury are the initial goals in management of AKI by restoring renal perfusion and hemodynamic stability. Treatment of intravascular hypovolemia when present is of primary importance and selection of the most appropriate resuscitation fluid (crystalloid vs colloid)[61] is critical when blood products are not indicated. Synthetic colloids (hydroxyethyl starch [HES], gelatin, and dextran) are associated with an increased incidence of AKI and should be avoided in patients at risk or who already have AKI.[62–64] With regard to allogenic albumin, the SAFE trial found no differences in 28-day mortality, new organ dysfunction, incidence of AKI, duration of dialysis, or other secondary end points when comparing normal saline with 4% albumin in a heterogeneous ICU population.[65] However, in a subgroup analysis of patients with traumatic brain injury, albumin was associated with increased mortality, whereas in a subgroup analysis of patients with severe sepsis improved survival was shown in those receiving albumin.[66,67] After considering these findings, KDIGO clinical practice guidelines for AKI recommend that isotonic crystalloids should be used ahead of synthetic and nonsynthetic colloids for intracellular volume expansion in patients at risk for or presenting with AKI (level 2B).[4]

Contrast-induced nephropathy (CIN), defined as a 25% increase in creatinine level within 3 days of intravascular administration of iodinated contrast media, affects between 7% and 11% of patients undergoing intravenous contrast administration. All critically ill patients should be considered at risk for CIN and preventive measures undertaken with volume expansion (level1A), use of iso-osmotic contrast (level 1B), and avoidance of large volumes of dye. Sodium bicarbonate's ability to prevent free radical production by alkalization of the renal tubule has not shown benefit compared with normal saline alone in multiple clinical trials but can be used for volume expansion with results equivalent to normal saline expected.[4,67,68] Oral N-acetylcysteine has shown some added benefit compared with saline alone and can be added with low cost and minimal pharmacologic risk (level 2D). Data on the use of statins to prevent CIN are still too preliminary to make recommendations at present (not graded).[4,19]

TREATMENT OF ACUTE KIDNEY INJURY

After the causes of AKI have been determined, treated, or removed, the treatment of AKI becomes largely supportive, with the intention of allowing the recovery of renal function. Oliguria and anuria are prevalent in patients with AKI, particularly after surgery and trauma, and controlling volume status becomes an important element of supportive care. In addition to decreased urine output, shock and capillary leak frequently lead to volume overload, which in turn increases morbidity, length of stay, and mortality.[69–71] The front-line treatment of volume overload is diuretics when all sepsis has been adequately treated and patients are resuscitated and hemodynamically stable[4,72] (grade 2C). Loop diuretics such as furosemide or bumetanide may stimulate urine output and shift fluid balance in a favorable direction but diuretics do not reduce mortality or need for RRT.[23,73] Several meta-analyses have shown no benefit in mortality or need for RRT when diuretics were given to patients with AKI in an attempt to convert oliguric AKI (<500 mL urine output per day) to nonoliguric (>500 mL urine output per day) AKI across multiple populations of ICU patients.[23,28,62,63] Furthermore, diuretics have been shown to increase the incidence of AKI in patients receiving intravenous contrast dye and also increase the risk of AKI and need for RRT in cardiac surgery patients.[23,64,65] In addition, the European Society of Critical Care Medicine and KDIGO recommend that diuretics should not be given to prevent or treat AKI or force return of renal function (level 1B).

MANAGEMENT OF ELECTROLYTE ABNORMALITIES

Hyperkalemia can occur rapidly in patients with AKI and may result in life-threatening complications. Patients with rhabdomyolysis, crush injury, and shock reperfusion syndrome are at greatest risk. Symptoms related to hyperkalemia occur when potassium levels increase to more than 7 mmol/L, which leads to cardiac and neuromuscular transmission abnormalities, but lower levels can trigger these manifestations in the acute setting. Typical signs of hyperkalemia are severe muscle weakness and peaked T waves and shortened QT interval on cardiac rhythm strips. Electrocardiogram (ECG) manifestations are more likely with rapid-onset hyperkalemia and the presence of concomitant hypocalcemia, acidemia, and hyponatremia. A review of medications should be done to identify drug causes of hyperkalemia (β-blockers, inhibitors of the renin-angiotensin-aldosterone system, potassium-sparing diuretics, heparin and its derivatives, trimethoprim, and nonsteroidal antiinflammatory drugs).[74,75] Severe abnormalities are best treated with RRT; however, issues with timing of initiation of treatment may prompt urgent medical treatment before RRT is started. Regardless of the potassium level, treatment should be initiated on any ECG changes or neuromuscular complications. Treatment should be focused on stabilizing the cellular membranes affected by the hyperkalemia, driving extracellular potassium intracellularly and hiding the potassium, and removing excess from the body when possible. Stabilization of the membrane is achieved with intravenous calcium gluconate or calcium chloride. To hide the potassium intracellularly, a combination of insulin and glucose are given.[76] The authors recommend a bolus of 10 units of insulin followed by 5 mL of 50% dextrose, which can reduce the potassium level by 0.5 to 1.2 mmol/L for approximately 4 to 6 hours and it can be repeated every 2 to 4 hours if awaiting RRT initiation.[77] Sodium bicarbonate works by increasing the systemic pH, triggering a release of hydrogen ions from cells and causing an influx of potassium into the cell. There are limited data on the value of sodium bicarbonate as a treatment of hyperkalemia but a few studies show that continuous infusion of sodium bicarbonate can reduce hyperkalemia in patients with a baseline metabolic acidosis in 4 to 6 hours.[76,78]

In AKI, profound metabolic acidosis results from impaired acid secretion and reduced bicarbonate production in the renal tubule. Acidosis is further propagated by increased production of lactic acid and ketoacids in the critically ill. Severe acidemia suppresses myocardial contractility, predisposes to cardiac arrhythmias, causes venous vasoconstriction while decreasing total peripheral vascular resistance, reduces hepatic blood flow, and impairs oxygen delivery. Treatment with boluses of hypertonic (8.4%) sodium bicarbonate can worsen intracellular acidosis (deceiving clinicians through improving blood pH [paradoxic acidosis]) and lead to hypernatremia and extravasation injury if not delivered into a central vein.[79] Furthermore, in patients who are oliguric/anuric and have volume overload, the large sodium load can exacerbate the volume overload. Sodium bicarbonate treatment should be reserved for severe acidosis (pH<7.1) while awaiting dialysis in patients in whom the cause of AKI is prerenal AKI caused by volume depletion, or a postrenal obstruction. In addition, bicarbonate can be used affectively in patients with AKI caused by rhabdomyolysis in order to prevent further renal injury.[80]

Monitoring of calcium levels is essential in AKI. When GFR declines phosphate excretion decreases, leading to an increase of serum phosphate level and a decline in free serum calcium level. Calcium replacement in symptomatic patients is extremely important until the underlying cause is addressed. Symptoms can include paresthesias, tetany, confusion, seizures, or QT prolongation. Treating the underlying hyperphosphatemia alleviates the hypocalcemic symptoms in many cases.[81,82] In the critically ill this is best done with RRT.

RENAL REPLACEMENT THERAPY

If volume overload, electrolyte abnormalities, acid-base status, or azotemia complicate patient care, RRT becomes the mainstay of treatment. Approximately 13% of all ICU admissions require RRT[83] and this need is an independent risk factor for mortality.[84] Specific evidence-based indications for initiating RRT have not been published because of the diversity and complexity of the disease process. The KDIGO guidelines recommend following the global picture considering trends in electrolytes, azotemia, acid-base status, and degree of volume overload. The use of absolute numbers to trigger initiation of therapy is also discouraged per KDIGO guidelines.[4]

Volume overload is perhaps the most nebulous indication for RRT. Oliguria or anuria greater than 72 hours, total body weight 10% more than admission weight, and pulmonary edema causing hypoxia in the presence of AKI have been cited as indications for RRT. Azotemia with blood urea nitrogen (BUN) levels greater than 80 to 100 mg/dL begins to interfere with wound healing and causes a decrease in the level of consciousness. Potassium levels greater than 6 mmol/L and pH less than 7.15 are generally accepted thresholds for RRT.

With regard to potential benefits to early initiation of RRT, the Artificial Kidney Initiation in Kidney Injury (AKIKI) study group in 2016 evaluated initiation of early continuous RRT (CRRT) in a prospective, multicenter, open-label, randomized trial conducted in 31 intensive care units in France. The goal of the study was to see whether early initiation of RRT improved outcomes. Patients were randomized to an early group (within 6 hours of diagnosis of stage 3 AKI) or to a delayed group that met the set of standard indications for RRT listed in **Table 8**.

There was no difference in mortality between the early and delayed groups. Almost half of the patients in the delayed group never required RRT, had a significantly lower rate of catheter-related blood stream infections (10% vs 5%; P = .03), and had earlier spontaneous diuresis ($P<.001$).[85] Two different meta-analyses by Wierstra and colleagues[86] and Bhatt and Das[87] found no improvement in survival for early initiation of RRT. However, in a single-center randomized control trial, Zarbock and colleagues[88] found that even earlier initiation of RRT (within 8 hours of diagnosis of stage 2) resulted in more patients with recovered renal function at 90 days versus late initiation (within 12 hours of diagnosis of stage 3; 53.6% vs 38.7%) and significantly reduced 90-day mortality (39.3% and 54.7%). The patients in the Zarbock and colleagues[88] study were started on RRT earlier than the AKIKI group with improved outcomes suggesting that very early initiation (stage 2) of RRT may be beneficial. Further research regarding timing of RRT is necessary to resolve the question about benefits of early initiation.

Intermittent hemodialysis (IHD) is the mainstay of RRT therapy in the United States in hemodynamically stable patients. IHD is performed every day or every other day depending on severity of illness and rapidly removes solutes across a semipermeable membrane using a transmembrane concentration gradient.[89] Because of rapid fluid shifts over a short course of therapy, IHD is limited by intravascular depletion and hypotension, which is detrimental to the recovery of AKI. Schiffl and colleagues[90] evaluated the outcomes of different dosing schedules of IHD in 160 ICU patients with AKI. Patients were randomized to receive daily or alternate-day IHD. Daily hemodialysis resulted in less hypotension, sepsis, gastrointestinal bleeding, and respiratory failure, and a significant decrease in mortality.[90]

Hybrid modality such as slow low-efficiency dialysis (SLED) is performed over an 8-hour to 12-hour time period with lower dialysate flow rates than IHD. The benefit of SLED is the ability to use standard IHD machines, excellent solute clearance, and little impact on hemodynamic stability. A recent meta-analysis showed that renal recovery, days to renal recovery, number of treatments required for each dialysis modality, and hemodynamic instability were not significantly different between the CRRT

Table 8
Artificial Kidney Initiation in Kidney Injury study group requirements for initiation of continuous renal replacement therapy

Indications for Initiation of RRT	
Oliguria/Anuria	Sustained for >72 h
BUN Level (mg/dL)	>80–100
Potassium level (mmol/L)	>6
pH	<7.15
Volume Overload	Pulmonary edema with increased Fio_2 requirements >10% body weight

Abbreviation: Fio_2, fraction of inspired oxygen.

and SLED treatment groups.[91] The disadvantages of SLED are lack of availability of dialysis support staff for extended time on hemodialysis and lack of familiarity within the critical care community.

Hemodynamically unstable patients may not tolerate the rapid volume shifts seen with IHD. CRRT was developed for critically ill patients in shock or with otherwise tenuous hemodynamic status. CRRT is performed 24 hours a day, typically 7 days a week. Several modalities can be deployed on a CRRT machine depending on specific patient needs.

The simplest modality is slow continuous ultrafiltration (SCUF), in which blood is pumped through a semipermeable membrane causing plasma (ultrafiltrate) to be removed or ultrafiltered from the blood (**Fig. 1**). This modality is useful in patients who are volume overloaded with normal electrolytes and BUN, but fail to respond to diuretics.

Continuous venovenous hemofiltration (CVVH) is a CRRT modality in which a replacement fluid is added to the blood in the dialysis circuit. As this additional volume of fluid passes through the filter, solute is "pulled" with the ultrafiltrate, known as solute drag. The transportation of additional solute across the dialysis membrane by dilution of the blood with replacement fluid is known as convection (**Fig. 2**). The molecules removed with convection can be bigger than those removed by hemodialysis, which makes this modality potentially useful in patients with myoglobinuria or drug intoxication. Continuous venovenous hemodialysis (CVVHD) does not require a replacement fluid but uses a dialysis solution (dialysate) that is pumped countercurrent to the blood flow on the fluid side (as opposed to the blood side) of the membrane, creating a concentration gradient that allows solute exchange by diffusion (**Fig. 3**). CVVHD is useful in small molecule removal with solutes such as electrolytes and urea.

Another CRRT modality is continuous venovenous hemodiafiltration (CVVHDF), in which dialysate and replacement fluid are both added to their respective

SCUF

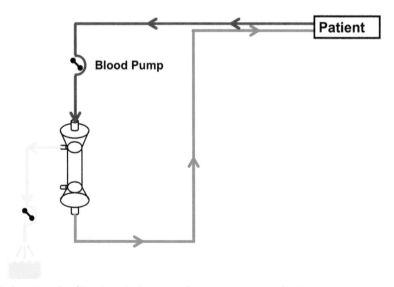

Fig. 1. SCUF, showing ultrafiltration via transmembrane pressure gradient.

CVVH

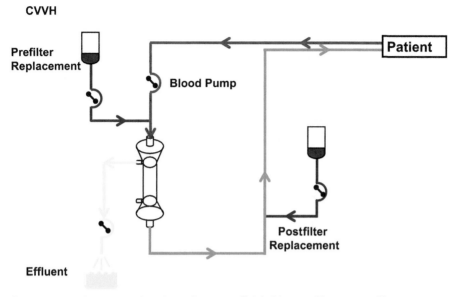

Fig. 2. CVVH using convection via replacement fluid either prefilter or postfilter.

compartments of the circuit, generating solute removal by both diffusion and convection. Fluid removal is achieved by ultrafiltration (**Fig. 4**).[92] The type of modality chosen depends on the individual patient's needs. SCUF is useful in patients with volume overload and relatively normal electrolytes and BUN that do not respond well to diuretics. When patients have electrolyte abnormalities and azotemia, CVVHDF is often the most efficient CRRT modality and is frequently used in most other cases. In a

CVVHD

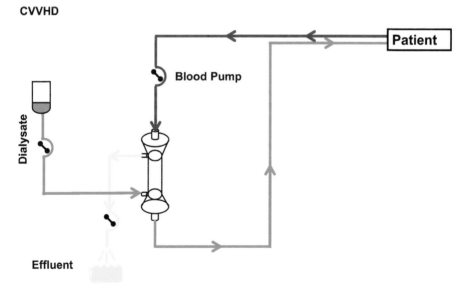

Fig. 3. CVVHD showing the diffusion of small solutes via the countercurrent of the dialysate.

CVVHDF

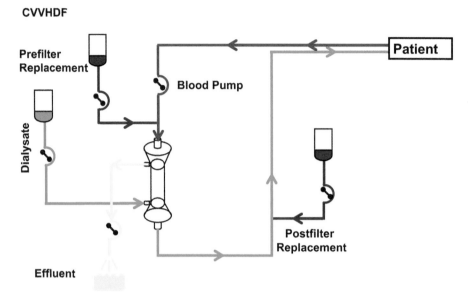

Fig. 4. CVVHDF combining components of ultrafiltration, hemodialysis, and convection.

single-center prospective randomized trial, Saudan and colleagues[93] compared CVVH and CVVHDF and showed decreased mortality with CVVHDF. However, no other prospective data have been reported regarding the optimal modality.[93]

The dose of CRRT is defined as the total volume of replacement fluid and dialysate given plus ultrafiltrate removed from the patient averaged per weight in kilograms per hour. A Cochrane Review completed in 2016 included 6 large studies with 3185 patients comparing a CRRT dose of less than 35 mL/kg/h versus greater than 35 mL/kg/h. There was no difference in mortality, recovery of renal function, or ICU days. There was higher incidence of hypophosphatemia with increased dose.[94] KDIGO recommends an average 24-hour dose of effluent volume in the range of 20 to 25 mL/kg/h when considering time off modality for filter changes, operating room procedures, and radiologic procedures (grade 1A).

To prevent clot formation within the filter of circuit, 3 options with regard to anticoagulation are available: heparin, regional citrate, or no anticoagulation. Systemic heparinization is easy to monitor and prevents filter thrombosis at the risk of bleeding complications. Regional citrate works by anticoagulating the circuit with an infusion of citrate, and by placing patients on a systemic calcium infusion to replace the calcium once the filtered blood is returned to the patient, which reduces risk of bleeding. Citrate is metabolized mainly in the liver, skeletal muscle, and renal cortex, making patients with acute liver injury/failure at high risk for hypocalcemia because they may not metabolize citrate normally. When compared in a multicenter randomized control trial there was no difference in renal outcomes and mortality between citrate and heparin. However, citrate was superior in safety, efficacy, and cost[95] (grade 2B). No anticoagulation may be an option for patients with liver or bone marrow failure who may already be coagulopathic.

Because renal recovery occurs over weeks to months, timing of cessation of RRT can be a nebulous end point. Return of native urine output is generally a good sign but recovering renal tubules may lack normal function and the ability to concentrate urine. Because of antidiuretic hormone unresponsiveness of the distal tubule and collecting system, patients recovering from AKI can develop high-output renal failure and be at risk for dehydration. Volume status needs careful monitoring and excessive urine losses may require scheduled intravenous crystalloid replacement. Uchino and colleagues,[34] in a post hoc analysis of a multicenter prospective observational study, found that patients with urine output greater than 400 mL/d with no diuretics and greater than 2300 mL/d with diuretics had an 80% chance of successful discontinuation of CRRT. In contrast, preadmission CKD was a strong negative predictor (odds ratio, 0.54) for unsuccessful cessation.[34] In a single-center retrospective study, Frohlich[96] reviewed patients who had a 2-hour creatinine clearance (2h-CrCl) drawn within 12 hours of cessation as a predictor of successful discontinuation. A 2h-CrCl of 23 mL/min had a sensitivity and specificity of 75.5% and 84.4% respectively and an overall accuracy of 78.8%. CrCl is useful because it is unaffected by use of diuretic therapy, hypotension, or oliguria.[97] In both studies a lower serum creatinine level was marginally predictive of success.

SUMMARY

AKI encompasses a wide variety of disease processes and is a common but serious problem in surgical patients. Ever-present awareness of the causes, preventive strategies, work-up, and treatment is vital to the management of critically ill surgical patients. ATN precipitated by some type of shock is the most common cause of AKI and rapid correction of the source and restoration of volume status are of paramount importance in the management of patients at risk. When AKI has led to sufficient electrolyte, acid-base, or fluid abnormalities, some form of RRT is necessary. Hemodynamically stable patients can be managed with daily IHD, whereas patients on vasopressors are likely to benefit from CRRT with care taken to provide appropriate anticoagulation and dose. Recovery from AKI may be slow, taking weeks to months, with death and end-stage renal disease being the undesired outcomes.

REFERENCES

1. Ad-hoc working group of ERBP, Fliser D, Laville M, Covic A, et al. A European Renal Best Practice (ERBP) position statement on the Kidney Disease Improving Global Outcomes (KDIGO) clinical practice guidelines on acute kidney injury: part 1: definitions, conservative management and contrast-induced nephropathy. Nephrol Dial Transplant 2012;27(12):4263–72.
2. Eriksson M, Brattström O, Mårtensson J, et al. Acute kidney injury following severe trauma: risk factors and long-term outcome. J Trauma Acute Care Surg 2015;79(3):407–12.
3. Kidney Disease: Improving Global Outcomes (KDIGO) Acute Kidney Injury Work Group. KDIGO clinical practice guideline for acute kidney injury. Kidney Int 2012;(Suppl(2)):1–138.
4. Khwaja A. KDIGO clinical practice guidelines for acute kidney injury. Nephron Clin Pract 2012;120(4):c179–84.
5. Grade Working Group. Available at: http://www.gradeworkinggroup.org/. Accessed February 13, 2017.
6. Doi K, Yuen PS, Eisner C, et al. Reduced production of creatinine limits its use as marker of kidney injury in sepsis. J Am Soc Nephrol 2009;20(6):1217–21.
7. Kim WY, Huh JW, Lim CM, et al. A comparison of acute kidney injury classifications in patients with severe sepsis and septic shock. Am J Med Sci 2012; 344(5):350–6.

8. Thomas ME, Blaine C, Dawnay A, et al. The definition of acute kidney injury and its use in practice. Kidney Int 2015;87(1):62–73.

9. Star RA. Treatment of acute renal failure. Kidney Int 1998;54(6):1817–31.

10. Macedo E, Bouchard J, Soroko SH, et al. Fluid accumulation, recognition and staging of acute kidney injury in critically-ill patients. Crit Care 2010;14(3):R82.

11. Liu KD, Thompson BT, Ancukiewicz M, et al. Acute kidney injury in patients with acute lung injury: impact of fluid accumulation on classification of acute kidney injury and associated outcomes. Crit Care Med 2011;39(12):2665–71.

12. Guay J, Lortie L. Activation of the renin-angiotensin system contributes significantly to the pathophysiology of oliguria in patients undergoing posterior spinal fusion. Eur J Anaesthesiol 2004;21(10):812–8.

13. Kellum JA, Sileanu FE, Murugan R, et al. Classifying AKI by urine output versus serum creatinine level. J Am Soc Nephrol 2015;26(9):2231–8.

14. Lehner GF, Forni LG, Joannidis M. Oliguria and biomarkers of acute kidney injury: star struck lovers or strangers in the night? Nephron 2016;134(3):183–90.

15. Prowle JR, Liu YL, Licari E, et al. Oliguria as predictive biomarker of acute kidney injury in critically ill patients. Crit Care 2011;15(4):R172.

16. Md Ralib A, Pickering JW, Shaw GM, et al. The urine output definition of acute kidney injury is too liberal. Crit Care 2013;17(3):R112.

17. Pan HC, Wu PC, Wu VC, et al. A nationwide survey of clinical characteristics, management, and outcomes of acute kidney injury (AKI) - patients with and without preexisting chronic kidney disease have different prognoses. Medicine (Baltimore) 2016;95(39):e4987.

18. Chalkias A, Xanthos T. Acute kidney injury. Lancet 2012;380(9857):1904 [author reply: 1905].

19. Papadopoulos J. Drug-induced complications in the critically ill patient: a guide for recognition and treatment. Mount Prospect (IL): Society of Critical Care Medicine; 2012. p. 472.

20. Taber SS, Mueller BA. Drug-associated renal dysfunction. Crit Care Clin 2006; 22(2):357–74, viii.

21. Perazella MA. Drug use and nephrotoxicity in the intensive care unit. Kidney Int 2012;81(12):1172–8.

22. Bonventre JV, Yang L. Cellular pathophysiology of ischemic acute kidney injury. J Clin Invest 2011;121(11):4210–21.

23. Ejaz AA, Mohandas R. Are diuretics harmful in the management of acute kidney injury? Curr Opin Nephrol Hypertens 2014;23(2):155–60.

24. Ostermann M, Joannidis M. Acute kidney injury 2016: diagnosis and diagnostic workup. Crit Care 2016;20(1):299.

25. Li SY, Chuang CL, Yang WC, et al. Proteinuria predicts postcardiotomy acute kidney injury in patients with preserved glomerular filtration rate. J Thorac Cardiovasc Surg 2015;149(3):894–9.

26. Becker GJ, Garigali G, Fogazzi GB. Advances in urine microscopy. Am J Kidney Dis 2016;67(6):954–64.

27. Klahr S, Miller SB. Acute oliguria. N Engl J Med 1998;338(10):671–5.

28. Macedo E, Mehta RL. Prerenal failure: from old concepts to new paradigms. Curr Opin Crit Care 2009;15(6):467–73.

29. Nickolas TL, O'Rourke MJ, Yang J, et al. Sensitivity and specificity of a single emergency department measurement of urinary neutrophil gelatinase-associated lipocalin for diagnosing acute kidney injury. Ann Intern Med 2008; 148(11):810–9.

30. Pepin MN, Bouchard J, Legault L, et al. Diagnostic performance of fractional excretion of urea and fractional excretion of sodium in the evaluations of patients with acute kidney injury with or without diuretic treatment. Am J Kidney Dis 2007; 50(4):566–73.

31. Thadhani R, Pascual M, Bonventre JV. Acute renal failure. N Engl J Med 1996; 334(22):1448–60.

32. Steiner RW. Interpreting the fractional excretion of sodium. Am J Med 1984;77(4): 699–702.

33. Nejat M, Pickering JW, Devarajan P, et al. Some biomarkers of acute kidney injury are increased in pre-renal acute injury. Kidney Int 2012;81(12):1254–62.

34. Uchino S, Bellomo R, Morimatsu H, et al. Discontinuation of continuous renal replacement therapy: a post hoc analysis of a prospective multicenter observational study. Crit Care Med 2009;37(9):2576–82.

35. Endre ZH, Kellum JA, Di Somma S, et al. Differential diagnosis of AKI in clinical practice by functional and damage biomarkers: workgroup statements from the tenth Acute Dialysis Quality Initiative Consensus Conference. Contrib Nephrol 2013;182:30–44.

36. Carvounis CP, Nisar S, Guro-Razuman S. Significance of the fractional excretion of urea in the differential diagnosis of acute renal failure. Kidney Int 2002;62(6): 2223–9.

37. Hall IE, Coca SG, Perazella MA, et al. Risk of poor outcomes with novel and traditional biomarkers at clinical AKI diagnosis. Clin J Am Soc Nephrol 2011;6(12): 2740–9.

38. Pru C, Kjellstrand CM. The FENa test is of no prognostic value in acute renal failure. Nephron 1984;36(1):20–3.

39. Legrand M, Le Cam B, Perbet S, et al. Urine sodium concentration to predict fluid responsiveness in oliguric ICU patients: a prospective multicenter observational study. Crit Care 2016;20(1):165.

40. Maciel AT, Park M, Macedo E. Physicochemical analysis of blood and urine in the course of acute kidney injury in critically ill patients: a prospective, observational study. BMC Anesthesiol 2013;13(1):31.

41. Miller TR, Anderson RJ, Linas SL, et al. Urinary diagnostic indices in acute renal failure: a prospective study. Ann Intern Med 1978;89(1):47–50.

42. Benjamin IJ, Griggs RC, Wing EJ, et al. Andreoli and Carpenter's Cecil essentials of medicine. 9th edition. Philadelphia: Elsevier/Saunders; 2016. p. 1190, xxv.

43. Gamss R, Stein MW, Rispoli JM, et al. What is the appropriate use of renal sonography in an inner-city population with new-onset acute kidney injury? J Ultrasound Med 2015;34(9):1639–44.

44. Podoll A, Walther C, Finkel K. Clinical utility of gray scale renal ultrasound in acute kidney injury. BMC Nephrol 2013;14:188.

45. Schnell D, Darmon M. Bedside Doppler ultrasound for the assessment of renal perfusion in the ICU: advantages and limitations of the available techniques. Crit Ultrasound J 2015;7(1):24.

46. Kjeldsen L, Cowland JB, Borregaard N, et al. Isolation and primary structure of NGAL, a novel protein associated with human neutrophil gelatinase. J Biol Chem 1993;268(14):10425–32.

47. Singer E, Markó L, Paragas N, et al. Neutrophil gelatinase-associated lipocalin: pathophysiology and clinical applications. Acta Physiol (Oxf) 2013;207(4): 663–72.

48. Haase M, Bellomo R, Devarajan P, et al. Accuracy of neutrophil gelatinase-associated lipocalin (NGAL) in diagnosis and prognosis in acute kidney injury: a systematic review and meta-analysis. Am J Kidney Dis 2009;54(6):1012–24.

49. Koyner JL, Garg AX, Coca SG, et al. Biomarkers predict progression of acute kidney injury after cardiac surgery. J Am Soc Nephrol 2012;23(5):905–14.

50. Dinarello CA, Novick D, Kim S, et al. Interleukin-18 and IL-18 binding protein. Front Immunol 2013;4:289.

51. Parikh CR, Han G. Variation in performance of kidney injury biomarkers due to cause of acute kidney injury. Am J Kidney Dis 2013;62(6):1023–6.

52. Liu Y, Guo W, Zhang J, et al. Urinary interleukin 18 for detection of acute kidney injury: a meta-analysis. Am J Kidney Dis 2013;62(6):1058–67.

53. Grubb AO. Cystatin C–properties and use as diagnostic marker. Adv Clin Chem 2000;35:63–99.

54. Filler G, Bökenkamp A, Hofmann W, et al. Cystatin C as a marker of GFR–history, indications, and future research. Clin Biochem 2005;38(1):1–8.

55. Zhang Z, Lu B, Sheng X, et al. Cystatin C in prediction of acute kidney injury: a systemic review and meta-analysis. Am J Kidney Dis 2011;58(3):356–65.

56. Wang WG, Sun WX, Gao BS, et al. Cell cycle arrest as a therapeutic target of acute kidney injury. Curr Protein Pept Sci 2016. [Epub ahead of print].

57. Meersch M, Schmidt C, Van Aken H, et al. Urinary TIMP-2 and IGFBP7 as early biomarkers of acute kidney injury and renal recovery following cardiac surgery. PLoS One 2014;9(3):e93460.

58. Chawla LS, Davison DL, Brasha-Mitchell E, et al. Development and standardization of a furosemide stress test to predict the severity of acute kidney injury. Crit Care 2013;17(5):R207.

59. Koyner JL, Davison DL, Brasha-Mitchell E, et al. Furosemide stress test and biomarkers for the prediction of AKI severity. J Am Soc Nephrol 2015;26(8):2023–31.

60. Flechet M, Güiza F, Schetz M, et al. AKIpredictor, an online prognostic calculator for acute kidney injury in adult critically ill patients: development, validation and comparison to serum neutrophil gelatinase-associated lipocalin. Intensive Care Med 2017;43(6):764–73.

61. Yerram P, Karuparthi PR, Misra M. Fluid overload and acute kidney injury. Hemodial Int 2010;14(4):348–54.

62. Brunkhorst FM, Engel C, Bloos F, et al. Intensive insulin therapy and pentastarch resuscitation in severe sepsis. N Engl J Med 2008;358(2):125–39.

63. Rioux JP, Lessard M, De Bortoli B, et al. Pentastarch 10% (250 kDa/0.45) is an independent risk factor of acute kidney injury following cardiac surgery. Crit Care Med 2009;37(4):1293–8.

64. Schortgen F, Girou E, Deye N, et al. The risk associated with hyperoncotic colloids in patients with shock. Intensive Care Med 2008;34(12):2157–68.

65. Finfer S, Bellomo R, Boyce N, et al. A comparison of albumin and saline for fluid resuscitation in the intensive care unit. N Engl J Med 2004;350(22):2247–56.

66. SAFE Study Investigators, Australian and New Zealand Intensive Care Society Clinical Trials Group, Australian Red Cross Blood Service, George Institute for International Health, Myburgh J, Cooper DJ, Finfer S, et al. Saline or albumin for fluid resuscitation in patients with traumatic brain injury. N Engl J Med 2007; 357(9):874–84.

67. Subramaniam RM, Suarez-Cuervo C, Wilson RF, et al. Effectiveness of prevention strategies for contrast-induced nephropathy: a systematic review and meta-analysis. Ann Intern Med 2016;164(6):406–16.

68. Brar SS, Shen AY, Jorgensen MB, et al. Sodium bicarbonate vs sodium chloride for the prevention of contrast medium-induced nephropathy in patients undergoing coronary angiography: a randomized trial. JAMA 2008;300(9):1038–46.
69. Bouchard J, Mehta RL. Fluid accumulation and acute kidney injury: consequence or cause. Curr Opin Crit Care 2009;15(6):509–13.
70. Bouchard J, Soroko SB, Chertow GM, et al. Fluid accumulation, survival and recovery of kidney function in critically ill patients with acute kidney injury. Kidney Int 2009;76(4):422–7.
71. RENAL Replacement Therapy Study Investigators, Bellomo R, Cass A, Cole L, et al. An observational study fluid balance and patient outcomes in the Randomized Evaluation of Normal vs. Augmented Level of Replacement Therapy trial. Crit Care Med 2012;40(6):1753–60.
72. Ho KM, Power BM. Benefits and risks of furosemide in acute kidney injury. Anaesthesia 2010;65(3):283–93.
73. Oh HJ, Kim MH, Ahn JY, et al. Can early initiation of continuous renal replacement therapy improve patient survival with septic acute kidney injury when enrolled in early goal-directed therapy? J Crit Care 2016;35:51–6.
74. Lee JW. Fluid and electrolyte disturbances in critically ill patients. Electrolyte Blood Press 2010;8(2):72–81.
75. Buckley MS, Leblanc JM, Cawley MJ. Electrolyte disturbances associated with commonly prescribed medications in the intensive care unit. Crit Care Med 2010;38(6 Suppl):S253–64.
76. Blumberg A, Weidmann P, Shaw S, et al. Effect of various therapeutic approaches on plasma potassium and major regulating factors in terminal renal failure. Am J Med 1988;85(4):507–12.
77. Lens XM, Montoliu J, Cases A, et al. Treatment of hyperkalaemia in renal failure: salbutamol v. insulin. Nephrol Dial Transplant 1989;4(3):228–32.
78. Blumberg A, Weidmann P, Ferrari P. Effect of prolonged bicarbonate administration on plasma potassium in terminal renal failure. Kidney Int 1992;41(2):369–74.
79. Kraut JA, Kurtz I. Use of base in the treatment of severe acidemic states. Am J Kidney Dis 2001;38(4):703–27.
80. Ron D, Taitelman U, Michaelson M, et al. Prevention of acute renal failure in traumatic rhabdomyolysis. Arch Intern Med 1984;144(2):277–80.
81. Reber PM, Heath H 3rd. Hypocalcemic emergencies. Med Clin North Am 1995; 79(1):93–106.
82. Tohme JF, Bilezikian JP. Hypocalcemic emergencies. Endocrinol Metab Clin North Am 1993;22(2):363–75.
83. Hoste EA, Bagshaw SM, Bellomo R, et al. Epidemiology of acute kidney injury in critically ill patients: the multinational AKI-EPI study. Intensive Care Med 2015; 41(8):1411–23.
84. Elseviers MM, Lins RL, Van der Niepen P, et al. Renal replacement therapy is an independent risk factor for mortality in critically ill patients with acute kidney injury. Crit Care 2010;14(6):R221.
85. Gaudry S, Hajage D, Schortgen F, et al. Initiation strategies for renal-replacement therapy in the intensive care unit. N Engl J Med 2016;375(2):122–33.
86. Wierstra BT, Kadri S, Alomar S, et al. The impact of "early" versus "late" initiation of renal replacement therapy in critical care patients with acute kidney injury: a systematic review and evidence synthesis. Crit Care 2016;20(1):122.
87. Bhatt GC, Das RR. Early versus late initiation of renal replacement therapy in patients with acute kidney injury-a systematic review & meta-analysis of randomized controlled trials. BMC Nephrol 2017;18(1):78.

88. Zarbock A, Kellum JA, Schmidt C, et al. Effect of early vs delayed initiation of renal replacement therapy on mortality in critically ill patients with acute kidney injury: the ELAIN Randomized Clinical Trial. JAMA 2016;315(20):2190–9.

89. Hemodialysis Adequacy Work Group. Clinical practice guidelines for hemodialysis adequacy, update 2006. Am J Kidney Dis 2006;48(Suppl 1):S2–90.

90. Schiffl H, Lang SM, Fischer R. Daily hemodialysis and the outcome of acute renal failure. N Engl J Med 2002;346(5):305–10.

91. Kovacs B, Sullivan KJ, Hiremath S, et al. Effect of sustained low efficient dialysis versus continuous renal replacement therapy on renal recovery after acute kidney injury in the intensive care unit: a systematic review and meta-analysis. Nephrology (Carlton) 2017;22(5):343–53.

92. Cerda J, Ronco C. Modalities of continuous renal replacement therapy: technical and clinical considerations. Semin Dial 2009;22(2):114–22.

93. Saudan P, Niederberger M, De Seigneux S, et al. Adding a dialysis dose to continuous hemofiltration increases survival in patients with acute renal failure. Kidney Int 2006;70(7):1312–7.

94. Fayad AI, Buamscha DG, Ciapponi A. Intensity of continuous renal replacement therapy for acute kidney injury. Cochrane Database Syst Rev 2016;(10):CD010613.

95. Schilder L, Nurmohamed SA, Bosch FH, et al. Citrate anticoagulation versus systemic heparinisation in continuous venovenous hemofiltration in critically ill patients with acute kidney injury: a multi-center randomized clinical trial. Crit Care 2014;18(4):472.

96. Frohlich S, et al. Use of 2-hour creatinine clearance to guide cessation of continuous renal replacement therapy. J Crit Care 2012;27(6):744.

97. Herrera-Gutierrez ME, Seller-Pérez G, Banderas-Bravo E, et al. Replacement of 24-h creatinine clearance by 2-h creatinine clearance in intensive care unit patients: a single-center study. Intensive Care Med 2007;33(11):1900–6.

Decompensated Cirrhosis and Fluid Resuscitation

Erin Maynard, MD, FACS

KEYWORDS

- Cirrhosis • Albumin • Normal saline • Hepatorenal syndrome • Antidiuretic hormone
- Hyponatremia

KEY POINTS

- Understanding of the unique physiology of end-stage liver disease is imperative to resuscitation of the patient with cirrhosis.
- The effects of albumin resuscitation in the patients with cirrhosis are more than mere volume expansion.
- Decompensated cirrhotics are total body volume expanded but intravascularly volume deplete.

INTRODUCTION

Physician encounters with patients with cirrhosis have become prevalent, with 1 in 10 Americans having some form of liver disease. Despite advances in the treatment of hepatitis C, the incidence of liver disease has not decreased and according to the National Institute of Health 10% of children in the United States have nonalcoholic fatty liver disease.[1] Cirrhosis carries a significant increase in mortality with the Centers for Disease Control and Prevention citing it as the fourth leading cause of death of Americans between the ages of 45 and 54 and the twelfth leading cause overall.[2] In-hospital mortality is reportedly 44% to 74% in some studies with yearly costs approaching $13 billion.[3] Given the prevalence of liver disease it is likely that all surgeons independent of specialty will encounter a patient with cirrhosis with nearly 10% of patients with cirrhosis undergoing surgery in their last 2 years of life. The understanding of resuscitation of the decompensated patient with cirrhosis is vital to decreasing morbidity and mortality. This article enhances the understanding of the unique physiology of the patient with decompensated cirrhosis to guide their needs in fluid resuscitation in critical illness.

Disclosure: The author has nothing to disclose.
Department of Surgery, Oregon Health and Science University, 3181 SW Sam Jackson Park Road, Portland, OR 97239, USA
E-mail address: maynarde@ohsu.edu

Surg Clin N Am 97 (2017) 1419–1424
http://dx.doi.org/10.1016/j.suc.2017.07.010
0039-6109/17/© 2017 Elsevier Inc. All rights reserved.

PHYSIOLOGY OF LIVER DISEASE

Before discussing specifics of fluid resuscitation in patients with liver disease it is imperative to understand the unique physiology of the patient with cirrhosis (**Fig. 1**). Portal hypertension in the setting of cirrhosis leads to splanchnic and arteriolar vaso-dilation. The exact mechanism of this is not exactly understood but nitric oxide is thought to play an important role. This dilation leads to a significant decrease in sys-temic vascular resistance, decreasing the effective arterial blood volume and blood pressure, which leads to a cascading chain of events. In response to the decrease of effective circulating blood volume the sympathetic nervous system and the renin-angiotensin system (RAAS) increase to try to compensate along with excretion of endogenous vasopressin. The activation of the RAAS leads to an increase in release of antidiuretic hormone leading to sodium and water retention with a disproportionate amount of free water retention increasing plasma volume, which can result in signifi-cant hypervolemic hyponatremia. The increase in sympathetic nervous system leads to an increase in heart rate and overall increase in cardiac output, which increases splanchnic blood flow.

DETERMINATION OF VOLUME STATUS

Determination of volume status in the patient with cirrhosis is important but often diffi-cult to determine given that up to 50% of extracellular fluid may be in the extravascular space manifesting is ascites and edema.[4] Patients who seem total volume expanded may often be intravascularly volume depleted putting them at risk for hepatorenal syn-drome (HRS). Overresuscitation of the postoperative patient with liver disease can result in ascites and hyponatremia, which is difficult to treat.[5] In a study aimed to eval-uate the effect of plasma expansion with albumin in patients with cirrhosis with renal failure, global end-diastolic blood volume index but not central venous pressure served as an indicator of cardiac preload. When examining predictors of fluid respon-siveness, central venous pressure, global end-diastolic blood volume index, stroke volume index, and cardiac index were significantly lower than in nonresponders, where a systemic vascular resistance index was significantly higher.[6]

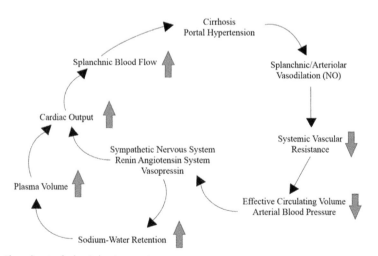

Fig. 1. Flowchart of physiologic events.

THE EFFECTS OF CIRRHOSIS ON ALBUMIN

Albumin is the most abundant protein in plasma and is exclusively synthesized in the liver. Besides regulating osmotic pressure, it has several other physiologic mechanisms that are altered in the setting of liver disease. Albumin serves as a carrier for water-insoluble molecules (eg, hormones, cholesterol, drugs, free fatty acids, and bilirubin); it plays a role in maintaining the competence of capillary permeability, which can increase in inflammatory states, such as sepsis; and acts as a free radical scavenger in its reduced form decreasing oxidative stress.[7] Although albumin synthesis has been demonstrated to increase during time of stress in patients without cirrhosis, synthesis can decrease 50% in the setting of cirrhosis. In addition to decreased protein synthesis patients with decompensated liver disease suffer from protein malnutrition from several sources (**Box 1**).[8] The additive effects of decreased synthesis of albumin, impaired intake of its precursors, and increased proteolysis creates a state of global hypoalbuminemia in those with cirrhosis that decreases effective circulating volume and oncotic pressure, which leads to renal sodium and water retention with third spacing of ascites and anasarca complicating their resuscitation. The contribution of hypoalbuminemia to mortality in liver patients is recognized in the Child-Pugh score (**Table 1**). Besides the overall decrease of albumin the function is also altered in patients with cirrhosis and has been demonstrated in several studies. The exact cause of this dysfunction is unknown but could be caused by saturation with bilirubin or structural modifications.

THE USE OF ALBUMIN IN FLUID RESUSCITATION

The use of albumin in critically ill patients without evidence of cirrhosis has been greatly debated and the subject of several studies. The Saline versus Albumin Fluid Evaluation (SAFE) study was a large double-blind randomized trial comparing 4% human albumin solution with normal saline in nearly 7000 intensive care unit patients. The results showed no difference in intensive care unit stay, number of failing organs, or mortality rates at 28 days. In the group with severe sepsis the mortality was less in the albumin infusion group (30.7% vs 35.3%) but this did not reach statistical significance. Given these findings and the expense of albumin compared with crystalloid the use of albumin has largely been discouraged in the patient without cirrhosis.

In the patient with cirrhosis the use of albumin has been largely based on its oncotic properties to increase effective circulating volume to stop the cascade of physiologic

---

Box 1
Sources of protein malnutrition

- Poor nutrition intake

- Anorexia from symptoms, such as early satiety from large-volume ascites and reflux

- Protein loss from large-volume paracentesis and metabolic alterations, including hormonal and nutrient utilization abnormalities, as in reduced glycogen stores creating an early fasting state that leads to concurrent breakdown of fat and amino acids

- Increased β-adrenergic activity, which leads to a hypermetabolic state creating insulin resistance, proteolysis, and amino acid use for gluconeogenesis

- Protein malabsorption secondary to increased gut permeability, reduced bile salts, and bacterial overgrowth

- Overall protein loss from reduced synthesis

Table 1
Child-Turcotte-Pugh classification

	1 Point	2 Points	3 Points
Encephalopathy	0	1–2	3–4
Ascites	None	Slight	Moderate
Bilirubin (mg/dL)	<2	2–3	>3
Albumin (g/dL)	>3.5	2.8–3.5	<2.8
PT prolonged (s)	1–4	5–6	>6
(INR)	<1.7	1.8–2.3	>2.3

Child's A = 5 to 6 points; Child's B = 7 to 9 points; Child's C = 10 to 15 points.
Abbreviations: INR, international normalized ratio; PT, prothrombin time.

events as depicted in **Fig. 1** and described previously. Three specific uses of albumin in patients with cirrhosis are discussed in more detail next.

Albumin Infusion After Large Volume Paracentesis

Diuretic-resistant ascites happens in up to 10% of patients with end-stage liver disease.[7] Although transjugular intrahepatic portosystemic shunt is an option for some, for many patients frequent large-volume paracentesis (LVP) is their only option. Paracentesis results in protein loss and large intracellular to extracellular volume shifts that results in vasoconstrictions and exacerbates the circulatory dysfunction described in **Fig. 1**. A randomized trial compared fluid resuscitation with albumin versus saline in the prevention of paracentesis-induced circulatory dysfunction. A total of 72 patients were randomized to receive either albumin or saline. Significant increases were found in plasma renin activity 25 hours and 6 days after paracentesis when saline was used with an increase in paracentesis-induced circulatory dysfunction in the saline group (33.3% vs 11.4%; $P = .03$). No difference was found in those patients with LVP less than 6 L.[9] Although most surgeons are not primarily involved in managing routine LVP in the setting of end-stage liver disease, the management of ascites plays a critical role in the acute care surgical settings in patients with ruptured umbilical hernias and ascites leak after laparotomy. Adequate resuscitation and control of excessive volume loss is critical in prevention of circulatory dysfunction to minimize mortality.

Management of Hypervolemic Hyponatremia

Hyponatremia (Na <130 mmol/L) is a common finding in cirrhosis and is an independent predictor of mortality, which is why it is now included in the Model of End Stage Liver Disease allocation system.[7] The first step in treatment is to determine whether the patient is hypovolemic or hypervolemic. Hypovolemic hyponatremia is less typical, and presents as a patient with low serum sodium in the absence of edema and ascites. This is often secondary to overdiuresis and the first step in management is to withhold diuretics and administration of normal saline.[7] There is no role or data to support the use of albumin in this setting.[10] Hypervolemic hyponatremia is the production of oversecretion of antidiuretic hormone leading to an unbalanced retention of water and sodium (see **Fig. 1**). The primary treatment of hypervolemic hyponatremia is free water restriction (<1000 mL/d). There are no data to support saline administration in this setting. The European Association for the Study of the Liver guidelines support the use of albumin in this situation to serve as potential volume expander to decrease RAAS activity based on B2 practice guidelines.[10] Hypervolemic hyponatremia can be iatrogenic after overresuscitation with crystalloid in the perioperative patient.[5]

Meticulous administration of fluids and free water restriction is paramount in avoiding this complication.

Management of Hepatorenal Syndrome

HRS defined by acute kidney injury in the setting of cirrhosis, no or minimal proteinuria, low sodium excretion (<10 mEq/L), and oliguria is a diagnosis of exclusion and is divided into HRS1 and HRS2.[10] HRS2 is the less severe kind and usually found in patients with diuretic refractory ascites. HRS1 is the more severe kind and is defined by a more than two-fold increase in creatinine in less than a 2-week period and is associated with significant mortality even with treatment or transplantation. HRS is a diagnosis of exclusion and prerenal acute kidney injury and kidney injury caused by acute infection should be ruled out. Both the treatment and prevention of HRS involves the use of albumin. Albumin has been shown in randomized trial to prevent HRS and improve survival in the setting of spontaneous bacterial peritonitis.[7] The hallmark of treatment of HRS1 is vasopressin or vasopressin analogue (eg, terlipressin) in addition to albumin administration. A randomized controlled trial in patients with HRS randomly assigned patients to either receive terlipressin (1–2 mg/4 hours) and albumin (1 g/kg followed by 20–40 g/d) or albumin alone. Primary outcomes were improvement in renal function and survival at 3 months. Results showed improvement of renal function in 43.5% of patients with combination treatment compared with 8.7% of patients treated with albumin alone (P = .017). Survival was not different between the two groups (27% vs 19% respectively; P = .7), reflecting the high mortality associated with HRS.[11] Terlipressin therapy alone was also studied with and without albumin in a prospective nonrandomized trial. Patients either received terlipressin (0.5–2 mg/4 hours), until complete response or for 15 days, or terlipressin along with intravenous albumin. Albumin administration was the only predictive factor of complete response (77% in patients receiving combination therapy vs 25% in the terlipressin alone group; P = .03), demonstrating that albumin plays an important role in the treatment of HRS along with vasopressin analogues.[5] HRS is seen in the postoperative patient given that anesthetic agents routinely increase splanchnic vasodilation and decrease hepatic blood flow. Postoperative patients with a rise in creatinine should be investigated for potential HRS and treated aggressively to minimize mortality.

SUMMARY

The critically ill patient with decompensated cirrhosis has a unique physiology and alterations in albumin that need to be understood to properly resuscitate them and minimize morbidity and mortality. Little data exist on specific resuscitation of the patient with cirrhosis as compared with those patients without liver disease. The effectiveness of albumin administration compared with saline administration in common settings, such as LVP, can be extrapolated to the care of the general surgical patient but further studies in this area are warranted.

REFERENCES

1. U.S. Department of Health and Human Services. National Institute of Diabetes and Digestive and Kidney Diseases. 2016. Available at: https://www.niddk.nih.gov/health-information/liver-disease/nafld-nash/definition-facts. Accessed July 19, 2017.
2. Centers for Disease Control and Prevention. 2016. Available at: https://www.cdc.gov/nchs/fastats/liver-disease.htm. Accessed July 18, 2017.

3. Horvath A, Leber B. Hospital mortality of cirrhosis: better, but still room for improvement! Liver Int 2013;33:809–10.

4. Davenport A, Argawal B, Wright G, et al. Can non-invasive measurements aid clinical assessment of volume in patients with cirrhosis? World J Hepatol 2013; 5(8):433–8.

5. Abbas N, Makker J, Abbas H, et al. Perioperative care of patients with liver cirrhosis: a review. Health Serv Insights 2017;10. 1178632917691270.

6. Umgelter A, Wagner K, Reindl W, et al. Haemodynamic effects of plasma-expansion with hyperoncotic albumin in cirrhotic patients with renal failure: a prospective interventional study. BMC Gastroenterol 2008;8:39.

7. Valerio C, Theocharidou E, Davenport, et al. Human albumin solution for patients with cirrhosis and acute on chronic liver failure: beyond simple volume expansion. World J Hepatol 2016;8(7):345–54.

8. Patel J, McClain C, Sarav M, et al. Protein requirements for critically ill patients with renal and liver failure. Nutr Clin Pract 2017;32(1):101S–11S.

9. Artigas A, Wernerman J, Arroyo V, et al. Role of albumin in diseases associated with severe systemic inflammation: pathophysiologic and clinical evidence in sepsis and in decompensated cirrhosis. J Crit Care 2016;33:62–70.

10. European Association for the Study of the Liver. EASL clinical practice guidelines on the management of ascites, spontaneous bacterial peritonitis, and hepatorenal syndrome in cirrhosis. J Hepatol 2010;53(3):397–417.

11. Martín-Llahí M, Pépin MN, Guevara M, et al. Terlipressin and albumin vs. albumin in patients with cirrhosis and hepatorenal syndrome: a randomized study. Gastroenterology 2008;134(5):1352–9.

Surgical Critical Care

Gastrointestinal Complications

Rowan Sheldon, MD, Matthew Eckert, MD*

KEYWORDS

- Intra-abdominal hypertension • Intra-abdominal pressure • Stress ulceration
- Abdominal compartment syndrome • Intestinal ileus • Olgilvie's Syndrome
- Enterocutaneous fistula • Pseudo-obstruction

KEY POINTS

- Intra-abdominal hypertension (IAH) represents an often under-recognized threat to the critically ill patient population.
- A wide range of associated causes, as well as difficulty attributing early organ dysfunction to intra-abdominal pressure (IAP), may lead to insidious progression.
- Recognition of risk factors, vigilant monitoring of abdominal pressures, early implementation of noninvasive measures to reduce IAP, and prompt decompressive laparotomy for refractory or progressive IAH are the keys to successful prevention and management of this condition.

Critical illness and injury affect the gastrointestinal tract almost uniformly to some extent. Complications of critical illness range from the sequelae of direct intestinal injury and repair to impaired motility, intra-abdominal hypertension (IAH), and ulceration, among others. Contemporary clinical practice has incorporated many advances in the prevention and treatment of gastrointestinal complications during critical illness. In this article, the epidemiology, risk factors, means of diagnosis, treatment, and prevention of some of these compilations are discussed.

STRESS ULCERATION

Extensive trauma, critical illness, and shock states may result in persistent relative hypotension and catecholamine release leading to prolonged splanchnic hypoperfusion. This can then be exacerbated by vasopressor requirements and overall low cardiac output. As a result, gastrointestinal vessels may fail to autoregulate or adequately compensate, resulting in mucosal ischemia. The cells then become dysfunctional, causing a decrease in bicarbonate release and lack of sufficient acid neutralization. As a consequence of this progressive intramucosal acidosis and hypoxemia, cell death outpaces cellular regeneration and ulceration occurs.

The authors have nothing to disclose.
Madigan Army Medical Center, Department of Surgery, General Surgery, MCHJ-CLS-G, Tacoma, WA 98431, USA
* Corresponding author.
E-mail address: matteckert1@gmail.com

Surg Clin N Am 97 (2017) 1425–1447
http://dx.doi.org/10.1016/j.suc.2017.08.002
0039-6109/17/Published by Elsevier Inc.

Epidemiology

Early studies surrounding the risk of stress-induced ulceration in the critically ill have demonstrated that some level of gastric ulceration will occur in nearly all patients requiring intensive care unit (ICU) care.[1] The critical question, however, is how often does this insult result in clinical significance. This becomes more difficult to assess due to variations in definitions. Maier and colleagues[2] studied 98 consecutive subjects who were critically ill, requiring intubation and ICU care for at least 72 hours without gastric feeding. Gastric aspirates yielded heme-positive results in 99%, with 12% being deemed grossly positive for blood. However, only 2% required a blood transfusion and 1% required an operation. Additional studies report the incidence of stress-induced bleeding to range from 0.05% to 2.3% of trauma patients, with the lower incidence being defined as requiring at least 2 units of blood transfusion and the higher incidence failing to define bleeding in its methods.[3,4] Despite the difficulty in interpreting the incidence, the increased morbidity and mortality of those who do develop bleeding is significant. A Canadian prospective multicenter cohort study encompassing 2252 subjects demonstrated a 48.5% mortality rate in the group with bleeding as opposed to 9.1% in the group that did not.[5] Although the higher associated mortality rate likely reflects the overall systemic burden of illness and injury in those with stress ulceration, the risk seems relevant in all critically ill surgical ICU patients.

Risk Factors

Stress ulceration is a result of hypoperfusion and vasoconstriction. Therefore, the 2 most prominent risk factors include persistent hypotension and vasopressor use. Mechanical ventilation also seems to play an important role in the biochemical pathway of this disease. The mechanism for this is proposed to be made up of 3 separate causes. First, the use of positive end-expiratory pressure (PEEP) is known to reduce cardiac preload, thereby exacerbating preexisting hypotension. The use of positive pressure ventilation has also been shown to result in the elevation of sympathetic nervous tone, resulting in exacerbation of vascular shunting by way of splanchnic vasoconstriction. Finally, newer data suggest that mechanical ventilation causes the release of interleukin (IL)-1b, IL 6, and macrophage inhibitory protein 2.[6] These proinflammatory cytokines augment the cascade of ongoing cellular damage and add to the already present mucosal damage. As a sum total, multiple studies have identified prolonged mechanical ventilation as an independent predictor of clinical bleeding and, thus, a target for prophylaxis. In fact, a study of 2252 consecutive subjects admitted to 1 of 4 affiliated medical-surgical ICUs suggested that the odds of developing a bleed after 48 hours of mechanical ventilation was as high as 15 times that of someone breathing spontaneously.[5]

Two populations that merit special attention are patients with traumatic brain injuries and burn injury. In patients with significant brain injury, the stress reactions previously noted are compounded by additional insult to the hypothalamic-pituitary-adrenal axis. Specific injury in this area has been noted to result in an upregulation of terminal parasympathetic activity. Initially proposed by Rokitansky in 1841 and clarified by Cushing in 1932, the cause is thought to be a disruption of the parasympathetic centers of the hypothalamus and its connections to the vagal nuclei in the medulla. Normally exhibiting a static inhibition of the vagal nuclei, the loss of this connection, therefore, causes an upregulation of the nerve and its actions. As a result, acetylcholine release on antral G-cells is disinhibited, yielding abnormally high acid secretion. Although typically thought to be part of a multifactorial cause of ulcer formation, the Cushing effect can be significant on its own. A review of the more than 2000 necropsies demonstrated the presence of hemorrhagic ulceration of the upper gastrointestinal tract in individuals who died of intracranial disorders to be more than twice that of individuals who died of other causes (12.5% vs 6.0%, $P<.001$).[7]

The physiologic changes in a burn patient are profound and rapid. A combination of severe hypovolemia and hypersecretion of catecholamines results in an exaggerated stress response capable of causing organ dysfunction and local ischemic changes. Unique to the burn patient, however, is that these changes occur in the absence of blood loss, thereby setting the stage for a marked hemoconcentration. Prior studies by Curreri and colleagues[8] identified markedly elevated factor V, VIII, platelet, and fibrinogen levels associated with focal vascular congestion and areas of coagulative necrosis within the gastric mucosa. As burn severity increases, there is a near linear increase in the incidence of gastrointestinal ulcer formation.[9] Thermal injury is further associated with a dose-response relationship with elevated cortisol.[10] This has been hypothesized to result in vago-adrenal stimulation, thereby increasing gastric acid secretion, potentiating an ulcerogenic state.[11]

Prevention

Indications for prophylactic acid reduction in the form of H2 receptor antagonists (H2RAs) or proton pump inhibitors (PPI) remains a point of contention. Multiple studies have demonstrated the physiologic efficacy of these medications' ability to maintain a gastric pH greater than 4. The clinical effect of this physiology has been less consistent. Although some studies have shown a significant risk reduction with either tٖrategy, others have demonstrated no effect. As a result, most major critical care societies recommend judicious use of stress ulcer prophylaxis. The current recommendation by the Eastern Association for the Surgery of Trauma is that stress ulceration prophylaxis only be used in a population with specific high-risk features[12] (**Box 1**).

It should be noted that these recommendations are only for patients without a primary reason for acid reduction, such as history of gastroesophageal reflux, duodenal ulceration, prior bariatric surgery, history of a gastrointestinal bleed, and so forth.

The best prophylaxis for stress ulceration is enteral feeding. Among the innumerable benefits of enteral feeding, it has also demonstrated a relative risk of developing stress ulceration of 0.3 compared with the use of parenteral nutrition.[13] Importantly, however,

---

Box 1
Acute risk factors in the development of stress ulceration

Mechanical ventilation (>48 hours)

Coagulopathy (INR >1.5, Plt <50k, aPTT >2 times normal)

Hypoperfusion (evidence of end-organ dysfunction)

High-dose corticosteroids (>250 mg/d hydrocortisone or equivalent)

Significant burn (second- or third-degree >35% TBSA)

Severe brain or spinal cord injury (GCS <9)

Multisystem trauma (ISS >15)

Sepsis

Abbreviations: aPTT, activated Partial Thromboplastin Time; GCS, Glasgow Coma Scale; INR, International Normalized Ratio; ISS, Injury Severity Score; Plt, Platelet; TBSA, Total Burn Surface Area.

the risk reduction of antiacid medication and enteral feedings is not additive. The use of enteral feeds in conjunction with H2RA or PPIs has demonstrated an increase in health care–associated pneumonia and all-cause hospital mortality.[14] Therefore, the resumption of feeds should be viewed as an indication to stop anti-ulcer medications in all patients for which there is no secondary rationale for acid reduction.

Management

When prophylaxis fails, the consequences to the patient run the spectrum from minor to catastrophic. The first priority, as with all ICU emergencies, is the management of the airway, followed by resuscitation and correction of any coagulopathy. The next step for acute gastrointestinal bleed in these patients is gastric lavage. Unlike patients presenting with de novo gastrointestinal bleeds, however, this step is not intended to be diagnostic. Instead, this is meant to remove clot, decrease gastric distention, minimize aspiration risk, and reduce local fibrinolytic activity of retained blood products.[15]

Pharmacologic intervention is then initiated. The agent of choice in this setting is somatostatin, given as a 250 μg bolus followed by 250 μg/h for 3 to 7 days. Somatostatin decreases splanchnic blood flow, thereby decreasing hemorrhage and encouraging clot formation. Pooled data from 14 trials totaling 1829 subjects found that the relative risk of continued or recurrent bleeding in subjects given somatostatin was 0.53 with a number needed to treat of 5.[16] In places where somatostatin is insufficient or where it may be harmful, as with renal failure and type 1 diabetes, the next pharmacologic agent to be used is vasopressin. Given at doses of 0.5 to 1.0 units/min, vasopressin activates peripheral V1 receptors, causing vasoconstriction. This helps to further augment hemostasis without causing significant risk of arrhythmia or cardiac ischemia. In several studies, vasopressin has been found as equally effective at enacting long-term cessation of gastrointestinal bleeding as more invasive methods such as embolization.[17] Although it was noted that the time to cessation was markedly longer for vasopressin, it still served as a useful adjunctive therapy. Finally, if the patient is not already on an acid-reducing medication, this should be initiated. Although studies have yet to demonstrate that PPIs help stop bleeding, they have been shown to decrease the risk of rebleeding with a risk ratio of 0.72.[18]

Despite that adequate resuscitation and gastric lavage yield cessation rates of 80% to 95%,[1,19] the gold standard for gastrointestinal bleeds remains upper endoscopy. In the setting of stress ulceration, esophagogastroduodenoscopy (EGD) can be both diagnostic and therapeutic. In this role, EGD performs 2 critical tasks: it can rule out other causes of bleeding (ie, peptic ulcer, esophageal varices, dieulafoy lesion, cancer) and it allows therapeutic intervention on larger bleeding vessels. Unfortunately, stress ulceration is typically a diffuse process that may require additional intervention (**Fig. 1**).

When ulceration occurs throughout the stomach, it may limit the utility of selective endoscopic intervention. Selective embolization and angiography may prove useful because it enables the vasoconstriction of a directed arterial bed. Vasopressin infusions of 0.4 U/min into the left gastric artery, or the celiac access, over the course of 48 to 72 hours have been shown to control bleeding in 73% of cases.[20]

Finally, surgery, although exceedingly rare, should never be forgotten in the unstable patient. Before embarking to the operating room, however, localization is imperative. It should go without saying that gastrointestinal tract bleeding will not be visible from the peritoneal cavity. In addition, it should be noted that surgical intervention for stress ulceration carries a substantial risk of mortality. Although the reason for this is unclear, it is likely a marker of the patient's underlying disease as much as the insult of surgery itself.

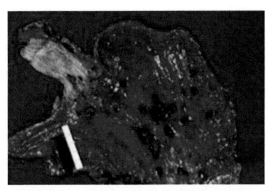

Fig. 1. Diffuse stress ulceration of the stomach. (*From* The University of Alabama at Birmingham Department of Pathology PEIR Digital Library© (http://peir.path.uab.edu/library/picture.php?/9176/search/12957m); with permission.)

Because stress ulceration is primarily a gastric disease, the options for surgical intervention are 4-fold: gastrectomy with oversewing a focal source of bleeding, subtotal gastric resection, gastric devascularization, and total gastrectomy.[15] The most limited of these methods is a gastrectomy with oversewing. This choice is an effective means of control only if specific sites of bleeding can be identified preoperatively and, as such, it is of limited value in many scenarios. With the diffuse distribution of disease typically seen, a subtotal gastrectomy with or without truncal vagotomy may offer more utility. Although logically this makes sense, studies have not born out a difference between these 2 operations. In a 1979 series of 60 procedures performed for stress ulceration, suture ligation, and subtotal resection had fundamentally identical outcomes with long-term hemorrhage control in 55% and 61%, respectively.[21]

Although the outcomes for more conservative operations is underwhelming, the results of more extensive operative approaches is bleak. Gastric devascularization is an approach whereby the left and right gastric and gastroepiploic vessels are ligated, leaving the stomach to live off of the short gastric vessels. Although data on this method are scarce, 1 study reported initial success rates of 100% with a rebleeding rate of 9% and a mortality of 38%.[21] For the sake of completeness, total gastrectomy should be discussed as the last respite for a desperate surgeon. Although it has been reported to be the most effective technique at stopping bleeding, survival after this procedure is currently case reportable. Nearly all case series involving patients requiring total gastrectomy for gastrointestinal bleeding due to stress ulceration report a mortality rate of 100%.[21–23]

Summary

Stress ulceration represents a ubiquitous disease with numerous gradations of severity. Although clinical significance is rare, the disease has proven difficult to combat. It is for this reason that physicians choose to give prophylaxis for a disease with an incidence of only 0.05% to 2.3%. A high index of suspicion and early recognition are mandatory to stave off significant complication.

ENTERIC FISTULAE

Enterocutaneous and other bowel-related fistulous disease represent some of the most difficult to manage problems within general surgery. They can arise from several inflammatory settings, including areas of prior surgical intervention, malignancy, radiation, inflammatory processes, and autoimmune disease. Traumatic fistulae can create specific challenges in the critically ill because the complexities of multisystem trauma are layered onto the underlying insult of the exposed alimentary tract. Like any other organ system in the body, penetrating objects can cause fistulous connections between 2 adjacent structures.

Epidemiology

Damage-control surgery created a paradigm shift in surgery with the transition from lengthy definitive procedures to an abbreviated operative intervention.[24,25] This, in turn, necessitated a manner in which a second-look operation could be performed with minimal morbidity, so the open abdomen was used with increasing frequency. The application of negative pressure wound devices to the abdomen has rapidly increased during this time but not without consequence. Numbers vary widely but reports of enteroatmospheric fistula after open abdominal management have ranged from 4.5% to 25%.[26,27] In a 2009 study following 2373 acute trauma laparotomies, subsequent enterocutaneous fistula formation was only reported in 1.5% (36 subjects). In this population, 75% were due to penetrating injuries and 56% were multiple. The distribution of these injuries spanned the gastrointestinal tract with the most common being the large bowel (69%), followed by the small bowel (53%), duodenum (36%), and stomach (19%).[28]

Risk Factors

The rate of formation of enterocutaneous or enteroatmospheric fistulae seems to be most correlated with the injury pattern. Previous attempts to correlate the type of anastomosis with the rate of fistula formation failed to demonstrate significance. Kirkpatrick and colleagues[29] closely followed 232 full-thickness small bowel injuries after trauma, comparing stapled, hand-sewn, and combined construction methods of repair. Although their population yielded a 10.6% rate of enteroatmospheric fistula formation, no method of anastomosis was found to be statistically superior to another.

A recent systematic review comparing hand-sewn and stapled anastomoses in 1120 subjects after emergency laparotomy requiring bowel resection incorporating a total of 1120 subjects found no differences in outcomes.[30] These data are consistent with the elective surgical literature that has suggested similar efficacy and safety. In a 2012 Cochrane database systematic review of randomized controlled trials, stapled and hand-sewn anastomoses demonstrated no difference in rate of clinical dehiscence, radiologic dehiscence, stricture, hemorrhage, reoperation, or infection.[31] The only 2 factors that have consistently demonstrated elevated risk of enteroatmospheric fistulae are the need for a damage control operation and associated pancreaticoduodenal injuries.[29]

Treatment

The management of these fistulae can cause significant problems in the setting of surgical critical care. Patients typically have multiple organ system dysfunction that places them at increased risk of physiologic insult and nutritional deficiency. The first treatment goal is adequate resuscitation of the patient to correct fluid and any electrolyte balance. This becomes especially important in proximal fistulae where the output may be high in potassium and bicarbonate. The next step in fistula management is the control, containment, and evacuation of intestinal effluent. Although this can be managed in enterocutaneous fistulae by the placement of an ostomy device, enteroatmospheric fistulae create an additional problem. Due to the lack of a surrounding structural support, the placement of a simple ostomy bag can prove difficult. Described techniques include a floating stoma involving the use of a plastic silo device to isolate the open wound (**Fig. 2**).[32]

Other clinicians have found vacuum-assisted closure devices to be useful in excluding the open source of effluent and promoting local granulation.[33,34] Once the fistula is contained and the effluent controlled, attention may be directed toward eventual closure. Several factors have been identified as relative predictors of whether a fistula will close with conservative management or if surgical intervention will be required (**Table 1**).

In all cases, the patient requires physiologic optimization to give them the best chance of primary success. Early studies demonstrated a doubling of spontaneous closure rate with nutritional supplementation.[35,36] Multiple ongoing trials are investigating whether there is any difference between total parenteral nutrition (TPN) and enteral feeding, but there is no question that nutrition plays a central role. The theoretic benefit of TPN is a reduction in fistula output. Multiple novel attempts to feed the gut, however, have been used, including direct intubation of the fistula and postfistula enteral feeding.[37] Although intriguing, the efficacy of these novel methods has not been well studied.

Octreotide is often also discussed in the context of regulating fistula effluent. Theoretically, the somatostatin analogue would provide a decrease in gastrointestinal motility and secretion, leading to decreased overall output. Although lower output fistulae have demonstrated greater incidence of primary healing,[38,39] studies surrounding the utility of octreotide have demonstrated mixed results. A 1992 multicenter trial testing TPN alone versus TPN and octreotide showed no increase in overall primary closure rate. It did, however, demonstrate a significant decrease in time to closure (13.9 vs 20.4 days).[40] A meta-analysis of 10 studies testing octreotide and other somatostatin analogues, however, failed to demonstrate a statistically significant increase in the success of nonoperative closure.[41]

Although nonoperative management is preferable in the critically ill, there is a limit to the utility of medical optimization. Medical management will fail in approximately 40% of cases, thereby mandating surgical intervention for definitive treatment.[42] Although

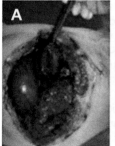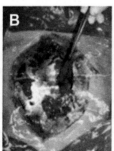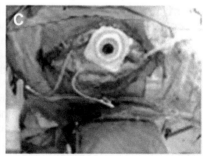

Fig. 2. Creation of the floating stoma for management of the open abdomen complicated by an intestinal fistula. (*A*) Large enteroatmospheric fistula. (*B*) Formalizing the fistula into a controlled ostomy with protective dressing covering the open abdomen. (*C*) Final application of ostomy appliance for control of fistula effluent and closed suction drainage of the open abdominal cavity. (*From* Manterola C, Flores P, Otzen T. Floating stoma: an alternative strategy in the context of damage control surgery. J Visc Surg 2016;153:419–24; with permission.)

Table 1 Factors increasing the likelihood of success in the primary closure of enteric fistulae	
Anatomic location	Esophageal, duodenal stump, jejunal
Tract length	>2 cm
Defect size	<1 square cm
Fistula output	Decreasing
Surrounding bowel	Healthy
Nutritional support	Well-nourished
Sepsis	Absent

Adapted from Fischer JE, Evenson AR. Gastrointestinal-cutaneous fistulae. In: Fischer JE, editor. Mastery of surgery. Philadelphia (PA): Lippincott Williams & Wilkins; 2007. p. 1401–8; with permission.

the timing and extent of operative closure has not been well studied, a bimodal distribution of surgical timing has been suggested. Some experts have suggested that early surgical intervention is warranted on fistulae with a low likelihood of success with conservative management. The benefits of this method suggest that the onset of the frozen abdomen can be avoided. Typically occurring by the end of the second postoperative week, the frozen abdomen places the bowel at increased risk of inadvertent injury and the potential for further complication.

If this window is missed or if conservative management is attempted and fails, then a delay of 6 to 12 months is said to be optimal. Although this delay is necessary for the adhesions of a frozen abdomen to soften and, thereby, decrease the risk of bowel injury,[43] prolonging time from injury is reported to have no increased success of primary closure. In fact, D'Hondt and colleagues[44] posit that in patients who are well-nourished and free from infection, any fistula that does not close within the first 6 weeks will mandate surgical intervention. It should be noted that the timing of surgery should be tailored to the patient. Early intervention may result in additional bowel injury. Prolonged waiting may result in ongoing nutritional and electrolyte losses, as well as the obvious quality of life concerns and ongoing medical care.

If patients present with an open abdomen that will prove difficult to close in the setting of a concomitant enteroatmospheric fistula, the first step is often to place a split-thickness skin graft over the exposed viscera. Although this offers no structural support for the abdominal wall, it effectively covers the exposed bowel, thereby minimizing water losses and infectious complications.[45] Deciding when to operate then becomes a matter of gestalt and experience. A simple manual pinch test with gentle distraction can easily demonstrate whether the bowel has begun to separate from its surrounding attachments (**Fig. 3**).

Given the difficulties with management of these fistulae, the obvious preference is prevention. In this context, prevention has mainly relied on strict adherence to good surgical principles. During the primary operation, the trauma surgeon should carefully manipulate the bowel so as to avoid serosal injury. Protection of the bowel should then continue into the postoperative period with the ready application of temporary abdominal closures and bowel protection devices. Attention to detail when applying these temporary closure systems will help prevent further bowel injuries. Avoidance of placing abrasive dressing surfaces under suction directly to the bowel surface is paramount. The use of atraumatic materials or specially designed sponges for intestinal contact is recommended. These suggestions are difficult to study but have gained wide support for this difficult problem.[46,47]

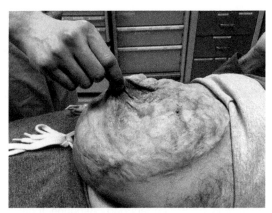

Fig. 3. Pinch test to determine readiness of split-thickness skin graft for removal following prior graft closure of damage control open abdomen. (*Courtesy of* M. Eckert MD FACS, Tacoma WA USA.)

Summary

Enteroatmospheric fistulae are a very difficult to manage problem in the trauma and surgical critical care population. The formation of these defects are difficult to predict and more difficult to prevent. They are highly morbid and their treatment becomes resource-intensive very quickly. As such, these patients are best managed by a multi-disciplinary team of surgeons, wound care professionals, nutritionists, and nurses. Although the individual patient needs vary greatly, the general principles of fistula management should remain the same.

INTESTINAL ILEUS AND OGILVIE SYNDROME

As previously outlined, nutrition in the setting of surgical critical care is of paramount importance. In the patient who cannot actively partake in caloric intake, however, options for nutrition are enteric feeding access versus parenteral nutrition. Although the ease of use with parenteral nutrition is enticing, it is clear that enteral feeding of any type is clearly superior. Not only does the administration of parenteral nutrition carry additional substantial risks of central line–associated infections and mechanical complications, it is also associated with increased risk of pneumonia and other complications.[48] For these reasons, many investigators conclude that TPN is best reserved for patients with gut failure or clear contraindications to enteral feeding.[49] It is in this context, however, that the problem of a posttraumatic or critical illness–associated ileus is such an important entity.

Epidemiology

The more common cause of gut failure in surgical critical care is divided into small bowel adynamic ileus and large bowel pseudo-obstruction, known as Ogilvie Syndrome. The overall incidence is difficult to assess due to variability in reporting; however, in a large study of patients identified with Ogilvie, nonoperative trauma provided the most common inciting condition (11.3%).[50] Other additive factors included orthopedic trauma,[51] renal failure,[52] use of narcotics, and the development of electrolyte disturbances.[53]

Cause

Bowel motility is a parasympathetic function. The control of this function is 2-fold, with the vagus controlling function up and to the splenic flexure via the celiac plexus, and the S2 through S4 nerve roots controlling all distal function. Initial cases of the disease described by Sir William Ogilvie in 1948 were of 2 men with large retroperitoneal tumors invading into the celiac plexus. These findings and subsequent confirmatory research have found that dysfunction of 1 of these 2 nervous plexuses yield the aperistalsis and colonic dilation that lead to the symptoms of this disease.

There are myriad reasons why a patient may experience dysfunction of these nervous plexuses. Various metabolic and physiologic derangements have been identified as causative factors. The most prominent of these includes infection, myocardial infarction, child birth, pelvic surgery, neurologic dysfunction, and renal failure.[54] Although most of this disease is focused on the large bowel, there are predisposing factors that may result in the dysfunction of the small bowel as well. So-called adynamic ileus is typically due to dysfunction of spinal nerves that augment intrinsic motor function due to focal irritation or cord defect.

Initially, this disease was poorly understood. Although focal inflammation was thought to be heavily involved, it was unclear how an organ with intrinsic neuronal activity was so affected by a more regional process. Recent advances have demonstrated that the sympathetic nervous system has a significant neuromodulatory effect on inflammation in the intestines. Moreover, loss of sympathetic innervation is closely linked with increasing inflammatory states in acute and chronic diseases.[55,56]

The 2 most relevant causes in the setting of trauma are hematoma and spinal cord injury. Although peritonitis along the posterior abdominal wall from any cause (eg, blood, succus, foreign body) may cause similar symptoms, it is the retroperitoneal hematoma that classically causes adynamic ileus in the posttraumatic patient. The accumulation of blood within this space irritates the nervous plexuses that exit the spinal cord at the level of the fore and midgut, resulting in both local interruption of parasympathetic stimuli and regional alteration of sympathetic control. In the patient with a spinal cord injury, the local loss of sympathetic innervation is then combined with the orthopedic trauma to the surrounding vertebral column and possible loss of vascular control, thereby compounding the clinical picture.

Diagnosis and Management

Regardless of the cause, the presentation is fairly similar. Both adynamic ileus and Ogilvie syndrome will present with obstructive symptoms such as feeding intolerance, abdominal distention, abdominal pain, and hypoactive bowel sounds. Interestingly, patients have been noted to continue to pass flatus in some 40% to 50% of reported cases.[57] The notable difference will be the segment of bowel involved. Adynamic ileus most classically involves the ileum, whereas Ogilvie syndrome arises as an acute dilation of the large bowel. Although Ogilvie can lead to a secondary dilation of the small bowel, it will always start distally and, thus, small bowel involvement is not required as part of the diagnosis.

Regardless of the constellation of symptoms, plain radiographs will show bowel dilation, often with air fluid levels (**Fig. 4**A). The extent of bowel involvement will vary, but Ogilvie will nearly always involve at least the cecum and right colon.[58] Once the diagnosis of pseudo-obstruction is suspected, the primary decision point is the patient's overall clinical stability. If the patient demonstrates evidence of perforation, peritonitis, or ischemia, further ancillary studies are no longer appropriate and surgical intervention is warranted.

If the patient is clinically stable, the workup begins by investigating for other causes of pseudo-obstruction or mechanical obstruction. Testing for *Clostridium difficile* is highly advisable, especially in the setting of prior antibiotic administration. Ruling out mechanical obstruction can then be accomplished by means of a

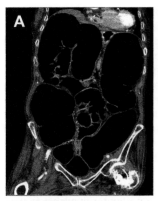 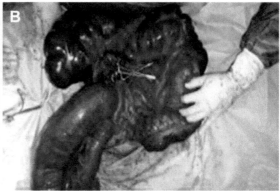

Fig. 4. (*A*) Coronal CT images of Ogilvie syndrome with pancolonic dilation. (*B*) Gross specimen of colonic Ogilvie syndrome at time of urgent resection. (*From* [*A*] By Milliways (Own work) [CC BY-SA 3.0 (http://creativecommons.org/licenses/by-sa/3.0)], via Wikimedia Commons. Available at: https://commons.wikimedia.org/wiki/File%3AOgilvie_ct_coronal. jpg; and [*B*] Gonzalez-Calatayud M, Gutierrez-Uvalle G. Pseudo intestinal occlusion: case report and literature review. Rev Med Hosp Gen Mex 2014;77(4):185–9; with permission.)

contrast-enhanced study. Although the classic test for this diagnosis was the water-soluble contrast enema, the contrast-enhanced CT has largely replaced it due to availability of CT, the ease of performing this study in patients without the need for bowel preparation,[59] and equal or increased sensitivity (96%) and specificity (93%).[60]

Once confirmed, the treatment of ileus and Ogilvie syndrome is divided into 3 distinct categories: supportive care, medical management, and procedural decompression. Supportive care is a step that should be instituted in nearly all patients because these interventions alone have been noted in to be highly effective at resolving symptoms. These interventions include taking nothing by mouth, nasogastric decompression, aggressive intravenous fluid resuscitation, electrolyte repletion, increasing mobility or frequent position changes, initiation of antibiotics if infection is suspected, and limitation of offending medications. The list of offending medications is lengthy, but those most commonly attributed include narcotics, anticholinergics, benzodiazepines, calcium channel blockers, stimulant withdrawal, and antiparkinson drugs. In 1 of the largest series, Wegener and colleagues[61] followed subjects with Ogilvie's syndrome and found that 70% of cases resolved with conservative management alone. Average time to response with these measures varies widely but has been reported to average between 3 and 5 days.[50,58]

There has been a great deal of interest in pharmacologic prokinetic agents that would aid in motility while not forcing contraction, as in the case of neostigmine, and raising the risk of perforation. The evidence for these interventions remains patchy and inconsistent but worthy of discussion.

The most commonly discussed medication is erythromycin. A macrolide antibiotic, erythromycin is known to stimulate gastric and small bowel motilin receptors, making it effective in the treatment of gastroparesis.[62,63] Although certain study models, specifically in rabbits, showed significant efficacy of erythromycin as a motility agent,[64,65] multiple studies have failed to demonstrate statistically significant differences in human colonic motility.[66,67] This has been explained by studies demonstrating a decreasing gradient of motilin receptors in humans from the stomach through the terminal ileum to the colon.[68,69] Despite these findings, case reports have suggested a correlation between erythromycin administration and resolution of symptoms.[70,71] Unfortunately, randomized controlled trials have yet to find prophylactic or therapeutic benefit, and erythromycin is associated with a significant (15%–20%) risk of side effects, including drowsiness, dystonic reactions, and agitation.[72]

A notable area of research is the utility of 5-hydroxytryptamine type 4 (5-HT$_4$) receptor agonists. These serotonin receptors have been noted to have varying roles along the cholinergic neurons, regulating peristalsis in the various portions of the gastrointestinal tract. One of these medications, cisapride, has shown efficacy in the treatment of Ogilvie syndrome.[73,74] Still another study researching the effect of antagonism of 5-HT$_4$ receptors again demonstrated that stimulation of these serotonin receptors increases colonic motility while slowing orocecal transit time.[75] Unfortunately, efficacy has come at the cost of patient safety because 5-HT$_4$ agonists have been linked to convulsive episodes[76] and notable cardiac arrhythmias, leading to death in at least 4 patients over a 3-year period.[77] Therefore, cisapride is no longer available for use as a prokinetic in the United States.

Two medications that warrant mentioning are the peripherally acting opiate antagonists, methylnaltrexone and almipovan. Although no studies have yet been published demonstrating their efficacy or lack thereof in patients who already have either ileus or Ogilvie syndrome, the proven improvement in bowel motility after colorectal surgery suggests that they may be promising targets for future study.

If a patient shows evidence of failing conservative management, certain pharmacologic therapies have demonstrated efficacy. The most prominent of these therapies in Ogilvie syndrome is either bolus or continuous infusion dosing of neostigmine. Initial studies performed in 1992 by Hutchinson and Griffiths[78] gave 2 mg of neostigmine to patients with demonstrated acute colonic pseudo-obstruction who failed 24 hours of conservative management. Their data only covered 18 administrations of the medication but yielded a 94% clinical response with only an 11% recurrence rate. In a more recent study, van der Spoel and colleagues[79] administered neostigmine at a rate of 0.4 to 0.8 mg/h for 24 hours, yielding a 79% response rate. As an acetyl-cholinesterase inhibitor, the medication can result in symptomatic bradycardia. This complication is rare, but atropine should be readily available. Additionally, neostigmine is metabolized by the kidney and is, therefore, contraindicated in patients with renal dysfunction. Finally, because the medication causes an intentional spasm of the colon, neostigmine carries the theoretic risk of perforation in the setting of pending ischemia or in patients with a missed distal mechanical obstruction.

In patients who fail both conservative and pharmacologic management, colonoscopic decompression may be required if marked colonic dilation threatens ischemia and perforation. It should be noted that colonoscopic intervention is markedly more difficult than standard diagnostic colonoscopic surveillance and should only be performed by experts. The reasons for this difficulty include an often tortuous colon and the inability to use insufflation or bowel preparation due to the increased risk of perforation. The incidence of perforation with decompressive attempts ranges from less than 1% to 4.5%[80–82] with an associated overall mortality rate of 1%.[83] Despite these risks, colonoscopic decompression with placement of a decompressive tube has shown an initial success rate of 61% to 95% with an ultimate clinical success after 1 or more attempts of up to 88%.[54,61,81,84]

Although each of these treatments can be instituted in a variety of contexts, close monitoring is a requirement for all patients because the risk of ischemia and perforation increases with worsening colonic dilation. This holds true not only for the size of colonic dilation in accordance with the law of Laplace but also for distention lasting greater than 6 days[54] or symptoms that worsen despite 48 to 72 hours of maximal medical therapy.[85] Each of these factors represents a statistically independent risk of perforation and should raise considerable concern and a re-evaluation of the current management strategy.

If the patient fails all of the previously strategies, surgical management offers the last option for treatment. In the nonurgent setting, a cecostomy may be considered. Percutaneous, laparoscopic, or open cecostomy allows for decompression of the dilated right colon in addition to the option for ongoing therapeutic intervention in the form of antegrade enemas. These interventions carry a fairly high complication rate. In a review of 67 subjects who underwent cecostomy placement at the Mayo Clinic, 45% developed a complication from their tube. Although no subject had to undergo a reoperation for their complication, problems included pericatheter leak, wound infection, tube dislodgement, colocutaneous fistula, and ventral hernia[86] (see **Fig. 4**).

The development of worsening abdominal pain, fever, leukocytosis, rising lactate, or suspicion of ischemia, peritonitis, or frank perforation mandates surgical intervention for pseudo-obstruction. Given the associated intestinal distention, a laparoscopic approach may be exceedingly difficult and the only likely appropriate intervention would be an emergent exploratory laparotomy. The extent of the bowel resected at this time should be tailored to the amount of colon involved in the underlying disease (see **Fig. 4**B). A primary anastomosis should be avoided in this situation because the viability of the resected margins cannot be guaranteed.[53] This development portends a poor prognosis for the patient and has been noted to carry an associated mortality of nearly 30%.[50] The high associated mortality rate is likely a combination of the effects of the intestinal disease and a marker of the severity of the patient's overall illness.[87]

Summary

Dysmotility of the large and small intestine may result from multiple causes, including mechanical obstruction and nonobstructive motility issues. After assessing for mechanical obstruction, it is important to follow a stepwise approach for diagnosis and treatment. Conservative measures are successful in almost all cases, with surgical intervention reserved for life-threatening complications.

ABDOMINAL COMPARTMENT SYNDROME

IAH and the development of the highly morbid abdominal compartment syndrome (ACS) represent a significant concern in the critical care management of many patients. Although first described in the nineteenth century, it was not until recently that significant research and clinical practice guidance was developed. Widespread recognition of this unique abdominal complication and its implications for multiorgan system effects has led to improved outcomes and the development of various treatment and prevention strategies. Understanding the concepts and importance of IAH begins with an appreciation of the range of intra-abdominal pressure (IAP), from normal to critical elevations (**Table 2**).

Although finite values for grades of elevated pressures are widely published, it is important to recognize that IAH or ACS represent a spectrum of disease. Therefore, negative effects, often clinically unrecognized early on, can have multisystem consequences throughout the pressure range. The normal IAP in a healthy individual is less than 8 mm Hg. Base-line health conditions outside of critical illness that are associated with an elevated IAP include obesity, pregnancy, ascites, and constipation. In the setting of trauma, sepsis or other systemic inflammatory conditions, the abdominal pressure may progressively increase. As pressure increases, the renal and visceral

Table 2
Grading system for intra-abdominal pressure

Pressure[a]	Grade
<8 mm Hg	Normal IAP
>12 mm Hg	IAH
12–15 mm Hg	Grade I
16–20 mm Hg	Grade II
21–25 mm Hg	Grade III
>25 mm Hg	Grade IV
>20 mm Hg + associated organ dysfunction	ACS

[a] Sustained IAPs.

Data from Kirkpatrick AW, Roberts DJ, Waele J, et al. Intra-abdominal hypertension and the abdominal compartment syndrome: updated consensus definitions and clinical practice guidelines from the World Society of the Abdominal Compartment Syndrome. Intensive Care Med 2013;39:1190–206.

perfusion is impaired, cardiac venous return decreases, intrathoracic pressures increase due to decreased diaphragmatic excursion, and jugular venous outflow decreases, leading to increased intracranial pressure along with numerous other multisystem effects.[88]

Progressive IAH may ultimately result in ACS, defined as a sustained IAP equal to or greater than 20 mm Hg with associated organ dysfunction.[89] ACS is a surgical emergency and mandates immediate intervention to reduce the abdominal pressure and halt further organ dysfunction. The development of this syndrome can often be prevented through early identification, monitoring, and intervention to reduce IAH. In the setting of critical illness with multisystem derangements, attributing new organ dysfunction to IAH or ACS can be difficult. Hence, a thorough understanding of potential manifestations and vigilant monitoring is important for surgeons and critical care clinicians.

Epidemiology

The concept of IAP was first described in 1863 by Mary and further explored by early investigators who described the relationship between intra-abdominal and thoracic pressures in both normal and pathophysiologic states.[90] Despite this early recognition of the potential detrimental effects of elevated IAP, it was not until the 1980s that researchers began to explore this syndrome in depth. A lack of consensus definitions and understanding of the negative effects of IAH or ACS, as well as variation in monitoring, likely contributed to the limited epidemiologic data available. It is not surprising that as recognition of this syndrome and its consequences improved, the incidence and complications were more frequently reported. Malbrain and colleagues[91] described an incidence of IAH in 27% of ICU admissions in a mixed medical-surgical population. Other investigators have reported similar findings when using the consensus definitions cited previously.[92,93]

Risk Factors

IAH has numerous well-described risk factors related to both underlying disease and injury patterns, as well as therapeutic interventions (**Table 3**).

Aggressive, large-volume resuscitation practices are among the better-understood high-risk scenarios. Crystalloid resuscitation strategies were the early mainstay of

Table 3
Risk factors for intra-abdominal hypertension and abdominal compartment

Disease or Injury	Iatrogenic
Pancreatitis	Massive transfusion
Major abdominopelvic trauma	Large-volume crystalloid infusion
Peritonitis or abdominal sepsis	Excessive pneumoperitoneum
Retroperitoneal hemorrhage	Prone positioning
Ascites or fluid collections	Peritoneal dialysis
Abdominal or retroperitoneal neoplasm	High mechanical ventilation pressures
Torso burns	Abdominal closure under tension
Ileus or pseudo-obstruction	Temporary abdominal closure under tension
Ruptured abdominal aortic aneurysm	

treatment of all types of hypovolemic and septic shock for much of the last century, only to be followed by aggressive practices of blood transfusion. Seeking to enhance the optimal physiologic recovery of critically ill surgical patients, the concept of supranormal resuscitation led to even more aggressive resuscitative practices. This strategy often combined large volumes of crystalloids and blood products, leading to progressive visceral and soft tissue edema, third-spacing of abdominal fluid, decreased abdominal wall compliance, and the development of IAH.[94] Subsequent prospective trials demonstrated no improvement with this resuscitation strategy and recognized its associated complications.

Prevention

Recognition of the potential risk factors for IAH or ACS, and regular monitoring of abdominal pressures, represent the critical steps in prevention. Physical examination of the abdomen is not adequate for assessing IAP.[95] Intrabladder pressure monitoring is 1 of numerous described monitoring methods but is likely the most widely used and easiest to perform. The development of commercial monitoring kits has facilitated this technique, but it is easily performed using a widely described method with a simple pressure transducer connected to a needle at the aspiration port of the urinary catheter.[96,97] Although bladder pressure is a surrogate for intra-abdominal cavity pressure, impaired perfusion of the abdominal viscera is the key factor for much of the organ dysfunction caused by IAH or ACS. Monitoring of the abdominal perfusion pressure (APP), where APP is the mean arterial pressure minus the IAP, with a goal of an APP greater than 60 mm Hg, provides an additional means to monitor this patient population.[98] Serial pressure measurements are recommended for those patients with risks factors for IAH or ACS. Although elevation of IAP may ensue during treatment of the patient's primary condition, serial monitoring aids the clinician in both the identification of ACS and the decision to implement abdominal pressure reducing measures.

A stepwise application of numerous nonsurgical measures to help reduce IAP has been described by the World Society for Abdominal Compartment Syndrome with assessment of supportive evidence (**Fig. 5**).[99]

These preventive measures are generally noninvasive, nonsurgical measures designed to increase space in the abdominal cavity and prevent further loss of abdominal wall compliance. Although preventive in the sense of avoiding progression to ACS, these steps represent the mainstay of management of IAH in almost all patients, with surgical management reserved for inadequate response or refractory elevation of IAP. In addition to the measures previously described, the strategy of damage-control resuscitation may prove essential to preventing progression to critical IAH or ACS.

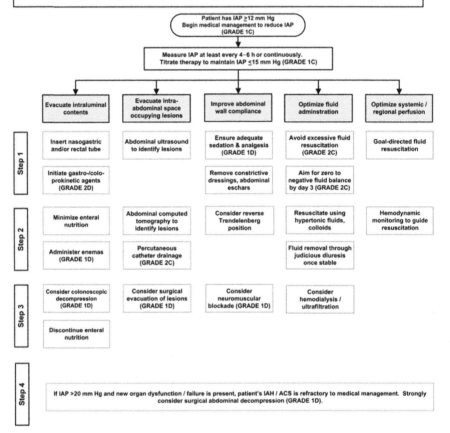

Fig. 5. Stepwise management algorithm for IAH. Evidence-based recommendations from the World Society of the Abdominal Compartment Syndrome. (*From* Kirkpatrick AW, Roberts DJ, Waele J, et al. Intra-abdominal hypertension and the abdominal compartment syndrome: updated consensus definitions and clinical practice guidelines from the World Society of the Abdominal Compartment Syndrome. Intensive Care Med 2013;39:1190–206; with permission.)

Using balanced blood product resuscitation, often driven by advanced bedside coagulation monitoring of the injured patient, and minimizing any crystalloid fluids has significantly decreased the incidence of IAH or ACS, as well as pulmonary morbidity.[100,101]

Management

When progressive IAH fails to respond appropriately to noninvasive measures, decompressive laparotomy is required to prevent the highly morbid complications of ACS. The widespread use of damage control laparotomy with planned management of the temporary open abdomen and delayed closure represent an important paradigm in the prevention of IAH or ACS complications. Application of the traditional Bogotá bag, negative-pressure wound therapy, and other methods of temporary closure allow decompression of the IAP, restoration of perfusion to critical organ systems of the abdomen, and decreased intracranial and intrathoracic pressures.[88] These procedures can be performed in the ICU for patients with labile hemodynamics who may not tolerate transfer to the operating room.

Once the abdomen has been decompressed with a temporary closure, attention shifts to supportive care of failing organ systems, source control of infectious etiologic factors, and treatment of any injuries contributing to IAH. As physiologic balance is restored, the patient may return to the operating room every 24 to 72 hours for washout of the abdominal cavity and assessment for potential closure. Indeed, the amount of time between the index decompressive laparotomy and the first take-back has been shown to predict primary fascial closure.[102] Once hemodynamic stability is achieved after damage control laparotomy, the use of small volumes of hypertonic fluids with strict limitation of other crystalloid solutions has been shown to increase both the success and time to abdominal closure.[103] Lesser amounts of isotonic crystalloid solutions overall seem to be closely linked to decreased risk of damage control laparotomy, as well as increased chances of abdominal closure once performed.[104]

Even the open abdomen with a temporary closure can develop recurrent ACS physiology and vigilant monitoring is imperative in these highest risk patients. Recurrent ACS has been reported after temporary dressing closures, including negative pressure wound therapy. The incidence of recurrent ACS has been reported as high as 50% in patients who underwent damage control laparotomy followed by closure under tension.[105] These patients frequently suffer increased rates of organ failure and require prolonged intensive care support. Therefore, in the critically ill or injured patient who has undergone decompressive laparotomy for IAH or ACS, continued monitoring of abdominal pressures and treatments as previously outlined are essential.

SUMMARY

IAH represents an often under-recognized threat to the critically ill patient population. A wide range of associated causes, as well as difficulty attributing early organ dysfunction to IAP, may lead to insidious progression. Recognition of risk factors, vigilant monitoring of abdominal pressures, early implementation of noninvasive measures to reduce IAP, and prompt decompressive laparotomy for refractory or progressive IAH are the keys to successful prevention and management of this condition.

REFERENCES

1. Miller TA, Tornwall MS, Moody FG. Stress erosive gastritis. In: Wells SA, editor. Current problems in surgery. St Louis (MO): Moseby; 1991. p. 459–509.
2. Maier R, Mitchell D, Gentilello L. Optimal therapy for stress gastritis. Ann Surg 1994;220(3):353–63.
3. Simons R, Hoyt D, Winchell R, et al. A risk analysis of stress ulceration after trauma. J Trauma 1995;39(2):289–93.
4. Cochard J, Leger A, Pinaquy C, et al. Gastrointestinal bleeding in trauma ICU patients: incidence and risk factors. Intensive Care Med 1997;23(Supplement 1):S140 [abstract: 195].

5. Cook D, Fuller H, Guyatt G, et al. Risk factors for gastrointestinal bleeding in critically ill patients. Canadian Critical Care Trials Group. N Engl J Med 1994; 330(6):377–81.

6. Bouadma L, Dreyfuss D, Ricard J, et al. Mechanical ventilation and hemorrhagic shock-resuscitation interact to increase inflammatory cytokine release in rats. Crit Care Med 2007;35(11):2601–6.

7. Karch S. Upper gastrointestinal bleeding as a complication of intracranial disease. J Neurosurg 1972;37(1):27–9.

8. Curreri P, Katz A, Dotin L, et al. Coagulation abnormalities in the thermally injured patient. In: Current topics in surgical research, vol. 2. New York: Academic Press, Inc, in press.

9. Choi Y, Lee J, Shin J, et al. A revised risk analysis of stress ulcers in burn patients receiving ulcer prophylaxis. Clin Exp Emerg Med 2015;2(4):250–5.

10. Sajdel-Sulkowska E, Kumar A, Clairmont G, et al. Elevated cortisol levels and changes in thymus metabolism in burn trauma. Burns 1978;5(1):136–42.

11. Pruitt B, Foley F, Moncrief J. Curling's ulcer: a clinical-pathology study of 323 cases. Ann Surg 1970;172(4):523–36.

12. Guillamondegui O, Gunter O, Bonadies J, et al. Practice management guidelines for stress ulcer prophylaxis. EAST practice management guidelines committee. 2008. Professional society guidelines; Available at: https://www.east. org/education/practice-management-guidelines/stress-ulcer-prophylaxis. Accessed February 1,2017.

13. Cook D, Heyland D, Griffith L, et al. Risk factors for clinically important upper gastrointestinal bleeding in patients requiring mechanical ventilation. Canadian Critical Care Trials Group. Crit Care Med 1999;27(12):2812.

14. Marik PE, Vasu T, Hirani A, et al. Stress ulcer prophylaxis in the new millennium: a systematic review and meta-analysis. Crit Care Med 2010;38(11):2222.

15. Nathens AB, Mair RV. Prophylaxis and management of stress ulceration. In: Holzheimer RG, Mannick JA, editors. Surgical Treatment: Evidence-based and problem-oriented. Munich: Zuckschwerdt; 2001. p. 1–13.

16. Imperiale T, Birgisson S. Somatostatin or octreotide compared with H2 antagonists and placebo in the management of acute nonvariceal upper gastrointestinal hemorrhage: a meta-analysis. Ann Intern Med 1997;127(12):1062–71.

17. Darcy M. Treatment of lower gastrointestinal bleeding: vasopressin infusion versus embolization. J Vasc Interv Radiol 2003;14(5):535–43.

18. Sachar H, Vaidya K, Laine L. Intermittent vs continuous proton pump inhibitor therapy for high-risk bleeding ulcers: a systematic review and meta-analysis. JAMA Intern Med 2014;175(11):1755–62.

19. Larson G, Schmidt T, Gott J, et al. Upper gastrointestinal bleeding: predictors of outcome. Surgery 1986;100:765–72.

20. Eckstein M, Kelemouridis V, Athanasoulis C, et al. Gastric bleeding: therapy with intra-arterial vasopressin and transcatheter embolization. Radiology 1984; 152(3):643–6.

21. Hubert J, Kiernan P, Welch J, et al. The surgical management of bleeding stress ulcers. Ann Surg 1980;191:672–9.

22. Quigless M, Bernard L. Total gastrectomy for stress ulceration of the stomach unresponsive to medical therapy. J Natl Med Assoc 1974;66(6):475–9.

23. Immediate results of emergency operation for massive upper gastrointestinal hemorrhage: a cooperative study by the Connecticut Society of American Board Surgeons. Am J Surg 1971;122:387–93.

24. Stone H, Strom P, Mullins R. Management of the major coagulopathy with onset during laparotomy. Ann Surg 1983;197:532–5.
25. Rotondo M, Schwab C, McGonigal M. Damage control: an approach for improved survival in exsanguinating penetrating abdominal injury. J Trauma 1993;35:375.
26. Barker D, Kaufman H, Smith L, et al. Vacuum pack technique of temporary abdominal closure: a 7-year experience with 112 patients. J Trauma 2000; 48(2):201–6.
27. Miller R, Morris J Jr, Diaz J Jr, et al. Complications after 344 damage-control open celiotomies. J Trauma 2000;48(2):201–6.
28. Teixeira P, Inaba K, Dubose J, et al. Enterocutaneous fistula complicating trauma laparotomy: a major resource burden. Am Surg 2009;75(1):30–2.
29. Kirkpatrick A, Baxter K, Simons R, et al. Intra-abdominal complications after surgical repair of small bowel injuries: an international review. J Trauma 2003;55(3): 399–406.
30. Naumann D, Bhangu A, Kelly M, et al. Stapled versus handsewn intestinal anastomosis in emergency laparotomy: a systemic review and meta-analysis. Surgery 2015;157(4):609–18.
31. Neutzling C, Lustosa S, Proenca I, et al. Stapled versus handsewn methods for colorectal anastomosis surgery. Cochrane Database Syst Rev 2012;(2):CD003144.
32. Subramaniam M, Liscum K, Hirschberg A. The floating stoma: a new technique for controlling exposed fistulae in abdominal trauma. J Trauma 2002;53(2):386–8.
33. Brindle C, Blankenship J. Management of complex abdominal wounds with small bowel fistulae: isolation techniques and exudate control to improve outcomes. J Wound Ostomy Continence Nurs 2009;36(4):396–403.
34. Medeiros A, Aires-Neto T, Marchini J, et al. Treatment of postoperative enterocutaneous fistulas by high-pressure vacuum with a normal oral diet. Dig Surg 2004;21(5–6):401–5.
35. Dietel M. Nutritional management of external gastrointestinal fistulas. Can J Surg 1976;19(6):505–9.
36. Thomas R. The response of patients with fistulas of the gastrointestinal tract to parenteral nutrition. Surg Gynecol Obstet 1981;153(1):77–80.
37. Slater R. Nutritional management of enterocutaneous fistulas. Br J Nurs 2009; 18(4):225–30.
38. Martinez J, Luque-de-leon E, Mier J, et al. Systemic management of postoperative enterocutaneous fistulas: factors related to outcomes. World J Surg 2008; 32(3):436–43.
39. Mawdsely J, Hollington P, Bassett P, et al. An analysis of predictive factors for healing and mortality in patients with enterocutaneous fistulas. Aliment Pharmacol Ther 2008;28:1111–21.
40. Torres A, Landa J, Azcoita M, et al. Somatostatin in the management of gastrointestinal fistulas. A multicenter trial. Arch Surg 1992;127(1):97–9.
41. Stevens P, Burden S, Delicata R, et al. Somatostatin analogues for treatment of enterocutaneous fistula. Cochrane Database Syst Rev 2013.
42. LaBerge J, Kerlan R, Gordon R, et al. Non-operative treatment of enteric fistulas: results in 53 patients. J Vasc Interv Radiol 1992;3(2):353–7.
43. Davis K, Johnson E. Controversies in the care of the enterocutaneous fistula. Surg Clin North Am 2013;93:2310350.
44. D'Hondt M, Devriendt D, Van Rooy F, et al. Treatment of small-bowel fistulae in the open abdomen with topical negative-pressure therapy. Am J Surg 2011;202: e20–4.

45. Cheesborough J, Park E, Souza J, et al. Staged management of the open abdomen and enteroatmospheric fistulae using split-thickness skin grafts. Am J Surg 2014;207(4):504–11.

46. Schecter W. Management of enterocutaneous fistulas. Surg Clin North Am 2011; 91:481–91.

47. Schecter W, Hirshberg A, Chang D. Enteric fistulas: principles of management. J Am Coll Surg 2009;209:484–91.

48. Kudsk K, Croce M, Fabian T, et al. Enteral versus parenteral feeding : effects on septic morbidity after blunt and penetrating abdominal trauma. Ann Surg 1992; 215:503–11.

49. Jeejeebhoy K. Total parenteral nutrition: potion or poison? Am J Clin Nutr 2001; 74(2):160–3.

50. Vanek V, Al-Salti M. Acute pseudo-obstruction of the colon (Ogilvie's syndrome). An analysis of 400 cases. Dis Colon Rectum 1986;29:203–10.

51. Tenofsky P, Beamer R, Smith R. Ogilvie syndrome as a postoperative complication. Arch Surg 2000;135:682–7.

52. Anuras S, Shirazi SS. Colonic pseudo-obstruction. Am J Gastroenterol 1984;79: 525–31.

53. Malone N, Vargas H. Acute intestinal pseudo-obstruction (Ogilvie's syndrome). Clin Colon Rectal Surg 2005;18(2):96–101.

54. Saunders M, Kimmey M. Systematic review acute colonic pseudo-obstruction. Aliment Pharmacol Ther 2005;22(10):917–25.

55. Polignano FM, Caradonna P, Maiorano E, et al. Recurrence of acute colonic pseudo-obstruction in selective adrenergic dysautonomia associated with infectious toxoplasmosis. Scand J Gastroenterol 1997;32:89–94.

56. Swaim MG, Blennerhassett PA, Collins SM. Impaired sympathetic nerve function in the inflamed rat intestine. Gastroenterology 1991;100:675–82.

57. Moons V, Coremans G, Tack J. An update on acute colonic pseudo-obstruction (Ogilvie's Syndrome). Acta Gastroenterol Belg 2003;66:150–3.

58. Delgado-Aros S, Camilleri M. Pseudo-obstruction in the critically ill. Best Pract Res Clin Gastroenterol 2003;17:427–44.

59. Jacob S, Lee S, Hill J. The demise of the instant/unprepared contrast enema in large bowel obstruction. Colorectal Dis 2008;10(7):729–31.

60. Godfrey E, Addley H, Shaw A. The use of computed tomography in the detection and characterization of large bowel obstruction. N Z Med J 2009;122(1395): 57–73.

61. Wegener M, Borsch G. Acute colonic pseudo-obstruction (Ogilvie's syndrome). Presentation of 14 of our own cases and analysis of 1027 cases reported in the literature. Surg Endosc 1987;1(3):169–74.

62. Patterson D, Abell T, Rothstein R, et al. A double-blind multicenter comparison of domperidone and metoclopramide in the treatment of diabetic patients with symptoms of gastroparesis. Am J Gastroenterol 1999;94:1230.

63. McCallum RW, Valenzuela G, Polepalle S, et al. Subcutaneous metoclopramide in the treatment of symptomatic gastroparesis: clinical efficacy and pharmacokinetics. J Pharmacol Exp Ther 1991;258:136.

64. Depoortere I, Peeters TL, Vantrappen G. Motilin receptors of the rabbit colon. Peptides 1991;12:89–94.

65. Costa A, De Ponti F, Gibelli G, et al. In vivo characterization of the colonic prokinetic effect of erythromycin in the rabbit. Pharmacology 1997;54:64–75.

66. Jameson JS, Rogers J, Misiewicz JJ, et al. Oral or intravenous erythromycin has no effect on human distal colonic motility. Aliment Pharmacol Ther 1992;6: 589–95.

67. Bradette M, Poitras P, Boivin M. Effect of motilin and erythromycin on the motor activity of the human colon. J Gastrointest Motil 2001;5:247–51.

68. De Ponti F, Malagelada JR. Functional gut disorders: from motility to sensitivity disorders. A review of current and investigational drugs for their management. Pharmacol Ther 1998;80:49–88.

69. Van Assche G, Thijs T, Depoortere I, et al. Excitatory effect of motilin on the isolated human colon. Gastroenterology 1995;108:A703.

70. Bonacini M, Smith OJ, Pritchard T. Erythromycin as therapy for acute colonic pseudo-obstruction (Ogilvie's syndrome). J Clin Gastroenterol 1991;13:475–6.

71. Armstrong DN, Ballantyne GH, Modlin IM. Erythromycin for reflex ileus in Ogilvie's syndrome. Lancet 1991;337:378.

72. Nelson R, Edwards S, Tse B, et al. Prophylactic nasogastric decompression after abdominal surgery. Cochrane Database Syst Rev 2007;3:CD004929.

73. Artal A, Freile E, Lanas A. Favorable response to cisapride in acute colonic pseudo-obstruction (Ogilvie's syndrome). Rev Esp Enferm Dig 1994;86(2): 615–8.

74. Bourhis F, Rolachon A, Bost R, et al. Acute colonic pseudo-obstruction (Ogilvie's syndrome): treatment with cisapride. Gastroenterol Clin Biol 1991;15(6–7): 559–60.

75. Sanger G, Banner SE, Smith M, et al. SB-207266: 5-HR4 receptor antagonism in human isolated gut and prevention of 5-HT-evoked sensitization of peristalsis and increased defaecation in animal models. Neurogastroentrol Motil 1998;10: 271–9.

76. De Otero J, Borrellas X, Codinas S, et al. A convulsive crisis in a patient with Ogilvie's syndrome treated with cisapride. Med Clin (Barc) 1994;102(7):278.

77. Wysowski D. Cisapride and fatal arrhythmia. N Engl J Med 1996;335:290–1.

78. Hutchinson R, Griffiths C. Acute colonic pseudo-obstruction: a pharmacological approach. Ann R Coll Surg Engl 1992;74(5):364–7.

79. van der Spoel J, Oudemans-van Straaten H, Stoutenbeek C, et al. Neostigmine resolves critical illness-related colonic ileus in intensive care patients with multiple organ failure – a prospective, double-blind, placebo-controlled trial. Intensive Care Med 2001;27(5):822–7.

80. Nivatvongs S, Vermeulen F, Fang D. Colonoscopic decompression of acute pseudo-obstruction of the colon. Ann Surg 1982;196:598–600.

81. Geller A, Peterson B, Gostout C. Endoscopic decompression for acute colonic pseudo-obstruction. Gastrointest Endosc 1996;44:144–50.

82. Bode W, Beart R, Spencer R, et al. Colonoscopic decompression for acute pseudo-obstruction of the colon (Ogilvie's syndrome) report of 22 cases and re-view of the literature. Am J Surg 1984;147:243–5.

83. Kahi C, Rex D. Bowel obstruction and pseudo-obstruction. Gastroenterol Clin North Am 2003;32(4):1229–47.

84. Harrison M, Anderson M, Appaleneni V, et al. ASGE standards of practice committee. The role of endoscopy in the management of patients with known and suspected colonic obstruction and pseudo-obstruction. Gastrointest Endosc 2010;71(4):669–79.

85. De Girgio R, Knowles C. Acute colonic pseudo-obstruction. Br J Surg 2009; 96(3):229–39.

86. Benacci J, Wolff B. Cecostomy. Therapeutic indications and results. Dis Colon Rectum 1995;38(5):530–4.

87. Jain A, Vargas H. Advances and challenges in the management of acute colonic pseudo-obstruction (Ogilvie Syndrome). Clin Colon Rectal Surg 2012; 25:37–45.

88. Cheatham ML. Abdominal compartment syndrome: pathophysiology and definitions. Scand J Trauma Resusc Emerg Med 2009;17:10.

89. Bailey J, Shapiro MJ. Abdominal compartment syndrome. Crit Care 2000;4: 23–9.

90. Coombs H. The mechanism of the regulation of intra-abdominal pressure. Am J Physiol 1922;61:159–70.

91. Malbrain ML, Chiumello D, Cesana BM, et al. A systematic review and individual patient data meta-analysis on intra-abdominal hypertension in critically ill patients: the wake-up project. World Initiative on Abdominal Hypertension Epidemiology, a Unifying Project (WAKE-Up!). Minerva Anestesiol 2014;80: 293–306.

92. Vidal MG, Ruiz WJ, Gonzalez F, et al. Incidence and clinical effects of intra-abdominal hypertension in critically ill patients. Crit Care Med 2008;36: 1823–31.

93. Reintam A, Parm P, Kitus H, et al. Primary and secondary intra-abdominal hypertension-different impact on ICU outcomes. Intensive Care Med 2008;34: 1624–731.

94. Balogh Z, McKinley BA, Cocanour CS, et al. Supranormal trauma resuscitation causes more cases of abdominal compartment syndrome. Arch Surg 2003;138: 637–43.

95. Kirkpatrick AW, Brenneman FD, McLean RF, et al. Is clinical examination an accurate indicator of raised intra-abdominal pressure in critically injured patients. Can J Surg 2000;43:207–11.

96. Katsios C, Ye C, Hoad N, et al. Intra-abdominal hypertension in the critically ill: inter-rater reliability of bladder pressure measurement. J Crit Care 2013;28: 886–92.

97. Malbrain ML. Different techniques to measure intra-abdominal pressure (IAP): time for a critical reappraisal. Intensive Care Med 2004;30:357–71.

98. Cheatham ML, White MW, Seagraves SG, et al. Abdominal perfusion pressure: a superior parameter in the assessment of intra-abdominal hypertension. J Trauma 2000;49:621–7.

99. Kirkpatrick AW, Roberts DJ, Waele J, et al. Intra-abdominal hypertension and the abdominal compartment syndrome: updated consensus definitions and clinical practice guidelines from the World Society of the Abdominal Compartment Syndrome. Intensive Care Med 2013;39:1190–206.

100. Duchesne JC, Kaplan LJ, Balogh ZJ, et al. Role of permissive hypotension, hypertonic resuscitation and the global increased permeability syndrome in patients with severe hemorrhage: adjuncts to damage control resuscitation to prevent intra-abdominal hypertension. Anaesthesiol Intensive Ther 2015;47: 143–55.

101. Weidemann HP, Wheeler AP, Bernard GR, et al. Comparison of to fluid-management strategies in acute lung injury. N Engl J Med 2006;354: 2564–75.

102. Pommerening MJ, DuBose JJ, Zielinski MD, et al. Time to first take-back operation predicts successful primary fascial closure in patients undergoing damage control laparotomy. Surgery 2014;156:431–8.

103. Harvin JA, Mims MM, Duchesne JC, et al. Chasing 100%: the use of hypertonic saline to improve early, primary fascial closure after damage control laparotomy. J Trauma Acute Care Surg 2013;74:426–30.
104. Joseph B, Zangbar B, Pandit V, et al. The conjoint effect of reduced crystalloid administration and decreased damage-control laparotomy use in the development of abdominal compartment syndrome. J Trauma Acute Care Surg 2014;76:457–61.
105. Duchesne JC, Baucom CC, Rennie KV, et al. Recurrent abdominal compartment syndrome: an inciting factor of the second hit phenomenon. Am Surg 2009;75: 1193–8.

Moving?

Make sure your subscription moves with you!

To notify us of your new address, find your **Clinics Account Number** (located on your mailing label above your name), and contact customer service at:

Email: journalscustomerservice-usa@elsevier.com

800-654-2452 (subscribers in the U.S. & Canada)
314-447-8871 (subscribers outside of the U.S. & Canada)

Fax number: 314-447-8029

Elsevier Health Sciences Division
Subscription Customer Service
3251 Riverport Lane
Maryland Heights, MO 63043

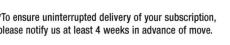